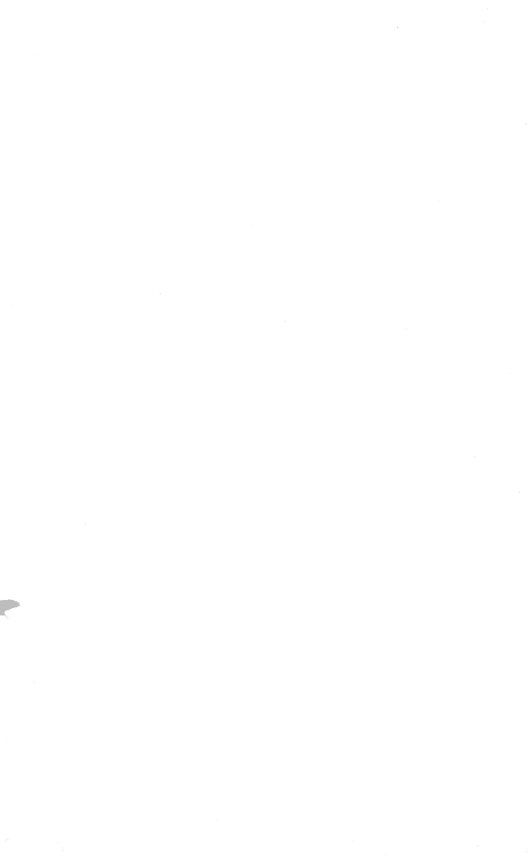

Biological Mediators
of Behavior and Disease:
Neoplasia

# Biological Mediators of Behavior and Disease: Neoplasia

Proceedings of a Symposium on Behavioral Biology and Cancer, held
May 15, 1981 at the National Institutes of Health, Bethesda, Maryland, USA

EDITOR:

## Sandra M. Levy, Ph.D.

Chief, Behavioral Medicine Branch, National Cancer Institute, National Institutes
of Health, Bethesda, Maryland, USA

Elsevier Biomedical
New York · Amsterdam · Oxford

Published by:

Elsevier Science Publishing Co., Inc.
52 Vanderbilt Avenue, New York, New York 10017

Sole distributors outside the USA and Canada:

Elsevier Science Publishers B.V.
P.O. Box 211, 1000 AE, Amsterdam, The Netherlands

Library of Congress Cataloging in Publication Data

Symposium on Behavioral Biology and Cancer (1981: National Institutes of Health)
    Biological mediators of behavior and disease, neoplasia.

    Bibliography: p.
    Includes index.
    1. Cancer—Immunological aspects—Congresses. 2. Cancer—Psychosomatic
    aspects—Congresses. 3. Stress (Physiology)—Congresses. 4. Cancer—
    Immunological aspects—Animal models—Congresses. I. Levy, Sandra M. II.
    National Institutes of Health (U.S.). III. Title. [DNLM: 1. Higher nervous activity—
    Congresses. 2. Neoplasms—Immunology—Congresses. 3. Behavior—Congresses.
    4. Neoplasms—Etiology—Congresses. 5. Central nervous system—Immunology—
    Congresses. 6. Stress, Psychological—Physiopathology—Congresses. 7. Stress,
    Psychological—Complications—Congresses. QZ 202 S979b]
RC268.3.S956   1981          616.99'4079       82-4966
ISBN 0-444-00708-3                             AACR2

Manufactured in the United States of America

# Contents

# PREFACE

This volume consists of an expanded set of original papers presented at a Behavioral Biology Working Group meeting held in the spring of 1981 at the National Cancer Institute, National Institutes of Health. The basic issue addressed by all the papers concerns possible regulating ties between behavior and cancer—especially human neoplastic disease. The distinguished group of contributors to this work reflect the true interdisciplinary nature necessary for such an inquiry, representing such fields as biochemistry, endocrinology, immunology, psychiatry, and psychology.

It would seem helpful to the reader to provide an overview of the research issues addressed in this volume. The balance of these introductory remarks will serve that end.

There were two domains of literature that were brought to bear on the question of behavior and neoplasia. One of these is concerned with the relationship of the central nervous system to immunological response factors. The other is concerned with immunological control of cancer as a disease process. While the issues can be viewed separately, ultimately they must be joined if in fact behavioral and emotional responses in humans affect the expression of neoplastic disease by immunological modulation. It was the task of the working group—and the aim of this volume—to examine the state of the evidence for this as well as for other possible linking pathways.

## LINKS BETWEEN THE CENTRAL NERVOUS SYSTEM AND IMMUNE SYSTEM IN ANIMAL AND HUMAN STUDIES

Ader, in his 1980 presidential address to the American Psychosomatic Society, concluded that immune processes are fundamentally homeostatic processes and can finally be understood only within the context of the complex host interacting with its environment. And ultimately, he argued, this integrated system of adaptive mechanisms is under the control of the central nervous system.

There is currently little dispute that the immune system and the central nervous system are inextricably linked (Rogers, et al., 1979; Amkraut & Soloman, 1975; Soloman & Amkraut, 1979). Recent work has indicated in fact a bi-directional, feedback relationship between the two systems. For example, Besedovsky, et al. (1977) reported results from a study that showed increased neural firings in the ventromedial hypothalamus in response to increased antibody production. And as will be discussed below, ablative studies involving destruction of portions of the hypothalamus drastically affect immune response.

Numerous lines of evidence in fact exist linking CNS effects (primarily by way of hypothalamic–pituitary–adrenal axis control) and immune response. In addition to ablative studies, investigative approaches have included pharmacological intervention (for the most part, mimicing hormonal effects in response to "stress") and conditioning approaches to immune regulation.

The role of the hypothalamus in mediating stress effects in the immune system has been reviewed widely in the literature (Sklar & Anisman, 1981; Stein, et al., 1979). For example, Stein, Schiavi, and Camerino (1976) reported a series of experimental ablative studies with guinea pigs examining the effect of anterior hypothalamic lesions on humoral immune response. It was found that such lesions had a protective effect against cases of anaphylactic shock in animals sensitized to ovalbumin. These researchers suggested that such a protective effect caused by hypothalamic lesion may be due to non-specific aspects of humoral immunity, such as diminished host susceptibility to histamine. In general, the hypothalamus is involved in the regulation of both endocrine and neurotransmitter processes, and cell-mediated immunity is also affected by this route (Balow, Hurly, and Fauci, 1975). (See chapter 7 in the present volume for a complete discussion of these studies.)

Hormonal release by the endocrine system is highly responsive to "emotional" and behavioral stress responses. The most frequently studied hormones are those of the pituitary–adrenal cortical system. The rapid release of ACTH in the stress reaction leading to corticosteroid synthesis release has been studied in various animal systems related to immune suppression (as well as occasionally, immune enhancement). For example, Balow, Hurly, and Fauci (1975) found that after chronic cortisone acetate treatment in guinea pigs, peripheral circulating lymphocytes showed a marked decrease in both antigen-induced migration inhibitory factor (MIF) and proliferation (although mitogen responses remained normal). Acute glucocorticoid administration was not associated with changes in cell-mediated lymphocyte function in this work.

Several other hormones (thyroid, testosterone, and growth hormones) and other agents (epinephrine and norepinephrine, for example) have all been shown to modulate immunocompetent cell levels—again, mostly by depressing—but occasionally enhancing—responsiveness. (See chapters 2 and 3 in this volume for further discussion of endocrine factors and immune response.)

A study of pharamacological control of T-cell cytotoxicity in humans linked with central nervous system regulation has been reported recently (Renoux, 1981). In this work, sodium diethyldethiocarbanate (DTC) induced recruitment and activation of both T-cells and NK cells, without direct effect on the B-cell line. This investigation reported activity of this pharmacologic agent as mediated through ". . . increased synthesis of T-cell specific hormonal factors, the levels of which are controlled by the brain neocortex" (Renoux, 1981).

Finally, perhaps the most impressive testimony to higher cortical control of the immune system emerges from the conditioning studies of Ader and his colleagues (Ader and Cohen, 1975; Cohen, et al., 1979; Rogers, et al., 1976). Employing a variety of control conditions, these researchers have shown that by pairing a saccharin drinking solution with an injection of cyclophosphamide (an immune suppressant), subsequent exposure to saccharin alone coupled with the introduction of an antigen (sheep erythrocytes) results in a lessened antibody response. This learning phenomenon has been demonstrated using both T-cell dependent and T-cell independent antigens (Wayner, et al., 1978). While in general, immune attenuation in these studies is relatively minor, nevertheless this conditioned phenomenon is consistent across investigations.

There have also been human studies (Palmblad, et al., 1977; Holm & Palmblad, 1976) of naturally occurring stress and immunity. For example, Bartrop, et al. (1977) investigated the effects of loss of a spouse in 26 bereaved persons compared to non-bereaved controls. Lymphocyte response to phytohemagglutinin and to concanavalin A were significantly suppressed at eight and six weeks, respectively. (However, there were no significant differences between the bereaved and controls in terms of T and B cell numbers, immunoglobulin, or delayed skin hypersensitivity.) These effects were time limited and mitogen induced response returned to normal by twelve months.

Palmblad and co-workers (1977) found no changes in proportion or total numbers of circulating T and B lymphocytes or monocytes after fasting in a healthy group of subjects. These investigators did find a significant decrease in DNA synthesis by lymphocytes stimulated in vitro by doses of pokeweed mitogen. (See Locke's chapter in this volume for a discussion of stress effects in humans attenuating natural killer cell activity.)

While the above overview is merely meant to be illustrative, it should at least be clear that CNS function modulates various immune parameters perhaps both directly by learned association, as well as indirectly through limbic-hypothalamic-pituitary-adrenal paths.

Equally important to the topic at hand, however, is the linkage between the immune system and neoplasia. This latter linkage is controversial and open to some dispute. The weight of the evidence, however, is in favor of some sort of immunological control of this disease process.

LINKS BETWEEN THE IMMUNE SYSTEM AND NEOPLASIA

When one is dealing with pathological processes across various fields of inquiry (from psychopathology to neoplasia), it may be possible to intervene therapeutically and demonstrate a clinically observable change in the pathological process by means essentially independent of original etiological factors. That is, it is perhaps a logical fallacy to assume that because one can alter a disease process, that the means of alteration reveals the original causation of the disorder. In terms of immunology and cancer, it might be possible to demonstrate clinically an alteration of cancer in some site by immunotherapeutic means (for example, by injecting a substance such as BCG--an attenuated tubercle bacillus—and eliciting a systemic response which potentialy includes cellular attack on the host's tumor), but this alteration of pathological process would not necessarily imply that the cancer arose because of immunological defect. And since the basic questions here were concerned wtih endogenous regulation of neoplasia, that is, questions of inherent control, the field of immunotherapy was not addressed directly.

While immunotherapy in the classic sense was not considered, several papers are concerned with the possibility of therapeutically enhancing immunological factors endogenously (by CNS control, for example) in order potentially to enhance surveillance against nascent tumor cell growth (see, for example, chapters, 2, 3, 9, and 10).

Experimental Tumorigenesis in Animal Models

There is currently a large literature demonstrating the effects of various forms of experimental "stress" (from caging conditions to electric shock) on tumor growth (and occasionally, tumor regression). (See Stoll, 1979, for a thorough review of this area.) For example, Riley (1975) reported significantly different latencies for mammary tumor development in three groups of C3H/HE mice carrying the Bittner virus. Parous animals housed under chronic stress conditions developed mammary tumors with a median latancy of 276 days in contrast with 358 days in non-parous animals housed under the same conditions and 506 days for non-parous animals housed under low stress, "protected" conditions. Ultimately, 100% of all three groups eventually developed tumors. A fourth group of animals, reared with virus-free foster parents and raised in a protected environment developed essentially no tumors. Hence, in this work there were interactive effects between "stress" and the pathogen—the latter being sufficient for tumor growth but with delayed effects in the low stress group.

As indicated above, however, stress has also been shown to inhibit tumor growth, as well as to have no effect on experimental tumorigenesis in the animals (Reznikoff & Martin, 1957; Rasmussen, et al., 1963). And while there have been reports in the literature of an increase in spontaneous tumors as a result of experimentally induced neurosis, (Corson, 1966), very few studies have been reported on the effect of stress on spontaneously arising tumors (except those arising from vertically transmitted viruses, such as used in Riley's work reported above).

With respect to immunologically-mediated stress effects on tumor growth, a recent study by Pavlidis and Chirigos (1980) reported impaired macrophage response in vitro to interferon and bacterial lipopolysaccharides in stress-restrained animals. These investigators also assessed the role of corticosteroids as mediators of the observed phenomenon by simultaneous administration in vivo of corticosteroids and interferon. Dexamethasone completely blocked the ability of interferon-treated macrophages to inhibit MBL-2 leukemic cell growth.

Pavlidis and Chirigos reported a time-dependent relationship between stress and inhibition of macrophage cytotoxicity. After in vivo administration of interferon, the mice injected one day prior to stress expressed less macrophage activation than the group injected at the initiation of stress. Sklar and Anisman (1981) discussed in detail the question of the timing of stress—coupled with the nature of the stress event—and the effects on tumor expression. Not only does it make a difference whether stress is applied before or after the transplantation of tumor cells, but the chronicity of the stress, itself, is a major parameter in study outcome. In general, with respect to physical stressors (such as shock), acute stress enhances tumor growth, but the effects decrease under conditions of chronic stress. In fact, neurochemical transmitters such as norepinephrine appear not only to recover function after acute depletion but over compensate for previous depletion in a rebound state (Anisman, 1978). Similarly, hormonal changes such as ACTH secretion and the release of corticosteriods sharply rise under conditions of acute stress, but decrease and return to normal with continued administration of the now chronic stress state.

Sklar and Anisman point out that while major parameters (such as the timing, sequencing, and nature of stress events related to experimental tumor growth) have been fairly carefully mapped out for endocrine and neurochemical transmitters, these same parameters have not been as systematically explored for immune function related to tumor growth. (See chapters 6 and 7, this volume, for a complete discussion of these issues.)

In general, although there has been a great deal of research activity related to tumorigenesis in animals mediated by endocrine and immune factors, the situation is far from clear at this point. The aggregate of experimental data suggests strongly that neuroendocrinological and immunological reactions to stress are capable of modifying experimental tumor initiation, growth, and even metastasis. (Although, again, occassionally the modulation is in the direction of inhibition of growth. For example, see Labarba,et al., 1969.)

It is always dangerous to generalize from animal models to human disease, although ultimately, the applicablity of tumor model systems to human neoplasia must be considered. Peters and Mason (1979) reported a survey of literature in which it was found that 95% of experimental studies involved the use of virally or chemically induced tumors which were allogeneic or doubtfully syngeneic to the host involved. In fact, most of the experimental data concerning stress and cancer have been obtained using tumor systems that are not readily applicable to the human situation. Chemical carcinogens have a rather weak effect in humans on the whole, and there is so far slim evidence for virally induced tumors in man. Therefore, the interpretation of the experimental animal work in this area must be based on an appreciation of the differential nature of the model systems related to tumor-host characteristics in humans.

Riley discusses some of these issues in chapter 8, this volume, and concludes that the selection of the proper tumor/host combination is critical. Both the syngeneic and allogeneic models prove to be rather impervious to stress or "psychological " effects, the former because of minimal host resistance in any case, and the latter because of the elicitation of a host rejection response unlike that occurring in most spontaneous tumor systems, and again, less likely to be mediated by "psychological " or stress response factors. On the other hand, slowly growing tumors that are under partial immunological control are capable of responding to the biochemical and cellular events induced by stress.

HUMAN STUDIES

Evidence that the immune system does mediate the expression of at least some cancers in humans is derived from naturally occurring correlates. Examples of such correlates include genetically caused immunological defects with higher than expected cancer incidence in such cases (such as a tendency to develop lymphoma and leukemia in cases of thymic deficient Di George Syndrone) and immune suppression through medical intervention with a resultant increase in neoplastic disease (such as post-chemotherapy leukemia). However, as Cochran (1978) and others have pointed out, these associations have to be interpreted with caution as these hematopoietic and lymphoid disorders may be the result of a regulatory defect rather than a true malignant process.

Clinically, it has long been apparent that human cancers do not advance at the same rate—despite similarity in histology and stage at diagnosis. Experimental systems may in fact be quite limited in revealing the nature of endogenous neoplastic control, especially the natural restraints to metastases and progression. Stoll (1979) questions why complete regression of metastatic disease is rare, but regression of small numbers of tumor cells in early stage cancer may be more common. He suggests that—in addition to local tumor factors such as vascularity, heterogeneity of tumor cells, and length of cell cycle—a small tumor burden is inhibited much more effectively by immune defenses. Cochran (1979) reports that tumors which histologically show an infiltrate of lymphocytes, plasma cells, and macrophages, have a better than average prognosis. This appears to be true for some sites only (breast, gastric, Hodgkins, and neuroblastoma). In a related study, Cochran (1969) found local recurrences less likely in such infiltrated tumors, suggesting a locally effective defensive role for the involved cells. Again, the extent of cellular infiltration tends to decrease as the cancer advances and metastasizes.

In recent years, the role for some form of host surveillance has been resurrected with emphasis placed on the role of activated macrophages and the discovery of naturally occurring (non-sensitized) cytotoxic cells, such as the Natural Killer (NK) cells (Herberman and Ortaldo, 1981). Such cells have spontaneous cytolytic activity against a variety of tumor cells, and there is increasing evidence that these cells may play an important role in cancer surveillance. (See chapter 10 in this volume by Herberman.)

Again, higher cortical control of such host antitumor activity is open to question. Herberman reports some data suggestive of CNS control. But systematic human studies, specifically linking emotional response with a specific immunological parameter such as NK activity, and correlated with disease course have not been carried out. (See Wunderlich's chapter 9 in this volume.)

There have been a few studies in this country and in England (Derogatis, et al., 1979; Pettingale, et al., 1977; Rogentine, et al., 1979) which have examined at a very gross level the character of psychological expression and course of neoplasia. Only the English group measured an immunological correlate (a serum immunoglobulin), under the rationale that circulating serum factors may interact with antigen or otherwise function as blocking complexes to cellular immune response against tumor cells. Methodologically, there were problems with each of these studies, but together, they do suggest an association between emotional suppression and more rapid diesease course. The next necessary step is the search for mechanisms underlying these relationships (but see Cunningham's chapter 4 for another view).

Currently, there is underway at NCI-NIH a prospective study of primary breast cancer patients (Levy, Lippman, and Herberman, 1980), where NK levels are also being measured repeatedly over time. NK levels are being measured against emotional response, and patterns of recurrence will be examined in these patients. If, in fact, peripheral blood NK activity correlates with disease progression, it should be apparent in this study's findings.

Again, the role of hormones mediating some human cancers, and the likely effect of emotional expression on hormonal release are fairly undisputed. For example, breast cancers with long absolute doubling times tend to have high estrogen receptor titers. Since these tumors have a high likelihood of responding to hormonal influences, it is possible that psychological factors might exercise hormonally-mediated control over growth rate (Miller and Spratt, 1979). Chapter 3 in this volume by Lippman specifically addresses psychological links to hormonally dependent tumors in clinical populations.

Structure of This Volume

The major issues outlined above were addressed in detail by the contributors to this work. Each scientist writing from his or her own research base, was asked to address the central issue: What are the mediating links between higher cortical function and neoplasia?

In fact, the papers that were presented cluster into two groups. The first four chapters are primarily concerned with addressing the state of the evidence in clinical studies. Chapter 4 by Cunningham expresses an antimechanistic view related to research in this area, and suggests a more "wholistic " approach to behavior and cancer.

Chapter 5 by Miller is in some ways a transition paper, taking a broader perspective on the question of stress and disease in both animal models and human populations. The balance of the chapters are primarily concerned with animal models related to neuroendocrine and immune control of tumor systems.

Each of the authors examines within his or her own specialized area the state of evidence linking the central nervous system, other biological systems, and neoplasia. Each also addresses the necessary next extension of research beyond the limits of current knowledge. I have also included portions of the transcribed discussion that occurred after the two groups of papers were presented. If in fact new knowledge and understanding arise out of learned discussion these comments seemed worthy of inclusion.


DEDICATION OF THE PRESENT WORK

As in any enterprise of this sort, many individuals played a role in its successful completion. I would like to express my gratitude to Dr. Norman Braveman for his initial efforts in organizing this meeting. I would like especially to thank my secretarial staff, Mrs. Phoebe Edwards and Mrs. Judith Musgrave for their untiring generosity in preparing the volume for publication.

Finally, I would like to dedicate this volume to William D. Terry, M.D., Chief, Immunology Branch, NCI. Without his encouragement and support, this volume—and indeed, the working conference that generated it—would not have taken place.

SL

REFERENCES

Ader, R. and Cohen, N. Behaviorally conditioned immunosuppression. Psychosomatic Medicine, 1975, 37, 333-340.
Amkraut, A. and Solomon, G. From the symbolic stimulus to the pathophysiologic response: Immune nechanisms. International Journal of Psychiatry in Medicine. 1975, 5, 541-563.
Anisman, H. Neurochemical changes elicited by stress. In H. Anisman and G. Bignami (Eds.), Psychopharmacology of Aversively Motivated Behavior. New York: Plenum Press, 1978.
Balow, J., Hurley, D., and Fauci, A. Immunosuppressive effects of glucocorticosteriods: Differential effects of acute vs. chronic administration on cell-mediated immunity. The Journal of Immunology, 1975, 114, 1072-1076.
Bartrop, R., Luckhurst, E., Lazarus, L., et al. Depressed lymphocyte function after bereavement. 1977, Lancet, 834.
Besedovsky, H., Sorkin, E., Felix, D., and Haas, H. Hypothalamic changes during the immune response. European Journal of Immunology, 1977, 7, 323-325.
Cochran, A. Man, Cancer, and Immunity. New York: Academic Press, 1979.
Cochran, A. Journal of Pathology, 1969, 97, 459-468.
Cohen, N., Ader, R., Green, N., and Borejerg, D. Conditioned suppression of a thymus-independent antibody response. Psychosomatic Medicine, 1979, 41, 487-491.
Corson, S. Neuroendocrine and behavioral response patterns to psychologic stress and the problem of the target tissue in cerebrovisoral pathology. Annals of the New York Academy of Sciences, 1966, 125, 890-918.
Derogatis, L., Abeloff, M., and Melisaratos, N. Psychological coping mechanisms and survival time in metastatic breast cancer. JAMA, 1979, 242, 1504-1508.
Herberman, R., and Ortaldo, J. Natural killer cells: Their role in defenses against disease. Science, 1981, 214, 24-30.
Holm, G. and Palmblad, J. Acute energy deprivation in man: Effect on cell-mediated immunological reactions. Clinical Experimental Immunology, 1976, 25, 207.
LaBarba, R., Martini, J. and White, J. The effect of maternal separation on the growth of ehrlich carcinoma in the balb/c mouse. Psychosomatic Medicine, 1969, 31, 129-134.
Levy, S., Lippman, M., and Herberman, R. Emotional response to breast cancer and its treatment. NCI-NIH Protocol 80-C-49, 1980.
Miller, T. and Sprate, J. Critical review of reported psychological correlates of cancer prognosis and growth. In B. Stoll (Ed.), Mind and Cancer Prognosis. NY: Wiley and Sons, 1979.
Palmblad, J., Cantell, K., Holm, G., et al. Acute energy deprivation in man: Effect on serum immunoglobulins antibody response, complement factors 3 and 4, acute phase reactants and interferon—producing capacity of blood lymphocytes. Clinical Experimental Immunology, 1977, 30, 50.

Pavlidis, N. and Chirigos, M. Stress induced Impairment of macrophage tumoricidal function. Psychosomatic Medicine, 1980, 42, 47-54.

Peters, L. and Mason, K. Influence of stress on experimental cancer. In B. Stoll (Ed.), Mind and Cancer Prognosis. NY: Wiley and Sons, 1979.

Pettingale, K., Greer, S., and Dudley, E. Serum IgA and emotional expression in breast cancer patients. Journal of Psychosomatic Research, 1977, 21, 395-399.

Renoux, G. Immunopharmacology of sodium diethyldithiocarbamate. Paper presented at the 8th International Congress of pharmacology, Tokyo, 1981.

Reznikoff, M. and Martin, D. The influence of stress on mammary cancer. Journal of Psychosomatic Research, 1957, 2, 56-60.

Riley, V. Mouse mammary tumors: Alteration of incidence as apparent function of stress. Science, 1975, 189, 465-467.

Rogentine, G., Van Kammen, D., Fox, B., et al. Psychological factors in the prognosis of malignant melanoma: A prospective study. Psychosomatic Medicine, 1979, 41, 647-655.

Rogers, M., Dubey, D. and Reich, P. The influence of the psyche and the brain on immunity and disease susceptibility: A critical review. Psychosomatic Medicine, 1979, 41, 147-164.

Rogers, M., Reich, P., Strom, T., and Carpenter, C. Behaviorally conditioned immunosuppression: Replication of a recent study. Psychosomatic Medicine, 1976, 38, 447-451.

Sklar, L., and Anisman, H. Stress and cancer. Psychological Bulletin, 1981, 89, 369-407.

Solomon, G. and Amkraut, A. Neuroendocrine aspects of the immune response and their implications for stress effects on tumor immunity. Cancer Detection and Prevention, 1979, 2, 197-223.

Stein, M., Keller, S., and Schleifer, S. Role of the hypothalamus in mediating stress effects on the immune system. In B. Stoll (Ed.), Mind and Cancer Prognosis. NY: Wiley and Sons, 1979.

Stein, M., Schiavi, R., and Camerino, M. Influence of brain and behavior on the immune system. Science, 1976, 191, 435-440.

Stoll, B. Mind and Cancer Prognosis. NY: Wiley and Sons, 1979.

Wayner, E., Flannery, G., and Singer, G. Effects of taste aversion conditioning on the primary antibody response to sheep red blood cells and brucella abortus in the albino rat. Physiology of Behavior, 1978, 10, 402-404.

Participants

Robert Ader, Ph.D.
Department of Psychiatry
University of Rochester
  School of Medicine and Dentistry
Rochester, New York  14642

Hymie Anisman, Ph.D.
Department of Psychology
Carleton University
Ottawa, Ontario  K1S 586

Joan Borysenko, Ph.D.
Department of Medicine
Harvard Medical School
Boston, Massachusetts

Norman Braveman, Ph.D.
National Institute on Aging
National Institutes of Health
Bethesda, Maryland  20205

Alastair J. Cunningham, Ph.D.
The Ontario Cancer Institute
Toronto, Ontario M4X

Bernard Fox, Ph.D.
National Cancer Institute
National Institutes of Health
Bethesda, Maryland  20205

Ronald Herberman, M.D.
National Cancer Institute
National Institutes of Health
Bethesda, Maryland  29205

Sandra M. Levy, Ph.D.
National Cancer Institute
National Institutes of Health
Bethesda, Maryland  20205

Marc Lippman, M.D.
National Cancer Institute
National Institutes of Health
Bethesda, Maryland  20205

Steven Locke, M.D.
Department of Psychiatry
Beth Israel Hospital
Boston, Massachusetts  02213

Neal Miller, Ph.D.
Rockefeller University
New York, New York  10021

Vernon Riley, Ph.D.
Department of Microbiology
Pacific Northwest Research Foundation
Seattle, Washington  98104

Marvin Stein, M.D.
Department of Psychiatry
Mount Siani School of Medicine
New York, New York  10029

John Wunderlich, M.D.
National Cancer Institute
National Institutes of Health
Bethesda, Maryland  20205

Biological Mediators
of Behavior and Disease:
Neoplasia

I

HIGHER CORTICAL FUNCTION AND NEOPLASIA :

CLINICAL STUDIES

# MODULATION OF NATURAL KILLER CELL ACTIVITY BY LIFE STRESS AND COPING ABILITY

STEVEN LOCKE* AND LINDA KRAUS**
*Department of Psychiatry and Division of Behavioral Medicine, Department of Medicine, Beth Israel Hospital, 330 Brookline Avenue, Boston, Massachusetts, 02215;  **Department of Neurology, Boston University School of Medicine, 80 East Concord Street, Boston, Massachusetts, 02118

The notion that excessive "stress" can alter host defenses and resistance to disease is widely believed. Surprisingly, there has been little direct evidence to support this belief. The pioneering studies of Hinkle, Holmes, and others over two decades ago first documented the association of recent stressful life change with subsequent illness onset in man (Hinkle and Wolff, 1958; Holmes et al. 1957). Reviews of research on the health consequences of life change stress have concluded that stressful life changes, such as family deaths, geographic relocations and job loss, predispose susceptible individuals to risk of later illness (Dohrenwend and Dohrenwend, 1974; Gunderson and Rahe, 1974; Jenkins et al. 1976; Rahe and Arthur, 1978). However, the pathophysiological mechanisms mediating this relationship remain largely unknown. A logical focus for investigation is the immune system, the body's main line of host defense.

Evidence that stress may influence the immune response has been provided by research in both animals and man. The research on the effects of stress on experimental tumors and infections in animals has been well reviewed elsewhere (La Barba, 1966; Friedman and Glasgow, 1966; Rogers et al. 1979; Amkraut and Solomon, 1974; Stein et al. 1976; Riley, 1981; Ader, 1981). This report will focus on human research into the stress-immune function relationship. Since we have been particularly interested in host defenses against cancer, our emphasis will reflect that interest.

## NATURAL KILLER ACTIVITY AND CANCER

The notion that the immune system is responsible for recognition, "surveillance", and destruction of neoplastic cell growth as proposed by Burnet (1970) and other workers (Thomas, 1959) has been the cornerstone of immunological research in cancer. Following the demonstration that certain lymphocyte subpopulations were capable of lysing tumor cells in vitro (Cerottini et al. 1970), attention focused on these cytotoxic T-lymphocytes as the enforcers of immune surveillance. Subsequent research has led to substantial criticism of this hypothesis (Prehn, 1974; Stutman, 1975; Melief and Schwartz, 1975). This criticism has focused on a number of specific findings not accounted for by observations of the cytotoxic lymphocyte subpopulations previously believed responsible for immune surveillance. These findings include: 1) mice congenitally lacking a thymus and thus devoid of cytotoxic T-lymphocytes (nude mice) are not more prone to neoplasms than their T-lymphocyte competent littermates; 2) tumor specific transplantation antigens, thought to be necessary for recognition of tumor cells by cytotoxic cells, have not been found on many spontaneous tumors; 3) depression of the immune system is not necessarily associated with an increased incidence of neoplasia. Consequently, the search for the mediators of "immune surveillance" has continued.

Recently, it has been observed that lymphoid cell subpopulations from normal animals are capable of selectively lysing tumor cells while leaving normal cells intact (Kiessling et al. 1975). This discovery has changed the view of immune mechanisms implicated in the host defense against neoplastic disease. These spontaneously occurring cytotoxic effectors, active against a variety of tumors, hemopoietic stem cells and viral-infected target cells, have been dubbed "natural killer" (NK) cells. NK cells have been reported in all mammalian species examined, including mice, rats, and men. They have been characterized as non-T, non-B, or "null" cells.

Much research and discussion has focused on the characteristics of these NK cells and their mode of cytotoxic action (Henney et al. 1978). Many studies have examined differences between NK cells and other cytotoxic subpopulations. One important finding in this regard is that there is no obvious requirement for shared histocompatibility between effector and target for cytotoxic activity by NK cells but rather a hierarchy of target susceptibility exists. This is in contrast to other cytotoxic lymphocytes (Zinkernagel and Doherty, 1974). Another finding is that NK activity is not antibody dependent: natural killing occurs spontaneously without the addition of any other substance to the test system. Many studies have also examined the similarities and differences between those cells called NK cells in man and in other species (Herberman and Holden, 1978). For the purposes of this discussion, the most important aspect of NK cells in all species in which they have been identified is their apparent ability to discriminate between normal and malignant cell types.

Currently, there is an intense effort underway to understand the in vivo relevance of natural killer cells. Most of our present knowledge in this area has come from studies in mice. Several investigators have noted that the nude mouse, which congenitally lacks a thymus, has a relatively lower susceptibility to spontaneous or carcinogen-induced tumors (Rygaard and Poulsen, 1969; Stutman, 1974; Outzen et al. 1975). Transplanted tumors in nude mice have also failed to grow while skin allografts and xenografts grow readily (Bonmasser et al. 1975; Rotter and Trainin, 1975). Nude mice have high NK activity and yet are athymic and lack mature T-cells (Rygaard and Poulsen, 1969; Stutman, 1974; Outzen et al. 1975). Herberman and Holden (1978) have found that 200 to 400 times more tumor implant is required to produce tumor growth in nude mice and some of these implanted tumors regressed spontaneously. When these tumor cells were tested as target cells they were found to be highly sensitive to NK-mediated lysis by spleen cells from nude mice but resistant to lysis by cells from AL/N mice (Herberman and Holden, 1978).

A recent observation by Hansson et al. (1979) provides further exciting suggestions for the role of NK cells in vivo. They found an NK sensitive subpopulation of T-cells in the thymus and found the frequency of these natural targets was inversely correlated to the level of NK reactivity in the thymocyte donor. Since T-cell lymphomas seem to be the most sensitive tumors as NK targets, this suggests that the autologous NK target may in fact correspond to the target cell for leukemic transformation. NK cells may therefore play a central role as a homeostatic control mechanism for this potentially neoplastic population.

A number of investigators have also attempted to examine the role of NK cell activity in malignant disease in man. Most of these studies have focused on cell lines derived from the same type of cancer as that of the patients studied. The results have been conflicting, partially due to wide variation in study design. To circumvent some of these problems, some investigators have used lymphoblastoid, myeloid, or similar target cells in comparing carcinoma patients and normal donors (Rosenberg et al. 1974; Pross and Jondal, 1975). Analogous to the decreased NK activity found in tumor bearing mice, McCoy et al. found that many patients with lymphomas, colon cancer, lung cancer, and melanoma had depressed reactivity against the lymphoblastoid cell line, F265, but the reactivity of breast cancer patients was within the normal range (McCoy et al. 1973). Takasugi et al. have further reported that reactivity of cancer patients declined with tumor progression (Takasugi et al. 1977). Cannon and his co-workers compared normal donors and breast cancer patients for NK cell activity against the myeloid cell line, K562 and against two breast cancer lines. They found the reactivity against K562 was similar for both groups but breast cancer patients had had higher levels of activity against breast cancer derived lines (Cannon et al. 1977). Other investigators have

also found that the incidence of NK activity in cancer patients varies with
the target cell line (Hepner et al. 1975). Pross and Baines (1976) found that
patients with malignant disease had decreased NK activity compared to normal
controls and that this decrease was highly significant for patients with either
treated or untreated metastatic disease or untreated CLL. Eremin et al. (1978)
examined NK activity of lymphocytes derived from peripheral blood and also from
lymph nodes including those draining a variety of solid tumors obtained from
woman with clinically localized mammary carcinoma. They found a wide range
of activity in both normal and cancer patient derived cells from both blood
and lymph nodes and no significant differences between the patients and the
normals. Behelak et al. (1976) compared normal and CLL donors for NK activity
against xenogenic normal target cells. He found activity in this type of
system with normal donors but no detectable activity in the CLL patients.

In conclusion, a variety of studies have been performed both in mouse and
in man, which yield an initial but persuasive body of evidence implicating NK
cells as an important component of the host surveillance network against neoplastic disease (Herberman and Holden, 1979; Marx, 1980). Recently, macrophages also have been observed to possess spontaneous cytotoxic activity
against tumor cells (Oehler et al. 1977; Keller, 1978; Chow et al. 1979),
though activation of macrophage cytotoxic activity by exposure to tumor cells
is slower than the NK cell response. Thus it appears likely that host
defenses against cancer are comprised of several thymus-independent natural
killing mechanisms. It is probable that the mechanism for recognition and
selective destruction of nascent tumor cell lines is different from the cytotoxic defenses against well-established tumors or metastases. In any case,
the evidence for the role of NK cells in protection from cancer is compelling
and provides a basis for a strong argument for continued study of variations
in NK activity.

Since recent studies have raised the possibility that behavioral factors
may influence susceptibility to or the clinical course of human cancer (Thomas,
1979; Bieliauskas et al. 1979; Greer et al. 1979), it seemed appropriate to
study the influence of stress and other behavioral factors on natural killer
cell activity.

HISTORY OF THE STUDY OF STRESS AND IMMUNITY IN HUMANS
The study of "stress" in humans is complicated by confusion and disagreement
about the definition of "stress". In contrast to research in animals where
stressors can be operationally defined and quantified, ethical constraints

inherent in the use of human subjects limit the nature of experimental designs and encourage the use of naturally occurring stresses. The psychoendocrinology of human stress has been thoroughly reviewed by Rose (1980). Examples of experimental stressors used in human stress research are listed below in Table 1. To avoid the ethical issues involved in studies of human stress, many investigators have chosen to take advantage of naturally occurring stresses such as those listed in Table 2. Consequently, there are few controlled experiments on human stress. Instead, the literature contains studies which make use of the various models of human stress listed in Table 3. Since "stress" has been used to mean both the "stressor" and the subjective, inner experience of distress (really, "strain"), we will try to define the term operationally where it is used in this paper.

TABLE 1

EXPERIMENTAL STRESSORS

| Physical/Biological | Psychological |
| --- | --- |
| Starvation | Sensory deprivation |
| Sensory deprivation | Isolation |
| Sleep deprivation | Films |
| Thermal | Attention tasks |
| Barometric | Performance tasks |
| Weightlessness | Stress interviews |
| Acceleration | Conditioned avoidance |
| Noise | |

TABLE 2

NATURALLY-OCCURRING STRESS

| | |
| --- | --- |
| Occupational stress | Physical illness |
| Military training | Bereavement |
| Academic training | Life change stress |
| Incarceration | Inhibited power motivation |
| Surgery | Examination stress |

The historical basis for studying the influence of stress on human immunity is derived from several sources. The most compelling basis for interest in researching this relationship comes from a heritage of centuries of clinical stories about people who became ill following stressful life circumstances. In the first psycho-immunologic investigation of disease susceptibility, Ishigami (1919) measured opsonization of tubercle bacilli among chronic tuberculous patients during inactive and active phases of the disease. He reported observing decreases in phagocytic activity in the patients' white blood cells during episodes of "emotional excitement." Ishigami postulated that the stress of "contemporary" life led to decreases in immune function and resultant increased susceptibility to tuberculosis.

In the past two decades, a large body of evidence has related the occurrence of stressful life change to disease onset (Rabkin and Struening, 1976; Dohrenwend and Dohrenwend, 1974; Gunderson and Rahe, 1974). The pioneering research of Holmes and Rahe has become well-known (Holmes and Rahe, 1967). They, in addition to others, have demonstrated the increased incidence of illness onset following periods of high life change density. The premise underlying this finding is that life changes require adaptation, and too much life change is, by itself, "stressful." Despite methodological problems inherent in life change stress research (Rabkin and Struening, 1976; Hurst et al. 1978; Jenkins et al. 1979; Cleary, 1974), the association of illness onset with previous life change stress is widely accepted. However, we now need to elucidate the mechanisms by which the subjective experience of "stress" (really, "strain") is translated into pathophysiological changes which increase disease susceptibility and precede the onset of gross illness.

The effort to understand the pathophysiology of human disease led naturally to attempts to understand the influence of stress on human immune function (see Table 3). Concerned about the stressful consequences of space flight, NASA included immunologic assessments in their medical evaluation of astronauts before, during and after exposure to the space environment and the launch and recovery process. During the Apollo spaceflight program blood samples obtained during the immediate post-recovery ("splashdown") phase had higher WBC counts than during the pre-launch baseline period. Lymphoblast transformation, a measure of lymphocyte responsivity to mitogens, was unchanged (Fischer et al. 1972). Later, during the Skylab program, a more extensive immunologic assessment occurred during the extended spaceflight missions. In those studies lymphoblast transformation was depressed on the day of recovery-- a particularly stressful day of the mission--but soon returned to baseline, pre-flight levels. WBC counts were also elevated at recovery as were the percentage of circulating T-lymphocytes and the absolute number of polymorpho-nuclear leukocytes. No changes were observed in the morphology or number of lymphocytes during the study period (Kimzey, 1975). Neuroendocrine measures confirmed that the day of splashdown was apparently especially stressful for the astronauts (Leach and Rambaut, 1974).

Considering that the astronauts were an elite class of test pilots care-fully chosen for their extraordinary capacity to function effectively under stress (Wolfe, 1979), these findings are remarkable. The combination of gravitational stress and, presumably, some anxiety, was associated with alterations in several parameters of cellular immune function. In fact, during the disastrous mission of Apollo XIII, which nearly ended in tragedy due to an explosion which crippled the spacecraft, two of the three astronauts developed acute infections!

Another approach to the study of humans under stress has been used at Sweden's Karolinska Institute. In a series of experiments beginning in 1975, Palmblad and his colleagues have used short-term exposure to experimental stressors in an attempt to detect alterations in human immune function. Of particular interest are those experiments in which the effects of stress on cellular immunity were studied. In the first of these, sleep deprivation and exposure to loud noise during a 77 hour continuous attention task ("vigil") were employed as the experimental stressor. Blood samples were obtained prior to, during and after the vigil. Significant differences in several parameters of cellular immunity were observed. Interferon production was increased both during and shortly after the vigil. Phagocytosis decreased transiently during the vigil, but later rose to above-baseline levels after the vigil (Palmblad et al. 1976). In a later study (1979), Palmblad and his colleagues measured lymphoblast transformation and two parameters of granulocyte function in individuals who were stressed by forty-eight hours of sleep deprivation. While lymphoblast transformation was depressed following sleep deprivation, no changes were seen in the other measures--granulocyte adherence and leukocyte alkaline phosphatase activity. These two studies, taken together, demonstrate the critical role timing and duration of stressor exposure play in determining the nature of stress-induced immune alterations. Furthermore, it is unlikely that all forms of experimental stress have the same impact on the neuroendo-crine and immune systems. Inconsistencies in findings from studies using experimental stressors in both animals and man have led to attempts at designing studies using naturally-occurring stress in normal populations or populations at high-risk.

The first study to examine the effect of prolonged exposure to a naturally-occurring life stress on cellular immunity was the pioneering study of immune function among recently bereaved spouses (Bartrop et al. 1977). These investigators measured lymphoblast transformation in 33 pairs of bereaved spouses and age/sex/race-matched controls. Blast transformation was depressed among bereaved spouses at 8 weeks post-bereavement but not at 2 weeks in comparison to the non-bereaved controls.

The results suggested that the duration of the bereaved state was related to the observed impairment in cellular immunity among the bereaved. Furthermore, the observed immunologic differences could not be accounted for by changes in thyroxine, prolactin, growth hormone or cortisol levels during the study period. However, the neuroendocrine assessment was limited by the small number of samples.

While Bartrop was unable to replicate his findings in a second series, Schleifer and his coworkers, in a more elaborate, semi-prospective study, reported a similar depression of lymphoblast transformation observed in samples obtained 5-7 weeks post-bereavement from a sample of husbands of women with terminal breast cancer. In the latter study, these men were followed prospectively over a period of months with multiple samples collected prior to and following their spouses' anticipated death. No differences were observed in WBC count, total lymphocyte count or in absolute or relative T- and B-cell counts between the pre- and post-bereavement conditions. Interestingly, the depression in lymphoblast transformation observed 5-7 weeks post-bereavement has since diminished over time and appears to be returning towards the baseline levels observed at the time of entry into the study (Schleifer et al. 1980). Again, the observed post-bereavement immune suppression could not be explained by simultaneous measures of neuroendocrine function.

These two studies of bereavement stress constitute some of the strongest existing evidence for immunosuppressive change occurring during prolonged exposure to a type of naturally occurring life stress--a major personal loss. In light of reports of increased illness susceptibility among the recently bereaved (Rees and Lutkins, 1967; Jacobs and Ostfeld, 1977), the findings from these studies suggest a primary psycho-immunologic mediating mechanism. Since the findings in both of these bereavement studies failed to support the possibility that the observed immunosuppression resulted from alterations in neuroendocrine function, a direct brain-immune system link is strongly suggested. Recent reports of direct anatomical (Bulloch and Moore, 1980; Williams et al. 1981) and functional (Stein et al. 1981; Besedovsky et al. 1977;

Besedovsky et al. 1979) links between the nervous system and the immune system lend credence to this suggestion.

## LIFE CHANGE STRESS, COPING AND HUMAN IMMUNE FUNCTION

Another approach to measuring the impact of naturally-occurring human stress uses self-assessed life change stress measured by self-report from inventories of recent life events.  Locke and Heisel (1977) first employed this measure to test the idea that life change stress might impair immune response to vaccination.  Using 124 human volunteers undergoing A/NJ/76 influenza ("Swine Flu") immunization as subjects, they observed no relationship between life change stress reported for the intervals for either the previous year or previous month and the rise in antibody titer following vaccination.  Further-more, the post-vaccination antibody titer was independent of mood and the interaction between stress and mood.  They concluded that if human immune function were susceptible to the influence of stressful life change, that the impact of stress on the cellular immune system should be studied (Locke and Heisel, 1977).[1]

Following up on the earlier study of life change stress and response to vaccination, Locke and colleagues again investigated the relationship of life change stress and coping to immune function using a more comprehensive assessment.  Previous stress research suggested that there are marked differences between individuals in response to stress and that even within the same individuals the responses to stress can be different at different times (Rose, 1980).  Accordingly, we have been concerned about not only the effects of stress on immunity, but also possible factors that might attenuate or exacerbate the effects of stress.  Coping has been of particular interest to us.  It would seem that to the extent that an individual has effective coping strategies and social and psychological resources to rely upon, stress should occasion less deterioration of health and well being.

The term coping has become a catch-word for a variety of activities and processes, at times used interchangeably with such terms as mastery, defense, and adaptation.  We use the term rather broadly to refer to all responses that might protect an individual from the deleterious consequences of an experience. The protective function can be exercised in a variety of ways:  By eliminating or modifying the conditions that give rise to stressful experience (Mechanic,

---

[1]Two other studies have since reported a similar failure to relate variations in response to vaccination to life change stress (Roessler et al. 1979; Greene et al. 1978).

1962); by perceptually controlling the meaning of the experience in a way that diminishes its problematic character (as suggested in work by Lazarus e.g., 1966); and by keeping the emotional consequences of the problems within manageable bounds (Mechanic, 1962).

Several studies suggest that coping can modify the effects of stress on both self-reported distress and physiologic correlates of emotional upset. For example, George Vaillant found in his long-term prospective study of adult male health that the effectiveness of psychological defenses in young men predicts the quality of health in later adult life (Vaillant, 1978). In another study, myocardial infarction patients who used denial as a defensive style had higher survival rates in the acute recovery period (Hackett and Cassem, 1970). Finally, in another study parents who were judged to have more effective defenses during the period of intense life stress resulting from a child's fatal illness, exhibited lower urinary 17-hydroxycorticosteroid excretion rates (a stress-related hormone) than parents judged to have less effective defenses (Wolff et al. 1964).

A major line of our research was concerned with the relationship of life change stress and coping to natural killer cell activity. In one study, 108 undergraduates who volunteered for a study of "the influence psychological factors have on people's immune response" completed a recent life change stress questionnaire. The questionnaire consisted of the 43 items introduced by Holmes and Rahe (1967) plus 48 items specific to undergraduate life. The subjects indicated events they had experienced in the past year, month, and two weeks. They also indicated the amount of readjustment required by each of these events using a standard method (Masuda and Holmes, 1967). The sum of each subject's readjustment scores for experienced events was used to define life change stress for that individual.

We measured adequacy of coping with the 58-item version of the Hopkins Symptom Checklist. The subjects rated the extent to which they had been bothered by each of the 58 symptoms in the past week on a 5-point intensity scale. The symptoms included those of anxiety, depression, and somatization. We reasoned that inadequate coping should be evidenced by a greater degree of self-reported psychiatric distress.

The subjects also provided blood samples which were assayed for natural killer cell activity. Natural killer (NK) activity is measured using a cytotoxicity assay (Brunner et al. 1968). The target cell is a human leukemia cell, K562, which has been radioactively labelled. When the target cell is damaged or destroyed, the radioactivity inside the cell leaks out into the surrounding liquid. The test subjects' blood is separated and the white blood cells isolated. These white blood cells are then incubated together with the radiolabelled target cells. After several hours, samples of the incubation medium are assayed for radioactivity. From the amount of radioactivity detected in the medium, the rate of destruction of the leukemic target cells can be calculated. Individuals vary considerably in natural killing capacity of their lymphocytes. However, a given individual's NK activity tends to remain fairly stable over time (Williams et al. 1980).

To assess the relationship of variations in stressful life change and coping on NKCA, subjects were divided into high and low stress groups and good and poor copers based on median splits of their scores on the life change stress questionnaire and the Hopkins Symptom Checklist, respectively. We observed no significant difference in natural killer cell activity between the high and low stress groups for any of the three time periods examined.

However, when "coping" as defined by self-reported psychiatric symptoms was taken into account, a different picture emerged: There was a significant interaction of life change stress over the past year and symptom level on NK cell activity. The high stress/high symptom group had the lowest values of natural killer cell activity while the high stress/low symptom group had the highest. The three-fold difference in mean NK cell activity between these two groups was statistically significant. This interaction between life change stress and symptoms on NKCA was not observed for the two shorter, more recent time periods studied.

We were concerned that the association between self-reported psychiatric symptoms and diminished NK cell activity might reflect an underlying organic illness. But this hypothesis was not supported by further examination. If subclinical viral or allergic illness is associated with diminished NK activity, then individuals reporting more somatic symptoms should have lower killer cell activity than subjects reporting primarily "mental" symptoms. One-way analyses of variance were performed on comparisons of NK activity between the high and low groups of each subscale of the HSCL-58. The subscale scores were categorized as "high" or "low" for each subscale using a median split. There was no apparent relationship between level of self-reported somatic symptoms and NK activity. In contrast, high scores (reflecting more pathology) on the "mental" subscales were associated with significantly lower NK activity. Therefore, the alternative explanation that the association between symptoms and NK activity was simply a reflection of an underlying illness was not supported by these analyses (Locke et al. 1978).

Another way to consider the effects of coping is to examine aspects of personality that would affect how a person grapples with a stressful experience. David McClelland has argued that people with a certain motive profile termed "inhibited power motivation" ineffectively cope with power-related stresses, events that challenge or block expression of their power needs, and as a result are more susceptible to disease. He and co-workers have found that people who are high in inhibited power motivation and who report a large number of power-related life stresses have lower levels of salivary IgA, a class of antibodies importantly involved in defense against upper respiratory tract infections (McClelland et al. 1980). Most recently, John Jemmott, McClelland, Joan and Myrin Borysenko and their collaborators found evidence that the effects of power-related stress may be more longlasting on subjects high in inhibited power motivation than among other subjects (Jemmott et al. 1981).

We were interested in whether this motive profile might affect NK activity. In collaboration with McClelland, we reanalyzed our data. The results indicated that people who were high in power motivation and who reported a high degree of power-related life stress had lower NKCA and WBC counts than all other subjects (McClelland et al. unpublished manuscript).

McClelland's findings add further support to the contention that relatively stable characteristics of personality are associated with variations in immune function. In our own work, we have observed a series of significant relationships among measures of psychopathology using the MMPI and NKCA. Among our study subjects described earlier, we consistently observed more deviant scores in the direction of psychopathology among those subjects falling in the lowest quartile of NKCA values in comparison to those falling in the highest quartile (Locke et al. 1979). This preliminary finding awaits replication. The possibility that psychopathology and immunocompetence are inversely related is an important idea which requires further study.

In summary, then, our preliminary findings suggested three possibilities:

1) The effects of stressful life change on immunity depend on critical timing factors such as duration and proximity of the stressor.

2) Life change stress has a differential influence on various components of the immune system.

3) The effects of life change on immunity can be modified by effective coping.

In research underway we are attempting to replicate and extend these findings. In a study presently underway we are examining an older, more heterogeneous sample, and are collecting repeated measures on them over the course of a six-month period. The data include blood samples for NKCA, and other measures of cellular immune function, saliva samples for salivary IgA, as well as an extensive series of questionnaires on life change stress, coping, social support, physical health, and such personality factors as inhibited power motivation and ego development.

Another approach to investigating the effects on immunity of naturally-occurring stressors is to study populations about to undergo an experience presumed to be stressful. Examples of such stressful experiences include military training, combat missions and academic examinations. In a recently reported study from Canada (Dorian et al. 1981), psychiatric residents were studied twice, 10-14 days before and twice, 10-14 days after a major qualifying examination. Studying and sitting for the Oral Fellowship Examination is especially stressful for the candidates since the ability to bill the national health care system hinges upon success on this exam. Anecdotal reports of the severity of this "examination stress" led to the design of this innovative and well-controlled study. The experimental subjects (exam candidates) were compared to a control group of physicians matched for age and sex but not undergoing the exam.

Lymphoblast transformation was signficantly diminished among those about to be examined compared to the matched controls. By two weeks after the stressor, blast transformation was higher among the experimental subjects. When the groups were further divided by level of reported distress, additional differences emerged. The high distress pre-exam group had diminished late rosette formation compared to a subgroup of low distress controls. Late rosette formation is a measure of circulating T lymphocyte number. Since rosette formation can be influenced by autonomic agents (Galant et al. 1976; Grieco et al. 1976) it is tempting to speculate that this observed difference between stressed, high distress experimentals and low distress controls might be autonomically mediated. Interestingly, once again it is hard to explain these findings as a function of differences in corticosteroid levels since the experimental subjects had lower plasma cortisol levels than the controls.

The major significance of this study lies in its innovative design. The "experiment of nature" approach is a stronger design than correlational studies since the prospective format and the inclusion of a control group permit both within-subject and between-subject comparison as well as inferences about causality. The study findings suggest that examination stress may be immunosuppressive, especially among those subjects who report high

levels of distress during the stressor. Thus, this study supports the
contention of Locke and co-workers that stress coupled with adaptive failure
may be associated with immunosuppression (Locke et al. 1978).

We have reviewed a number of studies supporting the idea that brain and
behavior can influence immunity. We will now address briefly the question of
how these influences could be mediated.

MEDIATING MECHANISMS

Recent research in humans and animals has caused us to rethink our
traditional views on immunomodulation. Several studies have undermined the
widely believed notion that nervous system influences on immune function are
mediated primarily by classical neuroendocrine mechanisms, i.e., the hypothalamic-pituitary-adrenal (HPA) axis. Three separate studies have failed to
demonstrate a relationship between serum cortisol, prolactin, growth hormone
or thyroxine and depression of cellular immune function observed in humans
under stress (Bartrop et al. 1977; Schleiffer et al. 1980; Dorian et al. 1981).
Even though the conclusions of these studies were limited by the small number
of samples, there is good reason to search beyond the HPA neuroendocrine
pathways for mediating mechanisms.

A number of possibilities invite speculation. A decade of research has led
to the discovery and characterization of receptors on both lymphocytes and
granulocytes for neurotransmitters and peptides. This field of immuno-neuro-
pharmacology has been thoroughly reviewed by Hall and Goldstein (1981).
Despite the progress, little is known about the putative immunoregulatory role
attributed to these substances. In a general sense, substances which increase
intracellular cyclic AMP levels tend to be immunosuppressive. Such substances
include: histamine, isoproterenol, theophylline, and cholera toxin. In
contrast, substances which increase intracellular cyclic GMP tend to be
immunoenhancing. These substances include phenylephrine, acetylcholine and
insulin. Furthermore, $\alpha$-adrenergic agonists tend to increase cellular immune
function while $\beta$-adrenergic agonists are suppressive (Strom and Carpenter,
1980). Thus Crary has shown an increase in the number and activity of
circulating suppressor T cells following subcutaneous injections of epinephrine
in human volunteers (Crary, 1981). In contrast, my coworkers and I have
observed increased natural killer cell activity in blood samples obtained
during infusion of physiological doses of norepinephrine in human volunteers
(cited in Locke, in press).

In addition to evidence for neurohumoral modulation of immune function, recent studies have reported the detection of direct autonomic innervation of lymphoid organs.  Two laboratories have demonstrated independently that the thymus gland is innervated by autonomic fibers.  Using modern histochemical methods, Bulloch and Moore (1981) demonstrated cholinergic fibers in the thymus originating in the nucleus ambiguus in the brainstem.  Williams et al., using histofluorescent methods and electromicroscopy, have reported the observation of adrenergic nerve endings, not associated with blood vessels, in the mouse thymus and spleen.  They further noted the close association of these nerve endings to thymic mast cells (Williams et al. 1981).  Finally, chemical sympathectomy with 6-hydroxydopamine has been shown to depress antibody responses in treated animals (Besedovsky et al. 1979; Tanaka et al. 1977; Hall et al. 1980).

The most recent exciting and controversial possibility is that there exists an endorphinergic division of the autonomic nervous system involved in homeostatic regulation.  There is preliminary evidence that this proposed system may influence the immune system.  The presence of receptors for β-endorphin and met-enkephalin on lymphocytes has been detected (Wybran et al. 1979; Hazum et al. 1979).  Met-enkephalin was found to increase the percentage of active T lymphocyte rosettes (Wybran et al. 1979).  Since some tumors have been found to contain extremely high concentrations of neuropeptides (Pullan et al. 1980), it is possible that certain neuropeptides are involved in immune regulation.  Furthermore, β-endorphin in pharmacologic doses causes degranulation of mast cells in rodents (Galli, S: unpublished observations).

The mast cell, related to the basophil leukocyte, sits at the interface between the immune and the nervous system.  Responsive to immunogenic, endorphinergic and autonomic agonists, the stimulated mast cell releases histamine, a potent neurotransmitter with powerful autonomic and immunologic effects. Mast cells are located in close proximity to blood vessels in the brain (Ibrahim, 1974) and in the thymus (Williams et al. 1981).  Interestingly, mast cells are also found in high density in those organs most susceptible to psychophysiologic disorders: lung, bowel and skin.  It is not surprising that they have been implicated as mediators in some of these disorders (e.g., asthma).  It has even been informally suggested by Dvorak (personal communication) that they serve as messengers between the CNS and tumors, shuttling back and forth, "translating" in both immunologic and autonomic languages for tumors.  This latter proposal is especially interesting since suppressor T cells are activated by histamine and have immunosuppressive effects on certain

cellular immune function. Obviously, the mast cell has an important role
that we only poorly understand at present.

Conclusions

    From this review, it is evident that psychosocial factors, including ex-
posure to certain experimental stressors, life change stress, bereavement
stress, examination stress and the stress of spaceflight, are associated with
alterations of specific parameters of human cellular immune function. These
alterations tend to be in the direction of immune suppression. However, there
is also evidence suggesting a differential effect of "acute" (short-duration,
recent) and "chronic" exposure to some stressors. Furthermore, it is possible
that the cellular and humoral limbs of the immune system may differ in their
responsiveness to long-term vs. short-term stress. The findings of fifteen
recent studies of the effects of both acute and chronic stress on human immune
function are summarized in Table 3.

TABLE 3

SUMMARY OF FINDINGS FROM RECENT STUDIES OF THE RELATIONSHIP OF STRESS TO HUMAN
IMMUNE FUNCTION

| STRESSOR | FINDINGS |
| --- | --- |
| SPACE FLIGHT AND RECOVERY (Fischer et al. 1972) | ↑ WBC counts during immediate post-recovery phase<br>no change in LT pre-vs. post-flight |
| SPACE FLIGHT AND RECOVERY (Kimzey et al. 1975) | ↓ LT day R+0 (splashdown)<br>↑ circulating T-cells day R+0<br>↑ WBC day R+0<br>↑ absolute PMN's day R+0<br>no change in lymphocyte number or morphology |
| SLEEP DEPRIVATION AND NOISE (Palmblad et al. 1975) | ↑ interferon production during and after stressor<br>↓ phagocytosis during stressor<br>↑ phagocytosis after stressor |

(Legend follows)

TABLE 3 (cont.'d)

<u>STRESSOR</u>                                   <u>FINDINGS</u>

LIFE CHANGE STRESS                       no relationship between antibody response
  (Locke and Heisel, 1977)              to influenza vaccination and LCS and/or
    mood

BEREAVEMENT                              ↓ LT 8 weeks post-bereavement but not at
  (Bartrop et al. 1977)                 2 weeks post-bereavement (matched
    controls)

LIFE CHANGE STRESS                       lymphocyte cytotoxicity negatively
  (Greene et al. 1978)                  correlated with LCS
    LT not significantly correlated with LCS
    antibody response to influenza vaccination
    not related to LCS

LIFE CHANGE STRESS                       NK activity diminished among poor copers
  (Locke et al. 1978)                   under stress
    more psychopathological traits among low
    NK individuals
    LCS during immune response related to anti-
    body rise following influenza immunization
    Moderate LCS group had higher antibody
    rise than low or high LCS groups

SLEEP DEPRIVATION                        ↓ LT after sleep deprivation
  (Palmblad et al. 1979)                no change in granulocyte adherence or LAP
    activity

LIFE CHANGE STRESS                       ↓ antibody response to influenza vaccination
  (Roessler et al. 1979)                among high life change stress subjects
    with low ego strength
    no main effect of LCS

(Legend follows)

TABLE 3 (cont.'d)

| STRESSOR | FINDINGS |
|----------|----------|
| ACADEMIC STRESS<br>(Kasl et al. 1979) | seroconversion to EBV and clinical infectious mononucleosis among susceptibles predicted by factors suggestive of academic stress |
| BEREAVEMENT<br>(Schleifer et al. 1980) | ↓ LT 5-7 weeks post-bereavement<br>no difference in WBC, total lymphocyte or absolute or relative T & B cell counts between pre- and post-bereavement |
| EXAMINATION STRESS<br>(Dorian et al. 1981) | ↓ LT pre-exam vs. matched controls<br>↑ LT post-exam vs. matched controls<br>↓ cortisol pre- and post-exam<br>high stress subjects had ↑% late rosettes pre-exam |
| LIFE CHANGE STRESS<br>(Cohen-Cole et al. 1981) | ANUG patients had more negative LCS and more depressive symptoms<br>↓ LT<br>↓ PMN leukotaxis<br>↓ phagocytosis |
| LIFE CHANGE STRESS<br>(McClelland et al. 1980) | WBC counts and NK activity diminished in individuals characterized by combination of high nPOW motive style and high power-related LCS |
| ACADEMIC STRESS<br>(Jemmott et al. 1981) | ↓ salivary IgA levels during high stress periods<br>only subjects with inhibited power motivation failed to return to pre-stress levels after stressor |

(see Legend, next page)

21

TABLE 3 (cont.'d)

Legend:  ANUG   acute necrotizing ulcerative gingivitis ("trenchmouth")
         EBV    Epstein-Barr Virus
         LAP    leukocyte alkaline phosphatase
         LCS    life change stress
         LT     lymphoblast transformation
         NK     natural killer
         nPOW   need for power
         PMN    polymorphonuclear leukocyte
         R+0    day of recovery or splashdown

We postulate that the initial response to a state of mild stress is a
transient activation of certain components of the immune system. When this
state of arousal is prolonged, the transient enhancement may deplete the immune
system, resulting in temporary, relative immunodepression. There appears to be
an interactive effect of the stressor magnitude and the individual's adaptive
capacity on the immune response; exposure to a severe stressor coupled with
adaptive failure due to ineffective coping can lead to immunosuppressive
changes, even during a short-term stress. Thus, it is not stress itself which
is immunosuppressive, but stress coupled with poor coping. Such poor coping
may be a trait-dependent characteristic or state-dependent, as in the case of
a loss so massive as to exceed an individual's normally adequate adaptive
capacity. In addition, other factors such as social support may be moderating
variables and augment psychobiological adaptation and, hence, immunocompetence
in the face of severe stress. These complex interactions still require further
study.

Most people would readily agree that stress can affect physical health, but
more research is needed if the pathophysiologic mechanisms underlying the
relationship of stress, emotions, and immunity are to be better understood.
What is now needed are more studies permitting both within and between subject
comparisons, utilizing non-stressed control groups and a naturally-occurring
stressor of sufficient magnitude to alter immunity. Furthermore, it would be
useful to compare the effects of short-duration (1-14 days) and long-duration
(3-12 months) stressors. Finally, investigators should attempt to standardize
their immunologic and psychometric assessments to permit across study
comparisons.

Future research should also address an interesting question not specifically
addressed in our work: What types of coping activities reduce the impact of
stress on immune function? Such research could help provide the basis for

22

developing interventions with people at risk for immunodepression secondary
to stress.

ACKNOWLEDGMENTS
This work has been supported in part by the following grants and awards:
Young Investigator Award, National Cancer Institute, Behavioral Medicine Branch,
#1 R23-CA-29155; National Institutes of Health, Division of Research Resources,
Biomedical Research Support Grants #5 S07 RRO5484 (McLean Hospital) and #5 S07
RRO5487 (University Hospital); National Institutes of Mental Health, Psychiatry
Education Branch Training Grant # MH-151892 and N.I.H. Grant # NS 14387.
The authors wish to acknowledge with special thanks the assistance of the
following people:  Drs. Joan Borysenko, Myrin Borysenko, J. Stephen Heisel,
Michael Hurst, John Jemmott, Bernard Ransil and R. Michael Williams made
significant conceptual contributions in the development of this work.  Barbara
Beake, Deborah Copeland, Marlene Dietrich, Susan Edbril, Mindy Einerson,
Antonia Halton, Toni Hoover, Martin Ionescu-Pioggia, Katie Philips and Lisa
Steele have provided valuable technical assistance.  Drs. Herbert Benson,
Stanley King, Peter Knapp, Robert Rose and Alfred Stanton have provided support
and encouragement.  Finally, Shari Greenblatt has provided valuable editorial
assistance in the preparation of this manuscript.

REFERENCES
Ader R (1981) Psychoneuroimmunology.  New York: Academic Press.

Bartrop RW, Luckhurst E, Lazarus L et al (1977) Depressed lymphocyte function
    after bereavement.  Lancet 1:834-836.

Behelak Y, Banerjee D, Richter M (1976) Immunocompetent cells in patients with
    malignant disease I.  The lack of naturally occurring killer cell activity
    in the infractionated circulatory lymphocytes from patients with chronic
    lymphocyte leukemia (CLL).  Cancer 38:2274-2277.

Besedovsky HO, Sorkin E, Felix D et al. (1977) Hypothalamic changes during the
    immune response.  Eur J Immunol 7:232-325.

Besedovsky HO, DelRey A, Sorkin E et al. (1979) Immunoregulation mediated by
    the sympathetic nervous system.  Cell Immunol 48:346-355.

Bieliauskas L, Shekelle R, Garron D et al.(1979) Psychological depression and
    cancer mortality. Psychosom Med 41:77-78.

Bonmasser E, Campanile F, Houchens D et al.(1975) Impaired growth of a radia-
    tion-induced lymphoma in intact or lethally irradiated allogeneic athymic
    (nude) mice.  Transplantation 20:343-346.

REFERENCES (cont.'d)

Brunner KT, Maule J, Cerottini JC et al. (1968) Quantitative assay for the lytic action of immune lymphoid cells on $^{51}$Cr-labelled allogeneic target cells in vitro: Inhibition by isoantibody and drugs. Immunol 14:181-196.

Bulloch K, Moore RY (1980) Nucleus ambiguus projections to the thymus gland: Possible pathways for regulation of the immune response and the neuro-endocrine network (Abstract). Anat Rec 196:25.

Burnet FM (1970) The concept of immunological surveillance. Prog Exp Tumor Res 13:1-27.

Cannon GB, Bonnard GD, Djeu J et al. (1977) Relationship of human natural lymphocyte-mediated cytotoxicity to cytotoxicity of breast-cancer-derived target cells. Int J. Cancer 19:487-497.

Cerottini JC, Nordin AA, Brunner KT (1970) Specific in vitro cytotoxicity of thymus derived lymphocytes sensitized to alloantigens. Nature 228:1308-1309.

Chow DA, Green MI, Greenberg AH (1979) Macrophage-dependent, NK-cell-independent "natural" surveillance of tumors in syngeneic mice. Int J Cancer 23:788-797.

Cleary PJ (1974) Life events and disease: A review of methodology and findings. Reports from the Laboratory of Clinical Stress Research (Karolinska Institute) 37:39-40.

Cohen-Cole S, Cogen R, Stevens A et al. (1981) Psychosocial, endocrine, and immune factors in acute necrotizing ulcerative gingivitis ("trenchmouth") (Abstract). Psychosom Med 43:91.

Crary B (1981) The effects of epinephrine administration on human lymphocytes. Unpublished doctoral dissertation, Tufts University, Boston.

Dohrenwend BS, Dohrenwend BP (1974) Stressful life events: Their nature and effects. New York: Wiley Press.

Dorian BJ, Keystone E, Garfinkel PE et al. (1981) Immune mechanisms in acute psychological stress (Abstract). Psychosom Med 43:84.

Eremin O, Ashby J, Stephens JP (1978) Human natural cytotoxicity in the blood and lymphoid organs of healthy donors and patients with malignant disease. Int J Cancer 21:35-41.

Fischer CL, Daniels JC, Levin WC et al. (1972) Effects of the space flight environment on man's immune system: II. Lymphocyte counts and reactivity. Aerospace Med 43:1122-1125.

Friedman SB, Glasgow LA (1966) Psychologic factors and resistance to infectious disease. Ped Clin N Amer 13:315-335.

Galant SP, Lundak RL, Eaton L (1976) Enhancement of early human E-rosette formation by cholinergic stimuli. J Immunol 117:48-51.

Greene WA, Betts RF, Ochtill HN et al. (1978) Psychosocial factors and immunity: Preliminary report (Abstract). Psychosom Med 40:87.

REFERENCES (cont.'d)

Greer S, Morris T, Pettingale KW (1979) Psychological response to breast cancer: Effect on outcome. Lancet 2:785-787.

Grieco MH, Siegel I, Goel Z (1976) Modification of human T-lymphocyte rosette formation by autonomic agonists and cyclic nucleotides. J Allergy Clin Immunol 58:149-159.

Gunderson EK, Rahe RH, eds. (1974) Life stress and illness. Springfield, Illinois: Thomas.

Hackett TP, Cassem NH (1970) Psychological reactions to life-threatening illness: Acute myocardial infarction. In Abram HS (ed.), Psychological Aspects of Stress. Springfield, Illinois:Thomas.

Hall NR, Goldstein AL (1981) Neurotransmitters and the immune system. In Ader R (ed.), Psychoneuroimmunology. New York: Academic Press, 521-543.

Hall NR, McClure JE, Hu SK et al. (1980) Effects of chemical sympathectomy upon thymus dependent immune responses. Society for Neuroscience (Abstract), in press.

Hansson M, Keissling R, Andersson B et al. (1979) NK cell sensitive T-cell subpopulation in thymus: Inverse correlation to host NK activity. Nature 278:174-176.

Hazum E, Chang KJ, Cuatrecasas P (1979) Specific nonopiate receptors for beta-endorphin. Science 205:1033-1035.

Henney CS, Tracey D, Durdik JM et al. (1978) Natural killer cells in vitro and in vivo. Am J Path 93:459-467.

Hepner G, Henry E, Stolback L et al. (1975) Problems in the clinical use of the microcytotoxicity assay for measuring cell-mediated immunity to tumor cells. Cancer Res 35:1931-1937.

Herberman RB, Holden HT (1978) Natural cell-mediated immunity. In Klein G, Weinhouse S (eds.), Advances in Cancer Research. Academic Press, 305-377.

Hinkle LE, Wolff HG (1958) Ecological investigations of the relationship between illness, life experiences and the social environment. Ann Int Med 49:1373-1389.

Holmes TH, Rahe RH (1967) The social readjustment rating scale. J Psychosom Res 11:213-218.

Holmes TH, Hawkins NG, Bowerman CE et al. (1957) Psychosocial and psychophysiologic studies of tuberculosis. Psychosom Med 19:134-143.

Hurst MW, Jenkins CD, Rose RM (1978) The assessment of life change stress: A comparative and methodological inquiry. Psychosom Med 40:126-141.

Ishigami T (1919) The influence of psychic acts on the progress of pulmonary tuberculosis. Amer Rev Tuberculosis 2:470-484.

REFERENCES (cont.'d)

Jacobs S, Ostfeld A (1977) An epidemiological review of the mortality of bereavement. Psychosom Med 39:344-357.

Jemmott JB (1981) Stress, social motives and immunity. Unpublished doctoral dissertation, Harvard University, Cambridge.

Jenkins CD (1976) Recent evidence supporting psychologic and social risk factors for coronary disease. New Eng J Med 294:987-994.

Jenkins CD, Hurst MW, Rose RM (1979) Life changes: Do people really remember? Arch Gen Psychiat 36:379-384.

Kasl SV, Evans AS, Niederman JC (1979) Psychosocial risk factors in the development of infectious mononucleosis. Psychosom Med 41:445-466.

Keller R (1978) Macrophage-mediated natural cytotoxicity against various target cells in vitro. I. Comparison of tissue macrophages from diverse anatomic sites and from different strains of rats and mice. Br J Cancer 37:732-741.

Kimzey SL (1975) The effects of extended spaceflight on hematologic and immunologic systems. J Amer Med Wom Assoc 30:218-232.

Kiessling R, Klein E, Wigzell H (1975) "Natural" killer cells in the mouse. I. Cytotoxic cells with specificity for mouse Maloney leukemia cells. Specificity and distribution according to genotype. Eur J Immunol 5:112-117.

Labarba RC (1970) Experimental and environmental factors in cancer. A review of research with animals. Psychosom Med 32:259-276.

Lazarus R (1966) Psychological stress and the coping process. New York: McGraw-Hill.

Leach CS, Rambaut PC (1974) Biochemical responses of the Skylab crewman. Proceedings of the Skylab Life Sciences Symposium, Vol II, p. 1.

Locke SE (in press) Stress, adaptation and immunity: studies in humans. Gen Hosp Psychiat.

Locke SE, Heisel JS (1977) The influence of stress and emotions on human immunity (Abstract). Biofeed Self Regul 2:320.

Locke SE, Hurst MW, Heisel JS et al. (1978) The influence of stress on the immune response. Annual Meeting, American Psychosomatic Society, Washington, D.C.

Locke SE, Hurst MW, Heisel JS et al. (1979) The influence of stress and other psychosocial factors on human immunity. Presented at symposium: The Current Status of Psycho-immunologic Research, 36th Annual Meeting, American Psychosomatic Society, Dallas, TX.

Masuda M, Holmes TH (1967) Magnitude estimations of social readjustments. J Psychosom Res 11:219-225.

Marx JL (1980) Natural killer cells help defend the body. Science 210:624-626.

26

REFERENCES (cont.'d)

McClelland DC, Floor E, Davidson RJ et al. (1980) Stressed power motivation, sympathetic activation, immune function, and illness. J Human Stress 6: 11-19.

McClelland DC, Locke SE, Williams RM et al. Power motivation, distress and immune function. Unpublished manuscript.

McCoy J, Herberman R, Perlin E et al.(1973) $^{51}Cr$ release cellular lymphocyte cytotoxicity as a possible measure of immunologic competence of cancer patients. Proc Amer Assoc Cancer Res 14:107.

Mechanic D (1962) Students under stress. New York: Free Press.

Melief CJM, Schwartz RS (1975) Immunocompetence and malignancy. In Becker FF (ed.), Cancer, a comprehensive treatise, vol. 1. New York: Plenum Press.

Oehler JR, Campbell DA, Herberman RB (1977) In vitro inhibition of lymphoproliferative responses to tumor associated antigens and of lymphoma cell proliferation by rat splenic macrophages. Cell Immunol 28:355-370.

Outzen HC, Custer RP, Eaten GJ et al.(1975) Spontaneous and induced tumor incidence in germfree "nude" mice. J Reticuloendothel Soc 17:1-9.

Palmblad J, Cantell K, Strander H. et al. (1976) Stressor exposure and immunological response in man: Interferon-producing capacity and phagocytosis. J Psychosom Res 20:193-199.

Palmblad J, Petrini B, Wasserman J et al. (1979) Lymphocyte and granulocyte reactions during sleep deprivation. Psychosom Med 41:273-278.

Prehn RT (1974) Immunological surveillance: Pro and con. In Bach FH, Good RA, (eds.), Clinical immunobiology, vol. 2. New York: Academic Press.

Pross HF, Baines MG (1976) Spontaneous human lymphocyte-mediated cytotoxicity against tumor target cells. I. The effect of malignant disease. Int J Cancer 18:593-604.

Pross HF, Jondal M (1975) Cytotoxic lymphocytes from normal donors. A functional marker of human non-T lymphocytes. Clin Exp Immunol 21:226-235.

Pullan PT, Clement-Jonas V, Corder R et al. (1980) Ectopic production of methionine-enkephalin and beta-endorphin. Brit J Med 280:758-759.

Rabkin JG, Struening EL (1976) Life events, stress and illness. Science 194: 1013-1020.

Rahe RH, Arthur RJ (1978) Life change and illness studies: past history and future directions. J Human Stress 1:3-15.

Rees WD, Lutkins SG (1967) Mortality of bereavement. Br Med J 4:13-16.

Riley V (1981) Psychoneuroendocrine influences on immunocompetence and neoplasia. Science 212:1100-1109.

REFERENCES (cont.'d)

Roessler RL, Cate TR, Lester JW et al. (1979) Ego strength, life change and antibody titers. Paper presented at Annual Meeting, American Psychosomatic Society, Dallas, TX.

Rogers MP, Dubey D, Reich P (1979) The influence of the psyche and the brain on immunity and disease susceptibility: A critical review. Psychosom Med 41: 147-164.

Rose RM (1980) Endocrine responses to stressful psychological events. Psychiat Clin N Amer 3:251-276.

Rosenberg EB, McCoy JL, Green SS et al. (1974) Destruction of human lymphoid tissue-culture cell lines by human peripheral lymphocytes in $^{51}$Cr release cellular cytotoxicity assays. J Nat Cancer Inst 52:345-352.

Rotter V, Trainin N (1975) Inhibition of tumor growth in syngeneic chimeric mice mediated by a depletion of suppressor T cells. Transplantation 20: 68-74.

Rygaard J, Povlsen CO (1969) The mouse mutant nude does not develop spontaneous tumors. Acta Pathol Microbiol Scand 77:758-760.

Schleifer SJ, Keller SE, McKegney FP et al. (1980) Bereavement and lymphocyte function. Paper presented at Annual Meeting, American Psychiatric Association, San Francisco, CA.

Stein M, Keller S, Schleifer S (1981) The hypothalamus and the immune response. In Weiner H, Hofer M, Stunkard AJ (eds.), Brain, behavior and bodily disease. New York: Raven Press.

Stein M, Schiavi RC, Camerino M (1976) Influence of brain and behavior on the immune system. Science 191:435-440.

Strom TB, Carpenter CB (1980) Cyclic nucleotides in immunosuppression - neuro-endocrine pharmacologic manipulation and in vivo regulation of immunity acting via second messenger systems. Transplant Proc 12:304-310.

Stutman O (1974) Tumor development after 3-methylcholanthrene in immunologically deficient athymic-nude mice. Science 183:534-536.

Stutman O (1975) Immunodepression and malignancy. Adv Cancer Res 22:261-422.

Takasugi M, Ramseyer A, Takasugi J (1977) Decline of natural non-selective cell-mediated cytotoxicity in patients with tumor progression. Cancer Res 37: 413-418.

Tanaka S, Ito T, Kashahara K et al. (1977) Suppression of the primary immune response by chemical sympathectomy. Res Comm Chem Pathol Pharmacol 16: 687-694.

Thomas CB, Duszynski KR, Shaffer JW (1979) Family attitudes reported in youth as potential predictors of cancer. Psychosom Med 41:287-302.

Thomas L (1959) Discussion. Cellular and humoral aspects of the hypersensitive states. New York: Hoeber-Harper.

REFERENCES (cont.'d)

Vaillant GE (1978) Natural history of male psychological health, IV: What kinds of men do not get psychosomatic illness. Psychosom Med 40:420-431.

Williams JM, Peterson RG, Shea PA et al. (1981) Sympathetic innervation of murine thymus and spleen: Evidence for a functional link between the nervous and immune systems. Brain Res Bull 6:83-94.

Williams RM, Kraus LJ, Inbar M et al. (1979) Circadian bioperiodicity of natural killer cell activity in human blood (individually assessed). Chronobiologia 6:172.

Wolfe T (1979) The Right Stuff. New York: Bantam Books.

Wolff CT, Friedman SB, Hofer MA et al. (1964) Relationship between psychological defenses and mean urinary 17-hydroxycorticosteroid rates. Psychosom Med 26:576-591.

Wybran J, Appelboom T, Famaey JP et al. (1979) Suggestive evidence for receptors for morphine and methionine-enkephalin on normal human blood T-lymphocytes. J Immunol 123:1068-1070.

Zinkernagel RM, Doherty PC (1974) Restriction of in vitro T-cell mediated cyto-toxicity in lymphocytic choriomeningitis virus within a syngeneic or semi-allogeneic system. Nature 248:701-702.

# HIGHER CORTICAL FUNCTION AND NEOPLASIA: PSYCHONEUROIMMUNOLOGY

JOAN Z. BORYSENKO, Ph.D.+
+Division of Behavioral Medicine, Department of Medicine, Beth Israel Hospital
and the Charles A. Dana Research Institute and the Thorndike Laboratory,
Harvard Medical School, Boston, Massachusetts

## INTRODUCTION

Data from both clinical and animal model studies have implicated stress, coping and expression of affect as potential modulators in the development and/ or progression of neoplasia. Stress, or the inability to make a satisfactory behavioral adjustment to an environmental demand, increases susceptibility to illnesses that are immunologically regulated. The theoretical mechanisms underlying compromise of immunity as a function of stress involve behaviorally mediated hormonal changes that in turn functionally inhibit immunocompetent effector cells of several sub-classes. The study of the relation between behavior and immunity comprises the growing field of psychoneuroimmunology. In this review, psychoneuroimmunology will be related to the study of neoplasia. First, there will be a very brief historical overview of clinical and animal studies concerning behavior, life stress, coping and the development and course of cancer. The endocrine-immune axis will then be explored in some detail. Finally, studies of disease susceptibility and specific inhibition of immunity following stress in animals will provide a background for the integration of psychoneuroimmunological research into clinical studies of neoplasia.

## BEHAVIORAL VARIABLES IN THE ETIOLOGY AND COURSE OF CANCER

Personality variables have been studied extensively as possible risk factors in cancer and modulators of disease progression. This area has been reviewed recently by Fox (1979) and by Borysenko, Benson and Borysenko (1981). Studies relating behavioral considerations to cancer etiology or course must take into account two sources of possible error. Firstly, in some instances, the disease process itself can affect emotions and personality (Fras, 1973). Psychiatric symptoms may result from metastases to the central nervous system or from metabolic or hormonal sequelae of the cancer. Thus, it can be difficult to ascertain whether psychological changes are related to the development or progression of a cancer or are alternatively a physical result of the disease.

Secondly, the diagnosis of cancer itself, the adjustment to a chronic illness, fear of treatment and recurrence can cause personality and behavioral changes in cancer patients. These two caveats are inherent difficulties in retrospective studies. Nonetheless, such studies were valuable in describing characteristics of cancer patients and generating hypotheses that could then be tested semi-prospectively, prospectively and in animal model systems.

Cancer patients have been characterized retrospectively as emotionally repressed (Bahnson, 1966), unable to modulate the expression of emotions (Kissen, 1967; Greer, 1975) and reacting with feelings of helplessness and hopelessness to episodes of life-stress and loss (LeShan, 1966; Greene, 1966). Semi-prospective investigations, where the diagnosis of an at-risk population is predicted on the basis of personality and emotional variables, have led to similar descriptions of the cancer patient (Kissen, 1963; Schmale, 1966. Horne, 1979). Unfortunately, there are few extant prospective studies in this area. Such studies, of course, would constitute the evidence required to substantiate a true causal relation between personality or expression of affect and the development or course of cancer. Fox (1979) critically reviews these studies. One such study, where the cohort was large enough to be significant, was that of Shekelle and Coworkers (1981). They assessed depression by the Minnesota Multiphasic Personality Index D scale in 2,020 employed men aged 40-55. Cause-specific mortality was then ascertained for the next 17 years. Eighty-two men who died of cancer had significantly higher D scores than those who had died from other causes or who had survived. Men with D as the highest scoring subscale had more than twice the rate of cancer death ($p < 0.001$) when compared to men whose highest score was on any other subscale. The results could not be accounted for when adjusted for age, smoking or alcohol consumption. Further, studies of this sort are required to establish the putative association between depression and development of cancer. Such studies should address possible biological mediators in terms of the hormonal and immunological correlates of depression.

The prognosis of various types and stages of cancer is based on actuarial data. However, patients of the same age, sex, equivalent physical status and undergoing similar therapy can fare very differently with the same type of tumor. Most cases cluster about a norm, but there will be a few outstanding examples of people who survive much longer than expected. Others die more quickly than predicted. In several studies, the inability to express anger or inappropriate modulation of anger have been correlated with poor prognosis (Blumberg, 1954; Stavraky, 1968; Greer, 1975; Abeloff, 1977). In a five-year prospective study of psychological factors relating to breast cancer outcome,

75% of women whose initial response following mastectomy indicated a "fighting spirit" or strong denial had a favorable outcome at five years (Greer, 1979). In contrast, only 35% of those women responding with either stoic acceptance or a helpless/hopeless outlook were disease-free at five years. Initial reactions of helplessness and hopelessness occurred in 88% of the women who had died in the five-year period. Only 46% of those disease-free at five years had had such a reaction. Since the focus of this study was on patients with early cancer, the possibility that depressive reactions were mediated by systemic effects of the disease was lessened. These data have now held through an eight-year follow-up.

Prospective human studies are difficult and costly to perform. Many investigators have thus concentrated their efforts on animal model systems. Two such investigators, Drs. Riley and Anisman, have discussed this area in depth as part of this symposium (chapters 5 and 6, respectively). Animal model systems allow manipulation of variables that cannot be controlled for in human studies. Animal colonies can be genetically homogeneous, age-matched, and host to a single chosen tumor type. Diet and environment can be meticulously controlled. When subjected to stress, the type, chronicity, timing relative to tumor implantation and ability of the animal to exercise control over the stress, can be precisely determined. As elegantly illustrated by these investigators, such variables are critical to experimental outcome.

Early Russian animal studies of psychological risk factors in cancer were based on Pavlov's work with conditioned reflexes. Experimental "neuroses" produced in dogs and mice by conditioning were associated with an increased incidence of spontaneous tumors. In strains of mice predisposed to a particular tumor, behaviorally-induced "neuroticism" accelerated tumor development. Furthermore, "neurotic" mice developed larger tumors with shorter latency than did control mice after implantation of a standard number of tumor cells (Kavetsky, 1966). Early animal studies concerning psychological variables and cancer have been reviewed by LaBarba (1970). In some instances stress-inducing manipulations exacerbate tumor take and/or growth, while in other instances they are retarded. The literature is difficult to evaluate because of differences in stressors, species, tumor lines, environmental conditions, timing of the stress relative to tumor implant and chronicity of stress. Such factors will be discussed in more detail below and are addressed at length by Anisman elsewhere in this volume (chapter 5).

In a well-controlled study, Riley demonstrated that the stress engendered by exposure to environmental cues in a standard animal facility decreased tumor latency in female $C^3H$ mice carrying the Bittner oncogenic virus (Riley, 1975).

One group of mice was housed in a standard animal facility, the other in a sheltered facility designed to produce minimal stress. By 400 days, 92% of the mice in standard housing had developed mammary tumors as expected, compared to only 7% of those in the sheltered facility. By 600 days, however, as the mice aged and became progressively immunodeficient, tumor incidence in the sheltered group rose to expected levels. Tumor latency was influenced significantly by differential environmental conditions related to stress and increased corticosterone levels.

The interaction between experimental stress and coping ability has been investigated by Sklar & Anisman (1979). A single 1.1 hour exposure to inescapable electric shock of 6 sec duration at 1 min intervals significantly decreased tumor latency, increased size and decreased survival time of mice previously injected with mastocytoma cells. Coping ability and its relation to tumor growth was then investigated in yoked-control experiments. Both the escape group and their yoked controls were exposed to the same shock duration, but the yoked-controls had no ability to control shock-offset. Shock simply terminated in a behaviorally noncontingent manner when the yoked escape mouse jumped a barrier in a shuttle box. Tumors in the yoked-control group developed significantly faster and led to an earlier death. The group that could escape, however, did not differ significantly in tumor growth or mortality from animals who had never been shocked. Chronic stress, however, did not exacerbate tumor growth. The differential effects of acute and chronic stress are apparently related to the time course of endocrine-immune interactions that are discussed later in this chapter.

In a series of differential housing experiments, social isolation enhanced tumor growth in mice (Sklar, 1980). It was the abrupt change in social conditions, rather than isolation per se, however, that was responsible for increased tumor growth. In mice who were reared in isolation and then switched to group housing following tumor implant, behavior modulated tumorigenesis. Specifically, some mice remained passive after the transfer while others engaged in fighting. The fighters had significantly smaller tumors than the non-fighters. Sklar and Anisman hypothesized that fighting may comprise an adaptive coping response. Indeed, fighting is known to prevent some of the neurochemical changes induced by stress, as well as to ameliorate the ulcerogenic effects of shock stress. These data parallel human studies. Stress alone does not lead to increased tumor growth. Rather, inability to cope with stress seems most important.

Clearly, the inability to cope with a stress that occurs 1-2 years before a cancer diagnosis in humans cannot represent a primary etiologic agent. Most cancers grow slowly and become manifest only after a long latent period which can be estimated from observed doubling times of similar cells in culture. Most clinically detectable tumors consist of at least $10^{10}$ cells. Thus, about five years are required for one transformed cell to proliferate into a detectable tumor in the median case. Fox (1978) cites five years as a conservative estimate for the latency of lung cancer, and 11 years for breast cancer. While the inability to cope with relatively recent stressful situations is not biologically compatible with a role as an etiologic variable, it is possible that chronic endocrine changes consistent with a life-history of deficient coping may have an etiologic role. There are currently no data bearing on this issue. Hormonal changes secondary to recent episodes of stress, however, may have an effect on the survival or growth of established tumors caused by diverse etiologic agents. Thus, the latency of a tumor and its subsequent growth could theoretically be affected by mechanisms to be described below.

PSYCHONEUROIMMUNOLOGY

Given a particular genetic composition, a number of environmental factors can modify the basic immunocompetence of the host to produce a temporary, acquired immunodeficiency. Some cases of immunodeficiency may lead to overt disease while other cases pass with no apparent sequelae. Physical factors leading to acquired immunodeficiency have been well studied and include trauma, malnutrition, infection, neoplasia irradiation and a variety of drugs that are used to depress the immune system following organ transplantation. Aging itself is associated with involution of the thymus and a concomitant decline in both cellular and humoral immunity. Perhaps the most prevalent and least well appreciated of the environmental modulators of immune competence, however, are behavioral factors.

The premise that the immune system can be compromised behaviorally, leading to a transient acquired immunodeficiency, underlies the rapidly expanding field of psychoneuroimmunology. The nomenclature reflects interest in exploring the causal connection between psychological events, endocrine secretion and modulation of immunity. Early animal studies in this area fit into the more general rubric of psychosomatics and later of stress and disease susceptibility, paralleling human research. Once the effect of behavioral factors on disease susceptibility was substantiated, the search for intermediary mechanisms began. These mechanisms currently comprise two categories: An indirect pathway whereby behavioral parameters affect immunity through hormonal changes and a putative direct pathway involving bidirectional communication between the central nervous system and the lymphoid organs.

## STRESS, ENDOCRINE RESPONSE AND IMMUNITY

Stress is equally hard to define either as a stimulus or as a set of physiological responses. Mason has emphasized the specificity of hormonal responses to different types of stress (1974). Furthermore, Frankenhauser (1976) has shown that an individual's ability or perceived ability to master (cope) with a stress, is a potent modulator of physiological response. These data preclude a reductionistic definition of stress as the nonspecific response of the body to any demand (Selye, 1950). Rather, stress comprises a variety of different physiological responses arising to various stimuli, modulated by the adaptive capacity of the organism. The specific nature of the stress and its controllability are critical issues in animal studies of psychoneuroimmunology. For instance, the fear response to aversive stimulation is easily conditioned. If rats are signaled prior to shock, they show fear only when the danger signal is on. In rats receiving the same total amount of shock, those who are signaled prior to its occurrence and can thus discriminate safe from unsafe conditions, have lower levels of corticosterone and a reduced incidence of stomach ulcers compared to those in a state of chronic fear (Weiss, 1970 and 1971).

Given the variability of stressful stimuli, the cognitive or learned component of control or coping in the subject, and the chronicity of the stress, physiological response is not stereotypic. There are, however, a basic core of integrated endocrinological changes induced by stress that support the "fight or flight" response originally described by Cannon (1926). The endocrine response to physical stress and/or emotional arousal is initiated in the hypothalamus. Neurosecretory cells discharge hypophysiotropic neuropeptides via the hypophyseal portal system to the adenohypophysis where these products modulate release of pituitary hormones. Hypothalamic efferent neurons simultaneously stimulate secretion of catecholamines from the adrenal medulla via the splanchnic nerves. Catecholamine release then initiates a secondary cascade of hormonal effects which serve to perpetuate the metabolic response to stress (Figure 1). The endocrine response to tissue damage or blood loss due to trauma is mediated by sensory stimulation via hypothalamic afferent neurons from the more caudal levels; these neurons convey visceroception and direct sensation of painful stimuli from the polysynaptic ascending systems involving the midbrain limbic system and thalamus. Reactions

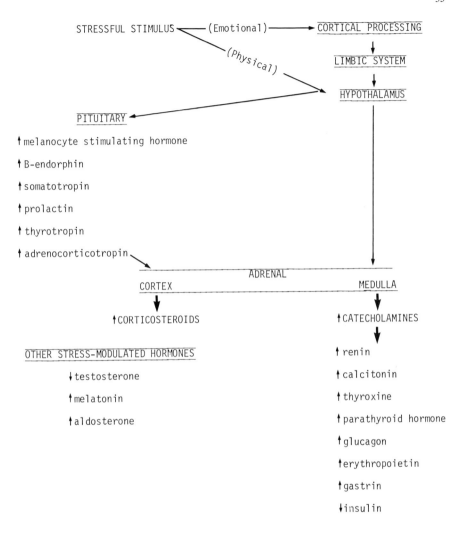

Fig. 1. Neuroendocrine sequelae of stress; the stereotypic response to stimuli arousing the need for "fight-or-flight."

to events that are stressful only in the context of past behavioral
experience, however, are likely to be mediated via afferent neurons arriving
from the neocortex either directly or by way of the limbic system.

The identification of hormones that are affected by stress has grown as
radioimmunoassay techniques for their detection have been perfected.  In
addition to corticosteroids and catecholamines which have been studied
historically in association with stress, more recently a number of other
hormones have also been identified.  Release of growth hormone (e.g.
somatotropin) (Brown, 1972), adrenocorticotropin (Mason, 1968), melanocyte-
stimulating hormone (Hirata, 1975), prolactin (Noel, 1972), thyrotropin
(Dewhurst, 1968), vasopressin, aldosterone, calcitonin, parathyroid hormone,
thyroxine, glucagon, renin, erythropoietin and gastrin have all been
associated with stress.  The last seven hormones mentioned are released in
response to sympathoadrenal stimulation which increases blood catecholamine
levels (for review see Landsberg, 1977 as well as chapter 10, this volume).

The catecholamines have been hypothesized to have a major role in the
integration of endocrine secretion (Landsberg, 1977).  Their release during
stress may allow an anticipatory change in hormonal milieu initiated by the
central nervous system.  With the exception of the thyroid hormones, none of
the other catecholamine regulated hormones are under direct pituitary control.
They are all normally subject to individual feedback loops which respond to
slow, sustained changes in the environment.  The secretion of all these
hormones is dependent on the adenylate cyclase 3',5'-cyclic adenosine
monophosphate (cAMP) system.  Since the catecholamines also activate the cAMP
system, a final common pathway exists whereby the usual regulatory pathways
can be overridden to produce an integrated hormonal response to stress
(Landsberg, 1977).  In general, the hormones released via the catecholamine
pathway potentiate circulatory and metabolic adjustments required for "flight-
or-flight."  This type of over-riding regulatory capacity is adaptive in that
it readies the system for immediate response.  On the other hand, sympathetic
arousal is easily conditioned.  A stimulus that is stressful only through
association can thus produce widespread hormonal changes through this pathway.
Since catecholamine output is known to vary as a function of the individual's
ability to cope with a stress (Frankenhauser, 1970), it is likely that
perceived control is an important modulator of all the catecholamine regulated
hormones.

Two hormones, insulin and testosterone decrease in response to stress.
Insulin decrease occurs as a direct result of catecholamine release and
enhances the primary metabolic effects of the catecholamines.  Insulin and

testosterone levels increase during recovery from stressful events and may contribute to restoration of homeostasis by promoting anabolic reactions to repair the stress-induced catabolism of body protein and fat stores (Mason, 1975). (For a complete discussion of potential endocrine effects on neoplasia, see chapter 10 by Lippman in this volume.)

Interest in hormonal regulation of the immune response is relatively recent, although it has been known for many years that acute stress causes a striking involution of the thymus (Dougherty, 1952). This involution can be mimicked by administration of adrenal and sex steroids. Conversely, adrenalectomy and gonadectomy induce increased growth of lymphoid tissue by removal of these inhibitory steroids from the system (Dougherty, 1964). Early ablation experiments also demonstrate the necessity for certain hormonal factors to maintain the integrity of lymphoid organs. Thyroidectomy and hypophysectomy, for example, culminate in lymphoid involution that can be partially prevented by selective replacement therapy with thyroid hormones and somatotropin.

The effect of adrenal corticosteroids on the lymphoid tissue of common laboratory animals and man has been well reviewed (Claman, 1977). Corticosteroids actually lyse lymphocytes in the thymic cortex of sensitive species such as the mouse, rat, rabbit and hamster, as well as inhibiting the metabolism of other lymphocytes. In "corticosteroid-resistant" species including humans and monkeys, corticosteroids inhibit lymphocyte metabolism, interfering with proliferation. Thus, with chronic stress, lymphoid organs progressively atrophy because cell division is retarded. In vitro, cortisol and to a lesser extent estradiol, progesterone and testosterone all inhibit the stimulation (blastogenesis) of human peripheral blood lymphocytes by mitogens. These steroids both decrease the rate of DNA replication and suppress recruitment of cells from the $G_0$ to the $G_1$ phase of the cell cycle (Mendelsohn, 1977). In addition to decreasing total number of lymphocytes, several specific immunological functions are also impaired by corticosteroids. Moreover, many of the inhibitory effects occur at very low concentrations (Bach, 1975), indicating that endogenous stress-induced elevations of steroids are capable of producing these effects.

In recent years, lymphocytes have been demonstrated to have membrane surface receptors for a number of different hormones. These include β-adrenergic catecholamines, E type prostaglandins, somatotropin, histamine, insulin, antidiuretic hormone and parathyroid hormone among others (for review see Bourne, 1974). All these hormones stimulate cell membrane adenylate cyclase and generate cAMP as a second messenger. Elevation in cAMP increases metabolism in immature cells, stimulating maturation. For instance, thymosin,

38

a hormone-like factor produced by thymic epithelial cells induces cellular
maturation marked by the appearance of a specific antigen (Thy 1-2) on T cell
precursors. This effect is mimicked by other agents that increase
intracellular cAMP (Bach, 1975). While such hormones stimulate proliferation
and differentiation of immature cells, they have a distinct inhibitory effect
on mature, immunocompetent cells. Both human and mouse lymphocyte reactivity
to mitogens is depressed by agents that raise intracellular cAMP. Similarly,
elevated cAMP inhibits immune cytolysis and interferon production by human
lymphocytes, histamine release by human basophils and antibody formation to
sheep red blood cells in mice (Bourne, 1974).

In many cAMP-sensitive systems, there is evidence for an opposing influence
of cyclic 3'-5' guanosine monophosphate (cGMP) (Figure 2). In the immune
system, cGMP appears to have enhancing effects that directly oppose the
inhibitory effects of cAMP. Antigen stimulated release of histamine from
basophils (Bourne, 1974), release of lysosomal enzymes from polymorphonuclear
leucocytes (Ignarro, 1974), proliferation of lymphocytes in response to
mitogens (Hadden, 1972) and lymphocyte mediated cytotoxicity (Strom, 1973) are
all augmented by cGMP. In addition, the cholinergic agonists carbachol and
dibutyryl cGMP, both of which raise intracellular cGMP levels, enhance "early"

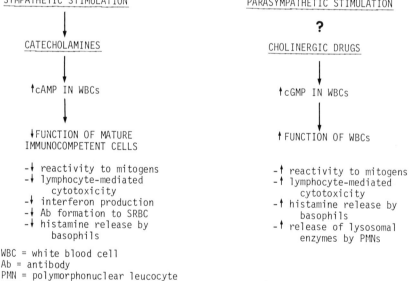

WBC = white blood cell
Ab = antibody
PMN = polymorphonuclear leucocyte
SRBC = sheep red blood cells (stimulating antigen)

Fig. 2. Modulation of immune function by autonomic activity through opposing
effects of the cyclic nucleotides cAMP and cGMP.

E rosette formation by human T lymphocytes. In contrast, early E rosette formation is inhibited by the β-adrenergic agonist isoproterenol or by dibutyryl cAMP, both of which raise intracellular cAMP levels (Galant, 1976; Grieco, 1976).

These results suggest that the autonomic nervous system has immunomodulatory effects, and that sympathetic stimulation with its attendant release of catecholamines has an overall inhibitory effect on the function of committed immunocompetent effector cells. Following prolonged stress, there are fewer circulating lymphocytes suggesting that the inhibitory effect of corticosteroids on lymphocyte proliferation outweighs the promoting effect of the catecholamines. Furthermore, the function of the existing pool of mature cells is subject to inhibition both by circulating epinephrine and corticosteroids. In addition to effects on lymphocytes, both agents also inhibit functions of macrophages, basophils, mast cells, neutrophils and eosinophils which all interact in either the afferent or the effector functions of the immune system.

It has been suggested that certain mediators of inflammation, vasoactive hormones and cAMP act as feedback regulators to control the extent of immune reactions (Bourne, 1974). In this regard, the immunoinhibitory effects of hormones released under conditions of acute stress would prevent the formation of auto-antibodies to components of tissue damaged by trauma. Hormonal regulation of immunity, however, must be considered in relation to other immunoregulatory pathways. Overall immune function is controlled at several levels. Heredity, cell-cell interaction and hormonal factors are different strata of regulation. One cannot be studied independently of the others. For instance, one type of lymphocyte, the suppressor cell, inhibits certain facets of immune responsiveness. Agents that increase intracellular cAMP inhibit the effector functions of most immune cells, including suppressor T cells (Weinstein, 1976).

Therefore, in systems regulated by suppressor cells, increase in cAMP should theoretically enhance some immune functions by inhibiting the suppressor mechanism. Recent studies in our laboratory, however, have shown that epinephrine injected into human subjects actually causes a transient increase in the population of circulating suppressor cells defined by the presence of $F_c$ receptors, and a parallel functional suppression of lymphocyte stimulation by mitogens (Crary, 1981). A high physiological dose of epinephrine was injected subcutaneously into normal human volunteers, and effects on peripheral blood lymphocytes were then assessed. Epinephrine injection was followed by a transient lymphocytosis. There was a striking, severalfold increase in a lymphocyte subpopulation characterized by azurophilic cytoplasmic granules. This lymphocyte subpopulation consisted of suppressor cells, identified by the presence of receptors for sheep erythrocytes and for the $F_c$ portion of IgG. The functional activity of these cells was determined by culture with a variety of mitogens. The proliferative response to all mitogens was suppressed at 15 and 30 min post injection relative to pre-injection values. Responsivity returned to baseline by 120 minutes. In a parallel assay, the generation of plasma cells in response to pokeweed mitogen stimulation was similarly suppressed. To determine if the observed increase in suppressor cell number and parallel inhibition of mitogen responsivity was a direct or indirect effect of epinephrine, peripheral blood was drawn from untreated volunteers. The mononuclear cells were then cultured with epinephrine. No effect on lymphocyte proliferation to mitogens was observed with cells exposed directly to epinephrine in vitro. Thus, the observed effects are likely to be mediated indirectly. These data indicate that epinephrine, in vivo, indirectly produces a striking, transient increase in peripheral suppressor cell number and activity.

Since it is likely that this apparent but unexpected increase in suppression is not mediated directly by epinephrine, but indirectly by some other agent triggered by epinephrine, the complexity of the system is obvious. Thus, further studies in intact organisms are required before generalizing the results from isolated in vitro systems to functions of whole organisms. The numerous possible cellular and hormonal interactions involved in controlling immune responsivity preclude simplistic interpretations of mechanisms mediating behavioral influences on immunity. Hormones other than the catecholamines and corticosteroids are clearly involved in immunomodulation, but their roles have not yet been well studied. Furthermore, the pattern of hormonal release varies as a function of different types of stress, chronicity of stress, and of the organism's ability to control the stress. These variables are of great importance in the ultimate understanding of stress, immunity and cancer.

## STRESS AND DISEASE SUSCEPTIBILITY IN ANIMAL MODEL SYSTEMS

Exposure to experimental stress generally decreases host resistance to diseases that are regulated immunologically. A variety of stressors have been evaluated in early studies. However, no direct measures of immune function were performed. Mice subjected to experimental stress by avoidance conditioning in a shuttle box or by physical restraint are more susceptible to infections with Herpes simplex virus (Rasmussen, 1957), Poliomyelitis virus

(Johnson, 1965), Coxsackie B virus (Johnson, 1963), and polyoma virus
(Rasmussen, 1969). Similarly, the stress of crowding markedly increases
susceptibility to Salmonella typhimurium (Edwards, 1977) and trichinosis
infection (Davis, 1958); predator-induced stress (cat vs. mouse) increases
infectivity with the parasite Hymenolepis nana in animals that have been
previously immunized (Hamilton, 1974). In a few cases, however, stress has
been demonstrated to protect against infection (Friedman, 1973). The nature
and chronicity of the stress, the time at which the infective agent is
introduced relative to the stress, the housing and social conditions of the
animals and the nature of the cellular interactions involved in the immune
response to the pathogen under investigation are critical to outcome. Overall,
cause and effect relations between stress and susceptibility to infection are
reproducibly demonstrable in adequately controlled experiments.

The comprehensive investigations of Riley (1981) have clarified some of the
seemingly contradictory effects of stress on immunity and disease in animals.
Rodents living in standard animal quarters are subject to noise, pheromones and
ultrasound distress signals from other animals undergoing capture or
manipulation. The corticosterone levels of such animals are 10 to 20 times
higher than those of rodents housed in a protected, low-stress environment
(Riley, 1975). Variables such as population density and proximity of males and
females that are usually uncontrolled are capable of modulating impressive
changes in corticosterone levels. When apparently "baseline" endocrine
parameters are in actuality already highly elevated, the effects of additional
experimental stress cannot be adequately assessed. It is thus of utmost
importance to keep animals in a low-stress, well-controlled environment.

In extensive, meticulously controlled experiments employing either virally-
induced or transplanted tumors, Riley has shown that stress (either living in
a standard animal facility or exposure to a mild, anxiety-provoking rotation)
consistently increases tumor growth. These effects can be mimicked by
injection of natural or synthetic corticosteroids into the animals. The
apparently contradictory results of some early animal experiments showing
inhibition of tumor growth by stress become understandable in view of the
timing of the stress relative to the tumor implant. Both tumor suppression and
tumor enhancement can be demonstrated in the same system as a function of the
timing of rotational stress or injection of corticosteroids (Riley, 1981).
Dexamethasone injection into mice seven days after implantation of a
lymphosarcoma promotes tumor growth; injection seven days before implantation
retards tumor growth. These differences probably reflect an initial hormonally
sustained immune inhibition followed by a rebound recovery and overshoot of

cell-mediated immune function. Immunologic rebound has been hypothetically attributed to sustained elevation in somatotropin and thyroid hormones which enhance lymphocyte proliferation (Baroni, 1971). Somatotropin is an obligatory factor in recovery of immune function following stress; it also directly antagonizes the lympholytic effects of corticosteroids.

## ANIMAL MODELS OF BEHAVIORAL STRESS AND IMMUNITY

In animal studies designed to evaluate specific immune functions following stress, deficiencies in both cell-mediated and humoral responses have been demonstrated. Decreased responsivity to mitogen stimulation (Gisler, 1974; Monjan, 1977), antigen stimulation (Joasod, 1976) and reduced lymphocyte cytotoxicity (Monjan, 1977) have been observed following stress. Prolongation in time to rejection of skin allografts (Wistar, 1960), reduced graft-vs.-host responsiveness, and diminished delayed hypersensitivity reactions (Pitkin, 1965) indicate suppression of cell-mediated immunity following stress in animals. When animals are stressed prior to or directly after immunization, there is also reduced antibody titer to flagellin, a bacterial antigen (Versey, 1960; Solomon, 1969), reflecting suppression of humoral immunity.

While stress is most frequently associated with immunosuppression, it can sometimes have an augmenting effect on the immune system (Mettrop, 1969; Folch, 1974). Again, some of these contradictory findings can be explained by differences in experimental design. The nature of the stress, its duration, and the interval between the stress and the immune measurements are extremely important. For example, mice subjected to chronic auditory stress show a biphasic response. During the first two weeks, there is a 50% decrease in lymphocyte cytotoxicity and mitogen responsivity, followed by a significant increase (above baseline) in the same immune functions for two weeks thereafter (Monjan, 1977). This is another example of rebound overshoot, indicating the importance of timing the stress relative to the measurement.

## INTERACTION BETWEEN THE CENTRAL NERVOUS SYSTEM AND THE IMMUNE SYSTEM

Studies involving specific hypothalamic lesions or electrical stimulation of hypothalamic regions suggest that the central nervous system influences immune responses directly. These data are reviewed by Stein and his colleagues elsewhere in this text (chapter 7). Mediating mechanisms underlying a potential reciprocal communication of the central nervous system and immune system are currently under intense investigation. Sympathetic and parasympathetic neurons arising from the hypothalamus that directly innervate both the thymus and spleen have been traced using the retrograde transport of horseradish peroxidase (Bullock, 1980; Williams, 1981). The mast cell, as described by Locke elsewhere in this work (chapter 1), may be the intermediary that transduces the nerve impulse into a chemical signal read locally by thymic or splenic lymphocytes. As in the case of hormonal modulation of immunity, sympathetic stimulation has immunoinhibitory effects. Chemical sympathectomy, for example, enhances the immune response to sheep erythrocytes in mice (Williams, 1981). Such studies provide evidence for a direct functional link between the nervous and immune system. Further evidence for a direct communication between the central nervous system and the immune system derives from the well-replicated finding that immunosuppression can be conditioned behaviorally in the rat (Ader, 1975; Rogers, 1976; Wagner, 1978).

## PSYCHONEUROIMMUNOLOGY AND CANCER

The inability to cope with the diagnosis, treatment and uncertainties of living with cancer may potentially affect prognosis through some of the mechanisms outlined above. Cancer is a group of diseases whose medical sequellae are accompanied by and sometimes dominated by the emotional reaction to the disease. Despite public education, cancer is still equated with disaster and death. Inherent in the phrase, cancer victim, is the dual dilemma of uncontrollability and unpredictability. In many cases, the onset of disease bears no apparent relation to controllable factors such as smoking or diet. Furthermore, the course of disease can be unpredictable. Even after clinical evidence of cancer is eradicated, the patient must live with the possibility of recurrence. In the vulnerable patient, anxiety that is unrelieved by adequate coping often progresses to depression.

The anxiety, novelty and unpredictability of living with cancer, where fear of recurrence is a prime concern, is the type of stimulus to which the individual does not "adapt out." There may be some individuals, presumably those who feel most helpless and lacking in control, who will continue to secrete epinephrine at a high rate (Frankenhauser, 1970). On the other hand, perceived mastery of the situation which would correlate with hope and a sense of control, should correlate with reduced epinephrine secretion. Likewise, the emotional condition of uncertainty can continue to provoke high cortisol secretion. It is also well known that hypersecretion of cortisol frequently accompanies endogenous depression. Approximately half such patients hypersecrete cortisol independent of stress responses (Sachar, 1980). Both corticosteroids and epinephrine have profound inhibitory effects on the immune system as reviewed above.

The role of the immune system in cancer is still poorly understood. The concept that cellular phenomena analagous to those involved in delayed hypersensitivity and allograft rejection are responsible for tumor cell killing has been seriously questioned (Baldwin, 1977). Recently, however, a subset of lymphocytes known as natural killer (NK) cells has been identified in mice and man (Herberman, 1975; Kenney, 1978; Herberman, 1979). These NK cells apparently have the innate ability to acquire cytotoxic properties spontaneously, without the need for prior sensitization, a property also referred to as spontaneous, lymphocyte-mediated cytotoxicity (Pross, 1976). These cells are being actively studied for a potential role in immunosurveillance against cancer cells and are discussed more fully by Herberman elsewhere in this volume. Macrophages are also capable of spontaneous antitumor activity (Haskill, 1975; Russell, 1977; Chow, 1979). In some systems, the elimination of small tumors is dependent on macrophages; in others on NK cell activity(Chow, 1979). It is apparent that in all probability, several different antitumor mechanisms exist which may operate preferentially against different tumors. Furthermore, some mechanisms may favor destruction of small cell foci such as nascent primary or metastatic cancers. Other mechanisms may operate with a larger cell load. As tumor immunology is elucidated, the interface between neuroendocrine and immune events can be further clarified.

Both natural killer cell activity and macrophage mediated cytotoxicity are inhibited by stress. Locke et al. as discussed in chapter one, demonstrated a significant decline in NK cell activity in students reporting high density life change stress, who also evidenced poor coping capacity. Stressful life events alone did not impair NK cell activity. Rather, the inability to cope was the discriminating variable. Long-term prospective studies would be necessary, however, to determine if individuals who have low NK cell activity as a function of poor coping demonstrate an increase in cancer incidence. The stress of inescapable physical restraint has been demonstrated to impair induction of macrophage-mediated cytoxicity by adjuvants in the mouse (Chirigos, 1979). In the same study, exogenous corticosteroids similarly suppressed the cytotoxicity of interferon-treated macrophages at physiological concentrations. In mice, the macrophage "natural" surveillance system is operative for only a few days after implantation of tumor cells (Chow, 1979). If mice are injected simultaneously with cancer cells and with silica particles to inhibit macrophage function, there is a significant increase in

the frequency of tumors produced. Thus, if natural surveillance is inhibited
at a critical period during the early growth of a tumor, the enlarging mass
may escape destruction. Following surgical removal of a cancer, tumor cells
are often shed into the tissue spaces and vasculature. Most of these cells
die, but some cells may remain to generate local recurrence or distant
metastases. The survival of tumor cells, and their ability to grow into
clones in the lungs of rats is enhanced either by stress or by the injection
of epinephrine (Van den Brenk, 1976). Growth enhancement can be prevented by
adrenalectomy.

Theoretically, increase in cortisol or epinephrine may increase tumor take
and/or growth, thus influencing either etiology or progression of neoplasia
through the above mechanisms. Unfortunately, no clinical study has yet
investigated the relation between affect, hormonal parameters, cell-mediated
immunity and disease progression. On the one hand, several studies have
related the inability to express hostility to the shortening of tumor-free
interval (Blumberg, 1954; Stavraky, 1968; Greer, 1975; Abeloff, 1977).
However, no hormonal or immunological measurements were incorporated in these
studies. On the other hand, a separate experimental literature concerning
motive style and an index of repressed aggression termed Activity Inhibition,
has addressed the endocrine-immune correlates of personality and expression of
hostility but without regard to cancer. McClelland et al. (1980) have studied
the relation between the Inhibited Power Motive Syndrome, urinary epinephrine
excretion, salivary Immunoglobulin A (IgA) levels and severity of upper
respiratory tract infection. The Inhibited Power Motive Syndrome consists of
a high need for Power (higher than the need for Affiliation) in combination with
high Activity Inhibition as reliably and reproducibly measured by the Thematic
Apperception Test. Individuals high in Activity Inhibition stringently control
the expression of negative feelings. Steele (1973) has shown previously that
such individuals have a higher resting urinary excretion rate of epinephrine
compared to controls who express different motive profiles. It is
hypothesized that such individuals may have chronically overactive sympathetic
nervous systems. McClelland et al. have also correlated the Inhibited Power
Motive Syndrome with higher urinary epinephrine excretion rates. In addition,
such individuals had a lower concentration of salivary secretory IgA than did
controls and reported more severe episodes of upper respiratory tract
infection (McClelland, 1980). In a prospective study of former Harvard
students, those showing the Inhibited Power Motive Syndrome in their thirties
had significantly higher blood pressures in their fifties than did other
subjects, controlling for initial blood pressures (McClelland, 1979). These

data arc similar to those of Harburg et al. (1973) correlating suppressed hostility with hypertension. In an extension of Locke's Study (1981), McClelland et al. (1981) found that students high in the need for power who reported a large number of power-related stresses, had both a leukopenia (decreased white blood cell count) and a dimunition of NK cell activity relative to other students studied.

Collectively, these data suggest that stress should not be viewed generically. What is stressful to one individual is not necessarily stressful to another. Power-related stress, in individuals who repress the expression of hostility, promotes a particular endocrinological shift consistent with increased activity of the sympathetic nervous system. This endocrine shift, in turn, correlates with decrease in the two immunological parameters that have been studied in relation to motive profile - salivary immunoglobulin A and NK cell activity. It is likely that the increase in severity of upper respiratory tract infection documented in individuals with the Inhibited Power Motive Syndrome when stressed (McClelland, 1980) is causally related to these endocrinological-immunological changes. It remains to be seen, however, if McClelland's construct of the Inhibited Power Motive is similar to reports of repressed hostility in the cancer literature, and if similar endocrinological and immunological measures correlate with poor cancer prognosis.

In summary, there are three possible levels where behavioral factors could influence either the development or progression of neoplasia (Figure 3). At a most basic level, endocrine changes produced by behavioral parameters could transform cells directly, producing an increase in spontaneously arising tumors. Other than the Russian studies of experimentally-induced neuroticism which have not been replicated (Kavetsky, 1966), there are no data in support of such a model. On a second level, behavioral parameters could inhibit immune function related to the destruction of tumor cells induced to transform by diverse etiologic agents. An original transformed cell multiplies to form a clone of cells which eventually becomes clinically detectable. It is still not well understood how some nascent tumors can escape immunologic scrutiny and continue to grow. Recent evidence, however, suggests that macrophages, NK cells and T lymphocytes can selectively destroy such small tumors. As we have discussed, behaviorally-induced endocrine changes can inhibit the function of all three types of anti-tumor effector cells. Thus, at this level, behavioral parameters could initiate a chain of events culminating in the escape of the growing tumor from immunological surveillance. On a third level, behavioral factors could promote endocrinological, immunological or other changes that lead to restored growth of a tumor that has been temporarily arrested.

| POSSIBLE LEVELS OF EFFECT | POSSIBLE MEDIATORS |
|---|---|

LEVEL I   DIRECT ETIOLOGIC AGENT     NEUROENDOCRINE CHANGES ?

↓

TRANSFORMATION

---

LEVEL II   FAILURE TO ELIMINATE     ↓IMMUNE SURVEILLANCE ?
NASCENT TUMORS

        natural killer cell
          activity
        macrophage function
        interferon
        cytotoxic T cells

---

LEVEL III   INCREASED GROWTH RATE     ↓IMMUNE FUNCTION ?
OF ESTABLISHED TUMORS     NEUROENDOCRINE CHANGES ?
OR RESUMPTION OF     TISSUE LEVEL CHANGES ?
ARRESTED GROWTH

---

Fig. 3. Three putative mechanisms by which behavioral factors could affect the etiology and/or progression of neoplasia.

Evidence for this third level of effect is purely circumstantial. Studies of bereaved individuals, for example, have shown increased mortality from cancer 6-18 months post-bereavement. Since most cancers have a much longer latent period, there would not be time for a tumor to form de novo and become lethally invasive. Such timing would be more consistent with the sudden increase in growth of a previously existing cancer. There are also many case reports documenting the sudden reappearance of cancers that had been presumed "cured," following surgery for an unrelated cause, or trauma. Both surgery and trauma are immunosuppressive secondary to endocrinologically mediated inhibition of lymphocyte and macrophage function.

Thus, it seems theoretically plausible that stress could upset the delicate host-tumor balance of an arrested neoplasm, leading to new growth and clinical detection. This type of hypothetical mechanism could account for the early retrospective observations where the diagnosis of a tumor followed 6-18 months after a significant lifestress. Future prospective studies could investigate this hypothesis by following a high-risk group of individuals such as bereaved spouses or retirees, and monitoring psychological, endocrinological, and immunological indices in the cohort. Since cancer incidence increases with age, it is probable that a significant number of such individuals would develop cancer during a 5-10 year study. We are now at a point where any further study of higher cortical function and neoplasia should include elucidation of potential intermediary mechanisms.

The need for integrative, multidisciplinary studies of affect, personality, endocrine and immune parameters is of paramount importance. Each individual discipline has contributed separate studies from which we infer that higher cortical function can modulate the progression of neoplasia. There are mechanisms we can invoke to explain this inference, but without large scale prospective clinical studies these mechanisms will remain hypothetical. It is likely that behavioral factors may have a greater modulatory influence on the progression of some cancers than others. The physiological correlates of behaviors implicated in modulation of neoplasia must be elucidated, and their interactions with various tumor types assessed. The ultimate goal would then be to change either the behavior or intervene in the physiology that it produces where such intervention would have a significant interaction with other factors determining prognosis.

REFERENCES

Abeloff, M.D. and Derogatis, L.R. (1977) Psychologic aspects of the management of primary and metastatic breast cancer. Prog. Clin. Biol. Res. 12, 505-516.

Ader, R. and Cohen, N. (1975) Behaviorally conditioned immunosuppression. Psychosom. Med. 37, 333-340.

Bach, J.F., Duval, D., Dardenne, M. et al. (1975) The effects of steroids on T cells. Transplant. Proc. 7, 25-30.

Bach, J.F., Dardenne, M. and Bach, M.A. (1975) Biochemical characteristics and biological activity of a serum factor produced by the thymus in mice and man. Ann. N.Y. Acad. Sci. 249, 186-191.

Bahnson, C.B. and Bahnson, M.B. (1966) Role of the ego defenses: denial and repression in the etiology of malignant neoplasm. Ann. N.Y. Acad. Sci. 123, 827-845.

Baldwin, R.W. (1977) Immune surveillance revisited. Nature 270, 557-559.

Baroni, C.D., Pesando, P.C. and Bertoli, G. (1971) Effects of hormones on development and function of lymphoid tissue. II. Delayed development of immunological capacity in pituitary dwarf mice. Immunology 21, 455-46.

Blumberg, E.M., West, P.M. and Ellis, F.W. (1954) A possible relationship between psychological factors and human cancer. Psychosom. Med. 16, 276-286.

Borysenko, J. (1982) Behavioral-physiological factors in the development and management of cancer. Gen. Hosp. Psych. 4, (in press).

Borysenko, J., Benson, H. and Borysenko, M. (1982) Fear, hope and cancer. Sci. Am., (in press).

Bourne, H.R., Lichtenstein, L.M., Melmon, R.L. et al. (1974) Modulation of inflammation and immunity by cyclic AMP. Science 184, 19-28.

Brown, G.M. and Reichlin, S. (1972) Psychologic and neural regulation of growth hormone secretion. Psychosom. Med. 34, 45-61.

Bullock, K. and Moore, R.Y. (1980) Nucleus ambiguus projections to the thymus gland: possible pathways for regulation of the immune response and the neuroendocrine network. Anat. Rec. 196, 25.

Cannon, W.B. (1926) The emergency function of the adrenal medulla in pain and the major emotions. Amer. J. Physiol. 33, 356-372.

Chirigos, M.A. and Schultz, R.M. (1979) Animal models in cancer research which could be useful in studies of the effect of alcohol on cellular immunity. Cancer Res. 39, 2894-2898.

Chow, D.A., Greene, M.I. and Greenberg, A.H. (1979) Macrophage-dependent, NK-cell-independent "natural" surveillance of tumors in syngeneic mice. Int. J. Cancer 23, 788-797.

Claman, H.N. (1977) Corticosteroids and lymphoid cells. New Engl. J. Med. 287, 388-397.

Crary, B., Borysenko, M., Sutherland, D. et al. Epinephrine administration causes a transient inhibition of responsivity to mitogens by human peripheral blood lymphocytes, (submitted).

Davis, D.E. and Read, C.P. (1958) Effect of behavior on development of resistance in trichinosis. Proc. Soc. Exp. Biol. Med. 99, 269-272.

Dewhurst, K.E., El Kabir, D.J., Harris, G.W. et al. (1968) A review of the effect of stress on the activity of the central nervous-pituitary-thyroid axis in animals and man. Confinia Neurologica 30, 161-174.

Dougherty, T.F. (1952) Effects of hormones on lymphatic tissue. Physiol. Rev. 32, 379-401.

Dougherty, T.F., Berliner, M.L., Schneeberg, G. et al. (1964) Hormonal control of lymphatic structure and function. Ann. N.Y. Acad. Sci. 113, 825-843.

Edwards, E.A. and Dean, L.M. (1977) Effects of crowding of mice on humoral antibody formation and protection to lethal antigenic challenge. Psychosom. Med. 39, 19-24.

Folch, H. and Waksman, B.H. (1974) The splenic suppressor cell: activity of thymus dependent adherent cells: changes with age and stress. J. Immunol. 113, 127-139.

Fox, B.H. (1978) Premorbid psychological factors as related to cancer incidence. J. Behav. Med. 1, 45-133.

Frankenhauser, M. and Rissler, A. (1970) Effects of punishment on catecholamine release and efficiency of performance. Psychopharmacologia 17, 378-390.

Frankenhauser, M. (1976) The role of peripheral catecholamines in adaptation to understimulation and overstimulation. In Servan, G. (ed.) Psychopathology of Human Adaptation. New York, Plenum, 173-192.

Fras, I. and Litin, E.M. (1967) Comparison of psychiatric symptoms in carcinoma of the pancreas, retroperitoneal malignant lymphoma and lymphoma in other locations. Psychosomatics 8, 275-277.

Friedman, S.B., Ader, R. and Grota, L.J. (1973) Protective effect of noxious stimulation in mice infected with rodent malaria. Psychosom. Med. 35, 535-537.

Galant, S.P., Lundak, R.L. and Eaton, L. (1976) Enhancement of early human E rosette formation by cholinergic stimuli. J. Immunol. 117, 48-51.

Gisler, R.H. (1974) Stress and hormonal regulation of the immune response in mice. Psychother. Psychosom. 23, 197-208.

Greene, W.H. (1966) The psychosocial setting of the development of leukemia and lymphoma. Ann. N.Y. Acad. Sci. 125, 194-201.

Greer, S. and Morris, T. (1975) Psychological attributes of women who develop breast cancer: A controlled study. J. Psychosom. Res. 19, 147-153.

Greer, S., Morris, T. and Pettingale, K.W. (1979) Psychological response to breast cancer: Effect on outcome. Lancet 13, 785-787.

Grieco, M.H., Siegel, I. and Goel, Z. (1976) Modification of human T lymphocyte rosette formation by autonomic agonists and cyclic nucleotides. J. Allergy Clin. Immunol. 58, 149-154.

Hadden, J.W., Hadden, E.M., Haddon, H.K. et al. (1972) Guanosine 3',5'-cyclic monophosphate: a possible intracellular mediator of mitogenic influences in lymphocytes. Proc. Nat. Acad. Sci. 69, 3023-3029.

Hamilton, D.R. (1974) Immunosuppressive effects of predator induced stress in mice with acquired immunity to Hymenolepsis nana. J. Psychosom. Res. 18, 143-150.

Harburg, E., Erfurt, J.C., Havenstein, L.S. et al. (1973) Socio-ecological stress, suppressed hostility, skin color, and black-white male blood pressure: Detroit. Psychosom. Med. 35, 276-296.

Haskill, S., Proctor, J.W. and Yamamura, Y. (1975) Host responses within solid tumors. I. Monocytic effector cells within rat sarcomas. J. Nat. Cancer Inst. 54, 387-393.

Herberman, R.B., Nunn, M.E. and Lavrin, D.H. (1975) Natural cytotoxic reactivity of mouse lymphoid cells against syngeneic and allogeneic tumors. I. Distribution of reactivity and specificity. Int. J. Cancer 16, 216-229.

Herberman, R.B. and Holden, H.T. (1979) Natural killer cells as antitumor effector cells. J. Nat. Cancer Inst. 62, 441-455.

Hirata, Y., Sakamoto, N., Matsukura, S. et al. (1975) Plasma levels of β-MSH and ACTH during acute stresses and metapyrone administration in man. J. Clin. Endocrinol. Metab. 41, 1092-1097.

Horne, R.L. and Picard, R.S. (1979) Psychosocial risk factors for lung cancer. Psychosom. Med. 41, 503-514.

Ignarro, I.J. and George, W.J. (1974) Mediation of immunologic discharge of lysosomal enzymes from human neutrophils with guanosine 3',5'-monophosphate. J. Exp. Med. 140, 225-238.

Joasod, A. and McKenzie, J.M. (1976) Stress and the immune response in rats. Int. Arch. Allergy 50, 659-663.

Johnsson, T., Lavender, J.F., Hultin, E. et al. (1963) The influence of avoidance learning stress on resistance to Coxsacki B virus in mice. J. Immunol. 91, 569-574.

Johnsson, T. and Rasmussen, A.F. (1965) Emotional stress and susceptibility to poliomyelitis virus infection in mice. Archiv. fur die Gesamte Virus Forschung 18, 392-397.

Kavetsky, R.E., Turkevich, N.M. and Balitsky, K.P. (1966) On the psychophysiological mechanisms of the organism's resistance to tumor growth. Ann. N.Y. Acad. Sci. 125, 933-945.

Kenney, C.S., Tracey, D., Dursik, J.M., et al. (1978) Natural killer cells: In vitro and in vivo. Am. J. Path. 93, 459-467.

Kissen, D. (1963) Personality characteristics in males conducive to lung cancer. Br. J. Med. Psychol. 34, 27-36.

Kissen, D. (1967) Psychosocial factors, personality and lung cancer in men aged 55-64. Br. J. Med. Psychol. 40, 29-43.

LaBarba, R.C. (1970) Experiential and environmental factors in cancer; A review of research with animals. Psychosom. Med. 32, 259-276.

Landsberg, L. (1977) The sympathoadrenal system. In S.H. Ingbar (ed.) The Year in Endocrinology, New York, Plenum, 304-309.

LeShan, L. (1966) An emotional life history associated with neoplastic disease. Ann. N.Y. Acad. Sci. 125,780-793.

Locke, S.E, Hurst, M.W., Heisel, J.S. et al. Stress, adaptation, and altered human natural killer cell activity, (submitted).

Mason, J.W. (1968) A review of psychoendocrine research on the pituitary-adrenal cortical system. Psychosom. Med. 30, 576-607.

Mason, J.W. (1974) Specificity in the organization of neuroendocrine response profiles. In Seeman, P., Brown, G. (eds.) Frontiers in Neurology and Neuroscience Research. Toronto, University of Toronto Press, 68-80.

McClelland, D.C. (1979) Inhibited power motivation and high blood pressure in men. J. Abn. Psych. 88, 182-190.

McClelland, D.C., Floor, E., Davidson, R.J. et al. (1980) Stressed power motivation, sympathetic activation, immune function, and illness. J. Human Stress 6,11-19.

McClelland, D.C., Locke, S.E, Williams, R.M. et al. (1981) Power motivation, distress and immune function. Unpublished manuscript, Department of Psychology and Social Relations, Harvard University.

Mendelsohn, J., Multer, M.M. and Bernheim, J.L. (1977) Inhibition of human lymphocyte stimulation by steroid hormones: cytokinetic mechanisms. Clin. Exp. Immunol. 27, 127-134.

Mettrop, P.J. and Visser, P. (1969) Exteroceptive stimulation as a contingent factor in the induction and elicitation of delayed-type hypersensitivity reactions to 1-chloro-2 and 4-dinitrobenzene reactions in guinea pigs. Psychophysiology 5, 385-388.

Monjan, A.A. and Collector, M.I. (1977) Stress-induced modulation of the immune response. Science 196, 307-308.

Noel, G.L., Suh, H.K., Stone, G. et al. (1972) Human prolactin and growth hormone release during surgery and other conditions of stress. J. Clin. Endocrinol. Metab. 35, 840-851.

Pitkin, D.H. (1965) Effect of physiological stress on the delayed hypersensitivity reaction. Proc. Soc. Exp. Biol. Med. 120, 350-351.

Pross, H.F. and Baines, M.G. (1976) Spontaneous human lymphocyte-mediated cytoxicity against tumor target cells. I. The effect of malignant disease. Int. J. Cancer 18, 593-604.

Rasmussen, A.F., Marsh, J.T. and Brill, N.Q. (1957) Increased susceptibility to herpes simplex virus in mice subjected to avoidance learning stress or restraint. Proc. Soc. Exp. Biol. Med. 96, 183-189.

Rasmussen, A.F. (1969) Emotions and immunity. Ann. N.Y. Acad. Sci. 164, 458-461.

Riley, V. (1975) Mouse mammary tumors: Alteration of incidence as an apparent function of stress. Science 189, 465-467.

Riley, V. (1981) Neuroendocrine influences on immunocompetence and neoplasia. Science 211, 1100-1109.

Rogers, M.P., Reich, P., Strom, T.B. et al. (1976) Behaviorally conditioned immunosuppression: replication of a recent study. Psychosom. Med. 38, 447-451.

Russell, S.W., Gillespie, G.Y. and McIntosh, A.T. (1977) Inflammatory cells in solid murine neoplasms. III. Cytotoxicity mediated in vitro by macrophages recovered from disaggregated regressing Moloney sarcomas. J. Immunol. 118, 1574-1579.

Sachar, E.J., Asnis, G., Nathan, R.S. et al. (1980) Dextroamphetamine and cortisol in depression. Arch. Gen. Psych. 37, 755-757.

Schmale, A.H. and Iker, H. (1966) The psychological setting of uterine cervical cancer. Ann. N.Y. Acad. Sci. 125, 807-819.

Selye, H. (1950) The physiology and pathology of the exposure to stress. Montreal, Acta Inc.

Shekelle, R.B., Raynor, W.J., Ostfeld, A.M. et al. (1981) Psychological depression and 17-year risk of death from cancer. Psychosom. Med. 43, 117-125.

Sklar, L.S. and Anisman, H. (1979) Stress and coping factors influence tumor growth. Science 205, 513-515.

Sklar, L.S. and Anisman, H. (1980) Social stress influences tumor growth. Psychosom. Med. 42, 347-465.

Solomon, G.F. (1969) Stress and antibody response in rats. Int. Arch. Allergy Appl. Immunol. 35, 97-104.

Stavraky, K.M., Buck, C.W., Loh, S.S. et al. (1968) Psychological factors in the outcome of human cancer. J. Psychosom. Res. 12, 251-259.

Steele, R.S. (1973) The physiological concomitants of psychogenic motive arousal in college males. Cambridge, MA. Doctoral Dissertation, Harvard University.

Strom, T.B., Carpenter, C.B., Garovoy, M.R. et al. (1973) The modulating influence of cyclic nucleotides upon lymphocyte-mediated cytotoxicity. J. Exp. Med. 138, 381-393.

van den Brenk, H.A.S., Stone, M.G., Kelly, H. et al. (1976) Lowering of innate resistance of the lungs to the growth of blood-borne cancer cells in states of topical and systemic stress. Br. J. Cancer 33, 60-78.

Versey, S.H. (1960) Effects of grouping on levels of circulating antibodies in mice. Proc. Soc. Exp. Biol. Med. 115, 252-255.

Wagner, E.A., Flannery, G.R. and Singer, G. (1978) The effects of taste aversion conditioning on the primary antibody response to sheep red blood cells and Brucella abortus in the albino rat. Physiol. Behav. 21, 995-1000.

Weinstein, Y. and Melmon, K.L. (1976) Control of immune responses by cyclic AMP of lymphocytes that adhere to histamine columns. Immunol. Comm. 5, 401-416.

Weiss, J.M. (1970) Somatic effects of predictable and unpredictable shock. Psychosom. Med. 32, 397-408.

Weiss, J.M. (1971) Effects of coping behavior in different warning signal conditions on stress pathology in rats.  J. Comp. Physiol. Psychol. 77, 1-13.

Williams, J.M., Peterson, R.G., Shea, P.A. et al. (1981) Sympathetic innervation of murine thymus and spleen:  evidence for a functional link between the nervous and immune systems.  Brain Res. Bull. 6, 83-94.

Wistar, R. and Hildemann, W.H. (1960) Effect of stress on skin transplantation immunity in mice.  Science 131, 159-160.

Published 1982 by Elsevier Science Publishing Co, Inc.
Sandra M. Levy, ed.
Biological Mediators of Behavior and Disease:
Neoplasia

INTERACTIONS OF PSYCHIC AND ENDOCRINE FACTORS WITH PROGRESSION OF NEOPLASTIC
DISEASES

MARC LIPPMAN, M.D.
Medical Breast Cancer Section, Medicine Branch, Clinical Oncology Program,
Division of Cancer Treatment, National Cancer Institute, National Institutes
of Health, Building 10, Room 6B02, Bethesda, Maryland 20205

INTRODUCTION

The notion that some human tumors might be profoundly dependent upon
hormonal factors for their growth was initially suggested by the pioneering
work of George Beatson ([1]Beatson 1896). Nearly a hundred years ago, he noted
that some women with breast cancer had objective regressions of their tumors
when treated by oophorectomy. These observations were the forerunner of
clinical and laboratory observations of paramount importance which established
that much of human neoplasia, including breast cancer, endometrial cancer,
prostatic cancer, leukemia, and lymphoma, as well as other tumors, are subject
to considerable growth regulation by the endocrine milieu.

In parallel, numerous studies have provided considerable evidence that environmental factors such as stress and the responses to those environmental
factors that are induced, such as anger and depression can profoundly alter the
endocrine milieu. It is the purpose of this chapter to attempt to summarize
the pathways by which psychic and endocrine factors can combine to influence
neoplastic cell growth. First, we will attempt to review the evidence
establishing the hormonal dependency of a major subset of human malignancies.
Second, information will be provided for understanding ways in which changes
in growth of tumors not classically felt to be hormone dependent may be
mediated by hormonal factors. Finally, we will provide some information
concerning how tumors themselves may alter the endocrine milieu and influence
either their own growth or those aspects of behavior affected by hormones.

56

A brief summary of important pathways in which psychic and endocrine factors may interact with human neoplasia is provided in figure 1. A brief consideration of the information summarized in this figure will provide a framework on which to consider the data to be reviewed later in this discussion. Clearly, the knowledge to an individual that he has been diagnosed as having cancer is extreme environmental stress. While this stressful event may evoke a wide range of emotional responses, there is no doubt whatsoever that stress itself

**INTERACTION OF PSYCHIC AND ENDOCRINE FACTORS
WITH PROGRESSION OF NEOPLASTIC DISEASE**

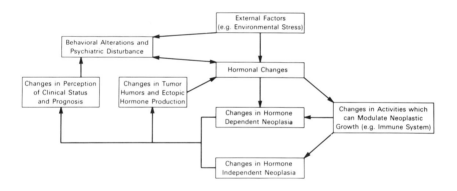

FIG. 1   Interaction of Psychic and Endocrine Factors with Progression of Neoplastic Disease

can induce profound effects on the hormonal environment. Many hormones are known to be affected. Best known, of course, are alterations in the hypothalamic-pituitary-adren axis resulting in highly significant changes in glucocorticoids ([2]Mason 1968). Endorphins are also known to be stimulated in many stressful environments ([3]Guillemin et al 1977). Significant effects on a host of other hormones, including growth hormone, catecholamines, prolactin, and testosterone have also been described ([4]Rose and Sachar 1981).

It is equally clear that a variety of psychiatric disturbances are also associated with profound hormonal changes. While outside the scope of this review, alterations in glucocorticoid secretion in depressive disorders as well as abnormalities of insulin, TSH response to TRH, and growth hormone responses have been described ([5]Sachar and Baron 1979). Conversely, profound effects on behavior are induced by alterations in the hormonal milieu. The behavioral and psychopathologic concomittants of thyroid disturbances, Cushing's syndrome, Addison's disease, disorders of calcium balance, etc., require little amplification. Thus, the combination of environmental factors, the individual's psychological makeup, and the response to disturbances in that environment can clearly alter hormonal factors in an interactive way.

Alterations in the endocrine milieu can alter growth of human neoplasia by two basic mechanisms: direct effects on hormone dependent neoplasia and indirect effects which may influence the growth of hormone dependent or hormone independent neoplasia. A basic description of endocrine factors directly mediating effects on hormone dependent neoplasia will form a major portion of this chapter. It is equally apparent, however, that changes in the endocrine environment of the organism can traumatically influence many other tissues and factors in the body responsible for tumor progression. Easily, the most obvious of these is the immune system. A host of hormones of which the glucocorticoids are simply the most often considered can alter inumerable aspects of immune function. In addition, however, effects on such factors as angiogenesis, platelet derived growth factor, the interleukins, and other growth factors may also occur. All of these latter factors may modulate nonneoplastic cell populations in such a way that tumor progression is altered. A striking example of such a phenomenon in terms of normal mammary gland development has to do with regression of mammary gland in male animals. It has long been appreciated that this is an androgen-mediated effect. However, a variety of elegant experiments have clearly demonstrated that the androgen effect is not a direct one. Androgens induce surrounding fibroblasts to secrete a mammary gland inhibitory factor which leads to mammary gland regression. Thus, the mammary cells have no direct response to the androgenic stimulus but breast tissue is observed to have a profound response to androgens. In analogous ways, hormonal effects on other non-neoplastic cell types may have the greatest potential influence on cancers not considered either classically hormone dependent or responsive to that particular hormone.

Changes in tumor growth rate of either hormone dependent or independent neoplasms can in themselves lead to profound responses. First, changes in perception of prognosis or clinical status on the part of the patient can dramatically alter behavior and psychiatric symptomatology. Stress responses will certainly be affected by direct observation of one's own clinical status. Clearly alterations in stress and behavior as already mentioned will introduce changes in the endocrine milieu.

Finally, many tumors secrete a variety of ectopic hormones and humors which can directly and indirectly induce hormonal changes. These can feed back on hormone dependent neoplasia or on non-neoplastic tissue and thus indirectly affect tumor growth. For example, the ectopic production of ACTH by lung cancer can result in marked elevations in plasma glucocorticoid concentrations with resultant modulation of the immune system.

Table 1  Hormones Produced Ectopically by Cancers

1.  ACTH and associated pro-hormones
2.  Lipotropin
3.  Chorionic gonadotropin and alpha chain
4.  Vasopressin
5.  Hypoglycemia producing factor
6.  Somatomedins
7.  Parathyroid hormone and parathyroid hormone-like peptides
8.  Prostaglandins
9.  Osteoclast activating factor
10. Erythropoietin
11. Hypophosphatemia producing factor
12. Growth Hormone
13. Prolactin
14. Gastrin
15. Secretin
16. Glucagon
17. Corticotropin releasing factor
18. Growth hormone releasing hormone
19. Somatostatin
20. Chorionic somatotropin

Thus, it can be seen that behavior and external factors can dramatically influence the endocrine environment leading to potential effects on tumor progression which in turn can feed back both positively and negatively on the psychic substrate to induce additional changes in the endocrine system. In many cases, the exact mechansims of these effects are not well understood. However, great attention has been given to the general area of hormone dependent neoplasia and considerable information is available concerning several classes of human tumors whose etiology, pathogenesis, and therapy is intimately related to the endocrine system. We will thus briefly review the data for those tumors in which hormonal manipulation effects can bring about substantial alterations in tumor growth rate and clinical status.

BREAST CANCER

Many of the most important clues concerning the hormonal dependency of breast cancer were initially derived from epidemiologic studies of risk factors. Many risk factors such as sex, age, age at menarche and menopause, age at first birth of a child, variations with coutry of origin, dietary factors and family history have been identified ([6]MacMahon et al 1973). Many of these factors are certainly interdependent; and, a substantial amount of information exists suggesting that the final common pathway for most, if not all, of these is eventually exerted via the endocrine system. These factors are most conviently divided into four groups: variations in risk associated with national origin, reproductive history, familial clustering, and the hormonal milieu.

As is well-known, there is a striking variation in breast cancer incidence rates in various areas of the world. For example, at age 50, the incidence of breast cancer is nearly 10 times higher in the United States than in Japan. This difference in incidence cannot be attributed to genetic factors since population studies have shown that Chinese or Japanese individuals living in Hawaii or San Francisco for several generations have the same rate of breast cancer as does the white population in that area ([7]Haenzel and kurihara 1968). Furthermore, the incidence of breast cancer is rising dramatically in post-World War II Japan. Obviously, environmental factors must be considered. Furthermore, more detailed analyses of these data yield interesting insights into breast cancer causation. For example, in countries with a high incidence of breast cancer, there is a continual increase in incidence with increasing age. On the other hand, in low-risk countries the rate of development of breast cancer actually may decrease after the menopause. This has suggested that two different etiologic types of breast cancer may exist; a pre-menopausal predominantly non-hormonally dependent variety and a post-menopausal variety with a long period of tumor promotion which is strongly influenced by the endocrine milieu ([8]DeWaard 1969). Unfortunately, a tremendous amount of information comparing differences in environmental factors such as diet is largely associative in nature rather than clearly pathogenic. For example, breast cancer incidence is strongly correlated with total food consumption, total fat consumption, total meat consumption, and higher rates of obesity. The transduction of these environmental differences into a mechanism which can account for 10-fold differences in breast cancer incidence has, however, proven elusive.

Recently an extremely provocotive set of observations by Henderson and colleagues ([9]Henderson et al 1981) has suggested that the endocrine variations in age at menarche, age of first birth, and age at menopause can account for nearly 80% of the difference in risk of breast cancer between high and low risk populations if relatively great weight is assigned to the years lying between menarche and age at first birth. Such a conclusion would clearly implicate environmental control of the endocrine milieu as the single most important risk factor in breast cancer since diet can profoundly influence age of onset of menses.

A second major area of epidemiologic investigation strongly implicating endocrine dependency of breast cancer is derived from an examination of reproductive history. If a relative risk of one is assigned to nulliparous women, then there is nearly a three fold variation in risk of breast cancer varying from 0.5 for women having their first child before the age of 20 to 1.4 to women giving birth after the age of 37. Interestingly, this protective effect of child birth prior to age 20 is persistent throughout life and is apparent even among women age 75 and older ([10]MacMahon et al 1970. This protective effect could be due to a pregnancy-induced alteration in the mammary gland leading to increased resistence to neoplastic transformation. Alternatively, a persistent post partum alteration in circulating hormone levels may be the mechanism of protection. Separating these two possibilities is clearly of substantial importance as either might suggest a means of substantially reducing breast cancer risk by prophylactic endocrine manipulations in young women. The latter mechanism could also be modulated by the CNS.

Contrary to popular notions, lactation per se does not appear to provide a significant protective effect against breast cancer ([11]Abramson 1966). It is interesting, however, that one recent study of Japan fisherwomen who nurse their children on only one breast revealed that there was a significant reduction of breast cancer on that side ([12]Ing et al 1977).

A critically important determinant of life-time breast cancer risk can be derived from examination of the family history of breast cancer. While some dispute exists concerning the exact risk ratios to be assigned, there is no question that first degree relatives with breast cancer (mothers and sisters) add significantly to the risk of breast cancer in other females in the family. In fact, there is nearly an eight-fold increase in breast cancer risk when a mother or sister has had bilateral breast cancer before reaching menopause ([13]Petrakis 1977) Further evidence for genetic factors may be derived from the weak association of breast cancer with certain HL-A antigens ([14]Petrakis 1971) and cerumen type. While such genetic factors might be expressed at a variety of levels, heritable differences in the endocrine milieu seem a likely locus. Thus, a comparison of high risk individuals with an appropriate control group might yield important insights into the hormonal background which predisposes to the development of breast cancer. At least two such studies, though well designed, have been somewhat disappointing ([15]Pike et al 1977; [16]Fishman et al 1978). Thus far, no convincing differences have been reported in prolactin gonadotropins, estrone, estradiol or estriol concentrations in serum from high and normal risk subjects although such claims have occasionally been made. One recent study has suggested a suppression of the night-time surge of plasma melatonin in some patients with breast cancer ([17]Tamarkin et al 1981). This observation will need further investigation.

Finally, the actual hormonal milieu has been examined in many women with breast cancer and compared to a variety of control populations in an effort to establish an important endocrine promotional factor in breast cancer. At the extremes, such data are absolutely convincing. For example, women having surgical castration for non-breast cancer reasons have a decreased life-time risk of breast cancer proportional to the years of menstrual life which are lost. It seems likely that estrogen is the direct causative agent since the protective effects of early ovariectomy are negated by administration of exogenous estrogens ([18]Feinleib 1968). Men, treated with estrogens, either as part of transexual procedures or as therapy for prostatic cancer, have increased risk of breast cancer. Numerous studies have suggested that women with a higher urinary estriol excretion, particulary as compared with estrogen and estradiol excretion have a decreased risk of breast cancer throughout their life. While these observations have been confirmed in several studies ([19]Miller 1978), these data cannot be attributed to an antiestrogenic effect of estriol ([20]Lippman et al 1977) as was originally thought, but rather are associated with some other, as yet undefined, abnormality of estrogen metabolism. Finally and of great interest, are the recent studies of Siiteri ([21]Siiteri et al 1981) which suggest that while estrogen concentrations are not abnormal in breast cancer patients, the amount of free estrogen in the circulation is elevated. This group has found evidence that increasing obesity is associated with an increased free concentration of estradiol. Furthermore, they have preliminary evidence that the estrogen binding protein in the serum of some breast cancer patients may be abnormal with a decreased affinity for estradiol. Thus, previous studies aimed at measuring total plasma estrogens would have missed this important difference in available ovarian estrogens.

Additional evidence for the endocrine regulation of breast tissue is derived from studies of exogenous estrogen administration. Thus far, multiple retrospective case control studies have failed to reveal a substantial alteration in breast cancer risk among oral contraceptive users ([22]Kelsey 1978; [23]Sartwell et al 1977). On the other hand, at least two studies have shown that prolonged use of oral contraceptives (greater than 8 and 5 years, respectively) ([24]Cassagrande et al 1976; [25]Craig et al 1974) were associated with an increased risk ratio. The data with post-menopausal estrogen administration are much less substantial for breast cancer than for endometrial cancer as will be discussed below. However, at least one study has shown an increase in risk of breast cancer related to long duration of use. Finally, breast cancer presenting during periods of elevated hormonal stimulation (pregnancy) tends to present at a more advanced clinical stage ([26]Anderson 1979). It is extremely important to bear in mind that subtle alterations in the endocrine milieu may require many years for their expression.

Thus, an overwhelming number of epidemiologic studies suggest that critical aspects of the endocrine milieu can influence the appearance and severity of human breast cancer in both males and females. Thus, it is far from surprising that many clinical studies aimed at altering the endocrine milieu in the hopes of altering breast cancer growth rates have been undertaken.

A review of the endocrine related biology of breast cancer is beyond the scope of this brief review. Suffice it to say that the most compelling evidence available for directly implicating endocrine factors in the regulation of human breast cancer is derived from isolated cell culture systems of human mammary carcinoma. The human and mammary nature of these cell lines has been extensively reviewed ([27]Lippman et al 1977). Direct addition of physiologic concentrations of hormones to human breast cancer cells can profoundly regulate growth and specific gene expression. It is worthwhile to mention the diversity of these hormones if only to point out the many potential pathways that both concentrations and activities of these hormones can be affected by the central nervous system. Hormones proven to affect breast cancer cells include estrogens, androgens, glucocorticoids, progestins, insulin, EGF, vasopressin, and iodothyronines and retinoids ([28]Lippman 1981). In addition, receptors have been demonstrated in human breast cancer cells for prolactin, Vitamin $D_3$ and calcitonin though definite responses to these hormones are not yet established.

## TREATMENT OF BREAST CANCER

In this section, we will review some of the endocrine manipulations which have been applied to human breast cancer, both early and late, which have been shown to influence growth rate and survival. The purpose of reviewing some of these therapies is to underline the fact that endogenous alterations in these hormones induced by CNS modulation (as described in the Introduction of this chapter) may bring about similar alterations in recurrence rates, tumor progression, and survival.

We will first examine early breast cancer. Given the lugubrious fact that many patients treated with curative intent will eventually recur and die from metastatic breat cancer, several studies attempted to alter recurrence rates by prophylactic endocrine therapy. Unfortunately, these efforts failed to demonstrate an important overall survival benefit in breast cancer patients treated with prophylactic oophorectomy ([29]Ravdin et al 1970) or ovarian irradiation ([30]Nissen-Meyer 1964). Many of these studies, however, were completed in the era before it was possible to detect biochemically (through the use of estrogen receptor analyses) those tumors which were more likely to be hormone dependent. Since it is appreciated that no more than about 1/3 of

breast cancer falls into the general category of estrogen dependency, it is
possible that the effect on a small minority of premenopausal patients likely
to benefit from such therapy would have been "washed out" by the proponderance
of patients in whom no benefit could be expected. Alternatively, the failure
to observe a benefit of endocrine therapy could have been based upon an
inadequacy of the therapy itself. Thus, a more recent prospective trial in
which ovarian irradiation was combined with partial adrenal suppression with
oral glucocorticoid administration has revealed highly significant survival
advantages for premenopausal patients so treated ([31]Meakin 1980). Finally,
hormonal therapy in combination with chemotherapy has yielded impressive
additional disease-free survival benefits in several patient populations
([32]Hubay et al 1980).

In addition to these obvious endocrine intervention studies, factors known
to be associated with increased estrogen concentrations (obesity) are associated
with a decreased disease-free interval in patients with breast cancer ([33]Donegan
et al 1978) This effect, as would be predicted, is seen primarily in that
proportion of patients that are more likely to have hormone dependent tumors
(e.g., the estrogen receptor positive patients) thus lending further credence
to the idea that subtle hormonal effects may strongly influence recurrence
rates. Advanced breast cancer has also been shown to respond to a variety of
endocrine manipulations. Several of these will be briefly described. It is
important to bear in mind that the actual mechansims by which these endocrine
therapies cause tumor regressions is not necessarily established. It is
difficult to administer a single hormone to an organism without altering the
concentrations and activities of a host of other factors. For example, the
pharmacologic administration of estrogens alters the concentrations of
prolactin, gonadotropins, glucocorticoids, androgens, and thyroid hormone. In

addition to these factors, a host of other specific growth activities of an as yet undefined nature may also be affected. For example, in a recent review of breast cancer cell growth in vitro ([28]Lippman 1981), it was shown that estrogens, androgens, glucocorticoids, progestins, Vitamin D-like sterols, prolactin, vasopressin, EGF, insulin, iodothyronines, and retinoids were all capable of strongly perturbing breast cancer cell growth. Therefore it is unreasonable to assume that alterations induced by a single endocrine treatment are necessarily mediated by that individual hormone. In fact, the hormonal therapy may not even act on the breast cancer cells directly, but rather through some more circuitous route. With this background in mind, a few of the endocrine therapies known to influence breast cancer cell growth can be discovered.

As already mentioned, Beatson first showed nearly one hundred years ago that oophorectomy benefited some patients with premenopausal breast cancer ([1]Beatson 1896). Using rigid criteria, the regression rate in unselected patients is about 25-30% ([34]Fracchia et al 1969). A median duration of this response is somewhat less than a year. Oophorectomy has been shown to be ineffective in women with low plasma estradiol levels which are indicative of loss of follicles from the ovary and consequent cessation of estradiol secretion

Adrenalectomy is also effective in the treatment of some patients with breast cancer. The precise mechanism of action of adrenalectomy is not known. The adrenal secretes large concentrations of androgen precursors of estrogens including androstenedione. These compounds can be converted peripherally to biologically active estrogens ([35]Grodin et al 1973), a reaction termed aromatization. This conversion can occur in many tissues including liver, brain, skin, hair follicle, breast and breast cancer. Overwhelmingly, however, adipose tissue makes the greatest contribution. This may explain why obesity is a risk factor for breast cancer as well as being associated with a shorter disease free interval and decreased survival. The positive correlation between the presence of estrogen receptor in tumor tissue and adrenalectomy provides support for the notion that the mechanism of action in most patients treated with adrenalectomy is a lowering of plasma estrogen concentrations. Interference with adrenal steroidogenous can be achieved by pharmacologic means with the use of the drug, aminoglutethimide ([36]Santen and Wells 1980). This spares the patient the need to undergo adrenalectomy.

Hypophysectomy has also been shown to be an effective therapy for many patients with metastatic disease ([37]Dao 1972). The mechanisms of action by which hypophysectomy causes breast cancer regression is not clear. In many cases, the mechanism is likely to be through a loss of ACTH secretion and adrenal suppression secretion since few responses to hypophysectomy have been reported following previous adrenalectomy. However, the removal of other pituitary growth factors including prolactin cannot be categorically ruled out. The notion that many human breast cancers are prolactin-dependent, however, appears unlikely. This is based upon the failure of prolactin-suppressing drugs (the ergoline derivatives, or l-DOPA) to induce regression in patients with breast cancer ([38]EORTC 1972).

The administration of high concentrations of androgens has also been shown to induce regressions in some patients with breast cancer ([39]Kennedy 1969). The mechanism of action of such androgen therapy is unknown. However, the use of less virilizing androgens such as calusterone or testolactone is apparently equally effective in producing regressions of disease ([40]Goldenberg 1969). The mechanism of such responses is of substantial interest in the context of this particular chapter since adrenal function can be profoundly altered by stress. The source of the majority of endogenous androgens in postmenopausal females is the adrenal gland, and their role in regulating breast cancer growth requires substantially more attention. In a mouse mammary tumor model system, Shionogi S115, androgens play a critical role in growth regulation ([41]Yates et al 1980).

One of the major paradoxes in the management of breast cancer is the benefit of administration of pharmacologic doses of estrogens to patients with metastatic disease. It is perplexing that the same hormone which in physiologic concentrations will stimulate growth can induce tumor regressions in up to 30% of patients with metastatic disease when administered in larger doses ([39]Kennedy 1969). Whether or not pharmacologic effects of estrogen are mediated directly at the level of the tumor is not currently known. Even more puzzling is the apparent withdrawal response observed in some patients following the cessation of therapy ([42]Kaufman and Escher 1961). Thus, patients having a tumor regression on estrogen therapy and then showing further progression of tumor will sometimes have a further regression of their tumor when the apparently ineffective estrogen treatment has been withdrawn.

Another class of steroid hormones, the progestins, have also been reported to induce remissions in patients with breast cancer ([43]Pannoti et al 1979). The mechanism of progestin action is also unknown although progesterone in certain animal systems appears capable of both lowering estrogen receptor concentrations and blocking estrogen receptor resynthesis following translocation of the receptor to the nucleus when bound to estradiol. Response rates in the 15-25% range for the administration of a variety of progestins has been reported. It should be recalled that progesterone concentrations in this therapeutic range occur normally only during pregnancy and the luteal phase of the menstrual cycle. Thus, endogenous progestin alterations are unlikely to be responsible for altering neoplastic cell breast cancer growth in the majority of patients with breast cancer. At these high concentrations, progestins also "promiscuously" interact with androgen and glucocorticoid receptors and thus may induce their effects indirectly. Of perhaps the greatest interest with respect to the issues which this chapter is concerned with are the effects of glucocorticoids on metastatic breast cancer cell growth. Remissions in up to 15% of patients have been reported with the massive administration of glucocorticoids ([44]Ker and Stewart 1966). Support for a multiplicity of mechanisms for such effects exists. First, glucocorticoids may directly inhibit breast cancer cell growth. This has been shown by examining the effects of glucocorticoids on human breast cancer cell lines in culture ([45]Lippman et al 1976). In this system, specific glucocorticoid receptors can be demonstrated in human breast cancer cells and glucocorticoids directly inhibit breast cancer cell growth by binding to these sites. Pharmacologic concentrations of glucocorticoids can also feedback on the hypothalamic pituitary axis and suppress the pituitary production ACTH. This can lead to a "partial andrenalectomy" with a lowered adrenal production of androgen precursors of estrogens. This effect may be responsible for the improved survival seen in early stage breast cancer patients treated with a combination of oophorectomy and exogenous glucocorticoid therapy previously described. Thirdly, glucocorticoids may modulate the immune system as described elsewhere in this volume. Clearly, a suppression of a population of immune cells which protect the tumor from normal immunologic mechanisms which might recognize it as foreign is also a possibility. Finally, glucocorticoids may well modulate the activity of other growth factors such as insulin or angiogenesis factors which are important in regulating tumor growth.

A variety of pharmacologic therapies which are critically important in the management of breast cancer by endocrine means (e.g. antiestrogen therapy) will not be discussed in this chapter. This is because such manipulations cannot be achieved as part of the body's response to stress or other psychic factors. Nonetheless, such manipulations do, of course, provide even more evidence for the endocrine dependency of human breast cancer. In summary, a host of convincing information establishes the responsiveness of human breast cancer to profound growth regulation by endogenously occurring hormones. These hormones can certainly be manipulated by therapeutic means but equally as clearly can be profoundly affected endogenously as part of the organism's emotional and psychic response to the knowledge of breast cancer or other life events. It is of the utmost importance to appreciate that while modest alterations of any single hormonal factor in response to psychic factors may fail to fully explain growth regulation of a hormone dependent tumor, much more significant effects may be seen when multiple small factors are considered as acting in concert. Finally, the information that many known endocrine factors can be substantially manipulated by emotional stimuli must lead to the conclusion that such regulation is equally possible for those growth factors which are yet to be identified.

Endometrial Cancer. The uterine endometrium is a classic example of a hormone dependent tissue. Its growth and morphology changes cyclicly throughout the menstrual life of a women in direct response to alterations in estradiol and progesterone concentrations. A wealth of endocrine and epidemiologic studies have strongly implicated steroid and peptide hormone abnormalities in the etiology of endometrial cancer. These have included chronic abnormal estrogen stimulation, disordered anterior pituitary function, diabetes, obesity, and infertility ([46]Dunn and Bradbury 1967). The inescapable conclusion from an analysis of all of these data is that prolonged or unopposed estrogen stimulation substantially increases the risk of developing endometrial cancer. The longer the endometrium is stimulated, as with the use of postmenopausal estrogen or in women with late menopause, the greater the risk of eventually developing endometrial cancer ([47]Antunes et al 1979). The increase in endometrial cancer among women with estrogen secreting tumors or the polycystic ovary syndrome al 1978) who have no luteal phase of the menstrual cycle emphasizes the role of progesterone induced endometrial sloughing as a protective mechanism. The higher rate of endometerial cancer in women without normal menstrual cycling treated with estrogens alone, as in Turner's syndrome, is further evidence supporting this idea. The causal role of continued unopposed estrogenic stimulation is further suggested by the high incidence of a history of irregular menses in women with endometrial cancer ([46]Dunn and Bradbury 1967). A reduction in premalignant changes such as endometrial hyperplasia is seen in women who resume normal cyclical ovarian function in response to ovarian wedge resection in the Stein-Leventhal syndrome ([49]Kaufman et al 1959) or in whom progesterone treatment at periodic intervals is begun.

Obesity is also a risk factor for endometrial cancer. As previously described for breast cancer patients, increased body fat is associated with an increased production of estrogen from androgen precursors. In addition, in premenopausal women, the association of obesity with anovulatory cycles and amenorrhea may provide the physiologic basis for increased risk. In postmenopausal women, the etiologic pathway is even more clear. After the menopause, the predominant blood estrogen is estrone, derived almost entirely from conversion of adrenal androgen precursors to estrogens in peripheral tissues. The rate of this conversion increases with age ([50]Hemsell et al 1974) and weight ([51]MacDonald et al 1978). As already mentioned, there is some evidence that in obese women alterations in plasma binding of estrogens may occur leading to even further elevations in plasma estrogen concentrations than would be presumed by direct measurement of the hormone.

Pharmacologic administration of estrogens in postmenopausal women is associated with at least a 4-9 fold increased risk of eventually developing endometrial cancer ([52]Feinstein and Horwitz 1978). Risk increases with both duration and dose.

Clearly, psychic factors can have an important interplay with these abnormalities of estrogen. For example, menstrual coordination in women living and many other factors are proven to induce menstrual abnormalities which may increase the risk of endometrial cancer. Obesity itself may reflect an emotional response to stress which may have, as a side effect, alterations in the endocrine milieu predisposing to cancer. Reduction in such a response to stress with concommitant weight loss may reduce the risk of either developing the disease or having a recurrence.

Endometrial cancer, once established, has also been shown to respond to endocrine therapy. In 1961, it was first reported that pharmacologic administration of progestogens could cause regression in about 1/3 of patients with endometrial cancer ([53]Kelley and Baker 1961); this has been confirmed in many other studies ([54]Bonte 1979). Endometrial cancer is primarily a disease of postmenopausal women. There are essentially no circulating levels of progestin like compounds in women of this age unless administered pharmacologically. Thus, it is unlikely that psychic factors are likely to directly result in tumor regression. Other hormones, however, may regulate endometrial growth. Estrogen can certainly stimulate mitoses in endometrial cancer cells and thus the mechanisms previously described in breast cancer may modulate endometrial cancer cell growth as well.

Carcinoma of the Prostate. Cancer of the prostate gland represents the first human maligna direct proof of hormonal dependency was demonstrated by experimental means. It is the second most frequenct cancer of men in the United States with the majority of cases occuring in men over the age of 70. It is critical to an understanding of the relative impact of endocrine factors on presentation and progression of this disease to appreciate that microscopic prostatic cancer can be found in a far greater proportion of men than those in whom the disease actually progresses to clinical attention. Thus, it is plausible to attempt to separate carcinogenesis per se from tumor promotion. It is in this particular prostate cancer. For example, the death rate is significantly higher in American blacks than in whites. However, American black men have an age standardized incidence rate about 6 times that of Nigerian black men, although the incidence of latent carcinoma is the same ([55]Jackson 1977). In that same study, it was reported that the fat intake of patients with carcinoma of the prostate exceeded that of age matched controls. Fat intake and possibly testosterone levels may act as critical conditioning factors in the progression from latent to clinical cancer. This critical role of the environment has been even further emphasized in a study involving Japanese men living in Hawaii who were found to have a higher incidence of clinical cancer than Japanese men living in Japan; once again, the incidence of latent cancer was the same ([56]Akazakis and Stennerman 1973).

Prostate is the target tissue upon which virtually all studies of androgen action have been performed. The pioneering work of Huggins ([57]Huggins and Clark 1940; [58]Huggins 1939), which the Nobel Prize was awarded, established the role of androgens in maintenance of the normal prostate and gave rise to the entire concept of androgen dependence. The subsequent demonstration that castration caused regression of prostatic cancer in men ([59]Huggins and Hodges 1941) initiated the era of hormonal management of cancer of the prostate. Exposure to androgens is clearly critical in the development of the disease. Individuals with inadequate production of testicular testosterone or insensitivity to testosterone do not develop prostatic cancer. Interestingly, however, concentrations of plasma androgens thus far have not been demonstrated to be different in patients with prostatic cancer versus the normal population

($^{60}$Hammond et al 1978).

In addition to testosterone, prolactin has been shown to play an important role in the prostatic growth of rodents. Hypophysectomy causes a more profound prolactin synergizes with testosterone in maintaining the normal male sexual accessory glands. Great caution should be employed in generalizing from these observations in rodents to humans. It should be recalled that in rodent models, prolactin is a critical hormone in the maintainence of breast cancer growth, whereas the role of prolactin in human breast cancer is far less established. On the other hand, responses to hypophysectomy in patients previously orchiectomized have been reported ($^{62}$Murphy 1971) as will be discussed below.

The endocrine therapy of prostatic cancer has been based on the concept that reduction of plasma androgens to low levels by orchiectomy should induce tumor regressions. However, it has been shown that estrogens can directly inhibit the effects of androgen on prostatic secretion in the absence of the pituitary gland ($^{63}$Goodwin et al 1961). These and other data imply a direct additional effect of estrogen on a prostate gland over and above its suppression of pituitary LH stimulation of testicular androgen production. Thus, a rationale can be developed for simultaneous use of orchiectomy and estrogens. It is beyond the scope of this chapter to review in detail the many studies examing differences in response rate and toxicity of prostatic cancer managed with either orchiectomy, estrogen administration, or both. It suffices to say that little convincing evidence exists to suggest clinically that an impressive additive effect exists for castration plus estrogen administration. On the other hand, some responses to estrogens have been reported in patients initially treated with orchiectomy who subsequently relapsed.

One of the difficulties, however, in evaluating the response to prostatic cancer has been the fact that overwhelmingly, the metastatic pattern of spread of this disease involves osteoblastic bone metastases. While reduction of acid phosphatase and relief of pain may be commonplace, the usual objective criteria of healing of lytic lesions and bone remodeling have been very difficult to orchiectomy or estrogen have ranged between 50 and 80% depending, to some extent, on the stage of disease and criteria used to evaluate response. The median duration of response has been approximately a year and a half, although occasional remissions can last substantially longer.

As described previously, the adrenal is often a source of androgen precursors. For this reason, suppression of adrenal production of androgens by exogenous glucocorticoids or via the use of adrenalectomy (medically or surgically) has been attempted. Such studies have generally yielded relatively low response rates ([64]Sandord et al 1976).

Based upon the fact that hypophysectomy will further interfere with adrenal function, as well as potentially remove other growth factors such as prolactin which may be important in human prostatic cancer, hypophysectomy has been attempted in a small series of patients. In some preliminary data ([62]Murphy 1971), a surprisingly high response rate to hypophysectomy varying between 40 and 63% has been seen. Thus, further evaluation of the role of pituitary hormones in prostatic cancer cell growth is required.

Glucocorticoid therapy has generally been ineffective in the management of prostate cancer. Thus, a major role for immune modulation in tumor progression in this disease has not been actively persued.

Leukemia and Lymphoma. Glucocorticoids influence the growth, differentiation, and function of virtually every tissue and organ system in the body ([65]Thompson and Lippman 1974). Among these diverse effects, inhibitory actions on lymphoid and hematopoietic tissues have long been appreciated ([66]Baxter and Forsham 1974). In fact, two of the earliest described effects of glucocorticoids in

man were lymphocytopenia and eosinopenia. Glucocorticoids produced marked
thymic atrophy in experimental animals. Thus, these steroids were initially
used with great enthusiasm when it was first discovered that they could kill
1972). The initial experience with childhood leukemia suggested response rates
of up to 70% in patients treated with glucocorticoids as a single agent.
Unfortunately, re-treatment results in substantially lower response rates.

It is now clear that most, if not all, glucocorticoid effects are mediated
by an interaction of either endogenously secreted or exogenously administered
glucocorticoids with specific glucocorticoid receptors found in the cytoplasm
of target cells. From the known affinity of these proteins for glucocorticoids,
an estimation of concentrations of hormone required to produce biological
effects can be made. There is a striking agreement between concentrations of
glucocorticoid required to saturate these receptor sites and concentrations required to induce biologic effects. Interestingly, the concentrations required
to inhibit leukemic lymphoblasts are only minimally above those normally found
circulating and are readily achievable during periods of stress. In fact, the
most impressive data available concerning ways in which psychic factors can
alter neoplastic progression can be found in the literature of spontaneous
remissions in leukemia following stressful events. Two of the best known are
the remissions of Bela Bartok, who upon receiving a commission from the Boston
Symphony Orchestra for his Concerto for Orchestra, had a spontaneous remission
of his leukemia. Dinu Lupati also had a spontaneous remission of his leukemia
while preparing for his final concert.

Glucocorticoids are also of extreme value in a variety of lymphoproliferative disorders including Hodgkin's disease and the non-Hodgkin's lymphomas.
The mechanisms of interaction of glucocorticoids with these malignant cells are
probably somewhat more complex than their direct effects on leukemic cells in

vitro would suggest. Obviously, glucocorticoids modulate many other aspects of the immune system and through these indirect means, eventual irradication of the disease may be achieved, once chemotherapy has reduced the malignant cell

Other Diseases. A smaller amount of evidence suggests that endocrine factors may be critical in the etiology, progression, or therapy of several other human malignancies, including ovarian cancer ([68]Hoover et al 1977), laryngeal cancer ([69]Saez and Sakai 1976), and malignant melanoma ([70]Fisher et al 1976). In each of these examples, some evidence for alterations in hormonal factors potentially regulated by psycho-neuro-endocrine pathways are plausible. However, due to the lack of solid data on hormonal dependency, they are not generally regarded as necesarily under direct hormonal control. It should be borne in mind, however, that given the scheme described in figure 1, many human malignancies not classically described as being directly hormone dependent may be profoundly affected by alterations in the endocrine milieu.

Ectopic Hormone Production. Cancer is capable of producing a variety of symptoms and effects which transcend those attributable to mass effects and invasion. It is only recently that some of these substances have been identified and some of the syndromes associated with such ectopic humor production have been identified. A list of hormones which have thus far been proven to be produced by cancers in provided in Table 1. Notable is the preponderance of polypeptide hormones on this list. Also interesting is the absence of certain hormones. Steroid hormones, including glucocorticoids have never been reported to be produced ectopically. It is worth stressing that in every case of ectopic hormone production thus far described, the hormone produced has been identical to the normally secreted hormone with respect to amino acid structure. Thus, it is far from surprising that profound biological effects may result from such hormonal production. This can profoundly influence cancer progression by several mechanisms. For example, in the ectopic ACTH production syndrome, the ectopic ACTH stimulates the otherwise normal adrenal to enormously excessive production of glucocorticoids and mineralacorticoids. altered host response to the tumor. Clearly, glucocorticoid effects on the immune system are only one way in which such ectopic hormone production may be manifested. In addition, the production of such ectopic hormones can be associated with many behavioral manifestations. Certainly, glucocorticoids, parathyroid hormone, and vasopressin can either directly or through the metabolic abnormalities they induce cause substantial behavioral effects which may be correlated with tumor progression. Under certain circumstances, the ectopic tumor production may be the major manifestation of the cancer itself. As shown in figure 1, these changes in tumors may either primarily or second-arily lead to hormonal changes which influence the growth of either hormone dependent neoplasia or less directly influence the growth of hormone independent neoplasia.

Even more perplexing than the known ectopic hormone syndromes are those paraneoplastic syndromes which have been attributed to humoral factors but for which direct isolation of the specific factor has not been possible. Amongst the critically important symptom complexes associated with certain malignancies are myopathies, myasthenic syndromes, dermatologic syndromes, digital clubbing and arthropathies, hematologic abnormalities, fever, central nervous system degenerative conditions, and cachexia. Each of these symptom complexes may regress completely with appropriate therapy of the tumor itself. Each of these symptom complexes can profoundly influence the individual's perception of his clinical status and prognosis and directly induce (via unknown mechanisms) behavioral alterations, and psychiatric disturbances. Not only can these psychic changes be correlated with the cancer, but they may (as displayed in figure 1) feed back on neuroendocrine pathways and thus produce further

derangements in the hormonal milieu. It is unfortunate that these syndromes

are so poorly understood with respect to their humoral etiology. Once again,

producing profound systemic responses with behavioral concommitants. This at

least raises the possibility that some of the information suggesting that

certain behavioral responses to tumors influence their progression may be in-

correct and the behavioral effects induced by the tumors themselves. A great

deal more information is critically needed in this area before many aspects of

the interactions of behavioral factors and tumor progression can be worked

out, at least with respect to causality.

REFERENCES

1. Beatson, G.T. (1896) Lancet 2, 104-107.
2. Mason, J.W. (1968) Psychosom. Med. 30, 576-607.
3. Guillemin, R., Vargo, T., Rossier, J, et al. (1977) Science 197: 1367-1369.
4. Rose, R.M., and Sachar, E.J. (1981) Psychoendocinology in Textbook of Endocrinology ed. by R.H. Williams, W.B. Sanders, Philadelphia pp. 646-671.
5. Sachar, E.J. and Baron, M. (1979) Ann. Rev. Neurosciences 2, 505-517.
6. MacMahon, B., Cole, P., Brown, J. (1973) J. Natl. Cancer Inst. 50, 21-36.
7. Haenzel, W., and Kurihara, M. (1968) J. Natl. Cancer Inst. 40, 43-68.
8. DeWaard, F. (1969) Int. J. Cancer 4, 577-586.
9. Henderson B.E., Cassagrande, J.T., Pike, M.E. (1981) in Hormones and Breast Cancer ed. Pike, M.E., Siiteri, P.K. and Welsch, C.W; Cold Spring Harbor Press, New York pp. 3-18.
10. MacMahon, B., Cole, P., Lin, T.M., Lowe, C.R., Merra, A.P., Rainihar, B., Salber, E.J., Valabras, V.G., Yuasa, S (1970) Bull WHO 43, 209-221.
11. Abramson, J.M. (1966) Israel J. Med. Sci. 2, 457-464.
12. Ing, R, Ho, J.H.C., Petrakis, N.L. (1977) Lancet 2, 124-127.
13. Petrakis, N.L. (1977) Cancer 39, 2709-2715.
14. Petrakis, N.L. (1971) Science 173, 347-349.
15. Pike, M.C., Cassagrande, J.T., Brown, J.B., Gerkins, V., Henderson, B.E. (1977) J. Natl. Cancer Inst. 59, 1351-1355.
16. Fishman, J., Fukushima, D., O'Connor, J., Rosenfeld, R.S., Lynch, H.T., Guirgis, H., Maloney, K. (1978) Cancer Research 38, 4006-4011.
17. Tamarkin, L., Danforth, D., Lichter, A., DeMoss, E., Chabner, B., Lippman, M.E. (1981) (submitted to Science).
18. Feinlieb, M. (1968) J. Natl. Cancer Inst. 41, 315-329.
19. Miller, A.B. (1978) Cancer Res. 38, 3985-3990.
20. Lippman, M.E., Monaco, M.E. and Bolan, G. (1978) Cancer Res. 37, 1901-1907.
21. Siiteri, P.K., Hammond, G. and Nisker, J.A. (1981) in Estrogens and Breast Cancer ed. by Pike, M.C., Siiteri, P.K. and Welsch, C.W., Cold Spring Harbor Press, New York, pp. 87-106.

22. Kelsey, J.L. (1978), Am. J. Epidemol. 107, 236-44.
23. Sartwell, P.E., Arthes, F.G., Tonascin, J.A. (1977) J. Natl. Cancer Inst. 59, 1589-92.
24. Cassagrande, J., Gerkins, V., Henderson, B.E., Mack, T., Pike, M.C. (1976) J. Natl. Cancer Inst. 56, 839-841.
25. Craig, M.J., Comstock, G.W., Geiser, P.B. (1974) J. Natl. Cancer Inst. 53, 1577-1581.
26. Anderson, J.M. (1979) Brit. Med. J. 1, 1124-1127.
27. Lippman, M.E., Osbourne, C.K., Knazek, R. and Young, N. (1977) New Eng. J. Med. 296, 154-159.
28. Lippman, M.E. (1981) in Hormones and Breast Cancer ed. by Pike, M.C., Siiteri, P., and Welsch, C.W. Cold Spring Harbor Laboratories pp. 171-184.
29. Ravdin, R.G. (1970) Surg. Gynecol. Obstet. 131, 1055-1064.
30. Nissen-Meyer, R. (1964) Clin. Radiol. 15, 152-160.
31. Meakin, J.W. (1980) in Endocrine Treatment of Breast Cancer ed. by Henningsen, B., Linder, F. and Steichele, C. Springer Verlag, Berlin pp.178-84.
32. Hubay, C.A. (1980) Surg. 87, 494-501.
33. Donegan, W.L., Hartz, A.J., Rimm, A.A. (1978) Cancer 41, 1590-1594.
34. Fracchia, A.A., Farrow, J.H., Depalo, A.J., Connolly, D.P., Huvos, A.G. (1969) Surg. Gynecol. Obstet. 128, 1226-1234.
35. Grodin, J.M., Siiteri, P.K., MacDonald, P.C. (1973) Endocrinol 36, 207-14.
36. Santen, R.J., and Wells, S.A. (1980) Cancer 46, 1066-74.
37. Dao, T.L. (1972) Ann. Rev. Med. 23, 1-18.
38. EORTC (1972) Europ. J. Cancer 8, 155-156.
39. Kennedy, B.J. (1969) Cancer 24, 1345.
40. Goldenberg, I.S. (1969) Cancer 23, 109-112.
41. Yates, J., Couchman, J.R. and King R.J.B. (1980) in Hormones and Cancer ed. by S. Iacobelli et al. Raven Press, New York pp. 31-39.
42. Kaufman, R.F. and Escher, G.C. (1961) Surg. Gynecol. and Obstet. 113, 635-640.
43. Pannoti, F., Martoni, A., DiMarco, A.R., Piano, E., Saccini, F., Beechi, G., Maltiol, G., Barbanti, F., Marra, G.A., Persiani, W., Cacciri, L., Spegnolo, F. Palenzona, D., Rocchetta, G. (1979) Europ. J. Cancer 15, 593-601.
44. Ker and Stewart (1966) Brit. J. Surgery 53, 151.
45. Lippman, M.E., Bolan, G., Huff, K. (1976) Cancer Res. 36, 4602-09.
46. Dunn, L.J., Bradbury, J.T. (1967) Obstet. Gynecol. 97, 465-471.
47. Antunes, C.M.E., Stolley, P.D., Rosensheim, D.B., Davies, J.L., Tonascia, J.A., Brown, C., Garcia, R. (1979) N. Eng. J. Med. 300, 9-13.
48. Nisker, J.A., Ramzy, I., Collins, J.A. (1978) Am. J. Obstet. Gynecol. 130, 546-50.
49. Kaufman, R.H., Abbott, I.P., Wall, J.A. (1959) Am. J. Obstet. Gynecol. 77, 1271-85.
50. Hemsell, D.L., Grodin, J.M., Brenner, P.F., Siiteri, P.K., MacDonald, P.C. (1974) J. Clin. Endocrinol. Metab. 38, 476-479.
51. MacDonald, P.C., Edman, C.D., Hemsell, D.L., Porter, J.C., Siiteri, P.K. (1978) Am. J. Obstet. Gynecol. 130, 448-55.
52. Feinstein, A.R. and Horwitz, R.I. (1978) Cancer Res. 38, 4001-4005.
53. Kelley, R.M. and Baker, W.H. (1961) New Eng. J. Med. 264, 216-222.
54. Bonte, J. (1979) Reviews on Endocrine Related Cancer 3, 11.
55. Jackson, M.A. (1977) Cancer Treat. Rep. 61, 167-172.
56. Akazakis, K and Stennerman, G.N. (1973) J. Natl. Cancer Inst. 50, 1137-1162.
57. Huggins, C. and Clark, P.J. (1940) J. Exp. Med. 72, 747-761.

82

58. Huggins, C. (1939) J. Exp. Med. 70, 543 556.
59. Huggins, C. and Hodges, C.V. (1941) Cancer Res. 1, 293-297.
60. Hammond, G.L., Kotturim, Vikko, P., Vikko, R. (1978) Clin. Endocrinol. 9, 113-21.
61. Grayback, J.T. (1963) Natl. Cancer Inst. Monograph 12, 189-199.
62. Murphy, C.P., Reynoso, G., Schoomees, R., Gailani, S., Bolerke, R., Kenny G.M., Murand, E.A., Schaldch, D.S. (1971) J. Urol. 105, 817-825.
63. Goodwin, D.A., Rasmussen-Taxdal, D.S., Ferreira, A.A., Scott, W. (1961) J. Urol. 86, 134-136.
64. Sandord, E.J., Drago, J.R., Rohner, T.J., Santen, R., Lipton, A. (1976) J. Urol. 115, 170-174.
65. Thompson, E.B., and Lippman, M.E. (1974) Metabolism 23, 159-202.
66. Baxter, J.D., and Forsham, P.H. (1974)
67. Claman, H.N. (1972) N. Eng. J. Med. 287, 388-397.
68. Hoover, R., Gray, L.A. Sr., Fraumeni, J.F. Jr. (1977) Lancet 2, 533-534.
69. Saez, S. and Sakai, F. (1976) J. Steroid Biochem. 7, 919-921.
70. Fisher, R.I., Neifeld, J.P. and Lippman, M.E. (1976) Lancet 2, 337-340.

# SHOULD WE INVESTIGATE PSYCHOTHERAPY FOR PHYSICAL DISEASE, ESPECIALLY CANCER?

ALASTAIR J. CUNNINGHAM
Ontario Cancer Institute, 500 Sherbourne Street, Toronto, Ontario, Canada
M4X 1K9

To give a reasoned answer to the question put by the title of this paper, we need first to ask whether events in the mind have any impact on the development or remission of cancer. And even before this, our attitude will be coloured by our beliefs on the effect mind has on the body generally, and on various kinds of physical disease. So we will begin by listing some of the evidence that mind and body are intimately connected and that mental states contribute to somatic disease. Then we will focus on cancer, discussing evidence that it is subject to some control by the body and ultimately by the mind. From there we need to enquire how the mind-cancer relationship can be most efficiently studied. Some speculations will finally be offered as to kinds of psycho-therapy that may prove worth investigating.

## 1. EFFECTS OF MIND ON BODY

The most familiar results of mental actions on body function are control of voluntary muscle by the central nervous system, and the effects on smooth muscle and viscera of autonomic nerves and neuroendocrine mechanisms (e.g., the general adaptation of stress, blushing, and sexual arousal). The ability of mind to control the body goes far beyond this, however. For example, by psychological conditioning of the "classical" or Pavlovian kind, animals or humans can be taught to make involuntary changes in such functions as urine flow or gastrointestinal motions in response to normally unrelated stimuli like scratching the skin, or even to verbal commands (Razran 1961).

Biofeedback is a form of "operant" conditioning by which individuals can learn voluntary control over local skin temperature, heart rate, certain brain wave patterns, smooth muscle contraction, blood pressure and the firing of individual nerve motor units (Basmajian 1979), things thought beyond conscious influence until recently. An attitude of expectation that an effect on the body (e.g., healing) will occur seems to contribute to bringing it about, e.g., it is well documented that an inert substance (placebo) can often produce beneficial results. A wide variety of conditions has been alleviated by placebos in some patients: anxiety, headache, hypertension, pain, hayfever, asthma, depression, arthritis, peptic ulcer (reviewed by Shapiro, 1968;

Brody, 1980; Benson and Epstein, 1975). "Faith healing" and "hex death", while less studied seem also to demonstrate the power of strong expectation or belief by an individual to facilitate his cure or death, respectively, in some cases.

Clinical hypnosis is a process of assisting a client to dissociate his conscious rational resistance to changes and to accept mentally, and translate into mental or physical action, the suggestions of a therapist. Bowers (1979) has reviewed the use of hypnosis for physical disorders such as relief of pain or asthma, removal of various allergic and skin conditions, including warts, and producing vascular changes. The field of psychosomatic disease is concerned with the ability of mental ideas and states to produce pathological changes in the body. Finally, exceptional individuals (yogis and others) have performed, in controlled surroundings, such feats as passing sharp objects through their flesh with little pain or bleeding, and walking on hot coals (at several hundred degrees centigrade) without burning. These feats should not be regarded as contradicting our knowledge of physiology: rather they provide experimental evidence that unusual mental states can allow ranges of physiological response broader than is commonly thought possible.

## 2. THE CONTRIBUTION OF MIND TO PHYSICAL DISEASE

Currently, conventional medicine tends to discount the role of the mind in somatic diseases, providing instead explanations at the level of molecules and tissues rather than considering the whole individual. This approach has proved quite successful (i.e., has led to cures) for many infectious diseases and for mechanical disorders amenable to surgery. Yet most of the remaining major health problems, at least in developed countries, are not simple in the sense of having a single, overwhelmingly obvious cause, but instead are essentially disorders of regulation, e.g., cardiovascular diseases, arthritis, chronic respiratory diseases, chronic pain, mental diseases, and appetitive disorders like smoking, alcoholism and obesity. Problems like these can hardly be said to have "a cause". Rather, they seem to involve defects in the balance of functions in the body: the concept of causality loses much of its meaning in such complex, multivariate, interacting systems. Cancer may be similar. Whenever regulation is defective, a contribution by the mind may be suspected since the central nervous system ultimately has some power to regulate all body functions (Fig. 1).

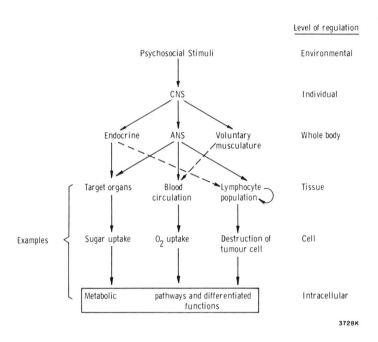

Fig. 1. Some pathways by which the mind may influence body functions.

Research on the contribution of the mind to physical disease can be grouped under two main headings: psychosocial aspects or the impact of different ways of perceiving and interacting with the world, and correlations between personality characteristics and disease susceptibility.

At the psychosocial level it appears that a sense of meaning to life, of belonging, and of some control over events is important to health (reviewed by Antonovsky, 1979). Cassel (1979) believes similarly that a perceived inability to cope with stress may be a fundamental cause of ill-health. Frequent and significant changes in a person's life also have been found in a number of studies to promote illness (e.g., Holmes and Rahe, 1967). Llynch (1977) discusses the voluminous evidence for an association between loneliness or bereavement and cardiovascular disease. Numerous experiments and observations on both animals and humans suggest that ill-health is increased under conditions where there is a lack of support and care from other members of the same species. Bartrop et al., (1977), have shown that the severe psychological stress of losing a spouse causes a substantial drop in the ability of T lymphocytes to respond to mitogenic stimulation; this work is particularly interesting because it suggests a mechanism connecting mental perception with susceptibility to disease.

Under a second heading, perhaps the best-known correlation between personality characteristics and disease comes from the work on susceptibility of type A individuals to coronary artery disease (reviewed by Chesney et al., 1981). Earlier, Ruesch (1948), Deutsch (1953) and others described an infantile personality structure which was felt to underly all psychosomatic conditions: traits included dependence and passivity, rigid and unrealistic ideals, and persistence of conflicts from earlier periods of development. Other workers attempted to identify personality elements that predisposed to particular psychosomatic symptoms (Dunbar, 1943; Alexander, 1950; Grace and Graham, 1952). For example, Grace and Graham found that hypertension was associated with personalities who were constantly prepared to meet threats, constipation with a grim determination to carry on despite difficulties, and duodenal ulcer with desire for revenge. Later writers (e.g., Engel, 1967) have concluded that there are typically several conflict issues in patients with psychosomatic disease and that the onset of these conditions is less specific than was earlier claimed. The large literature on personality characteristics of cancer patients is summarized in section 4, and has been critically reviewed elsewhere by Fox (1978).

## 3. IS CANCER SUBJECT TO SOME CONTROL BY THE BODY?

In the last section we have seen that there is a lot of evidence for important effects of mental state on physical health. We now want to ask whether this applies to cancer. The first step seems to be to enquire whether cancer cells are subject to any control at all, since once this is acknowledged, then the mind, as ultimate controller of body events, becomes a potential regulator of the disease. The next step is to ask what research evidence exists linking mental state and neoplastic disease (section 4), and the third, what clinical observations support this association (section 5)?

Opinions on the potential of the body to control cancer fall between two extremes. On the one hand is the idea that cancer is purely a disorder of cells; after appropriate mutation a clone of neoplastic cells simply grows autonomously until the host dies. At the other end of the spectrum lies the view that neoplastic changes in cells are not uncommon but that overt cancer only appears when there is a weakening of normal control mechanisms. Most biomedical scientists would probably take an intermediate position.

At what levels could cancer be controlled? There seem to be at least four kinds of mechanism which might regulate the growth of cancer cells, and be in turn subject to over-riding control by the central nervous system:

(1) Metabolic: Like their normal fellows, cancer cells need nutrients, ions and other materials from the extra-cellular fluid.

(2) DNA: The genetic lack of normal DNA repair enzymes leads to an increased rate of cancer in xeroderma pigmentosum (Fox, 1981) implying that DNA repair is a normal level of control.

(3) Tissue: Cancer cells are often not individually very different from normals, and so are subject to hormonal regulation. For example, some leukemic cells respond to erythropoietin in vitro; neoplasms of various organs (e.g., breast, prostate, some thyroid) are hormone dependent (Huggins, 1967). The normal control of tissue growth (c.f., regeneration of partly removed liver to the original size) is still poorly understood, but it is at this level that the failure of regulation may occur which permits neoplasms to grow.

(4) Immune system: The immune system would appear to be ideally suited for searching out and destroying even widely disseminated small tumors, and according to the immune surveillance hypothesis of Burnet (1970) it performs this function so effectively that we see only that small proportion of tumors which escape the monitoring process. In support of this, immune mechanisms have been shown to protect laboratory animals against spontaneous tumors in man. A disturbing finding, which speaks against the immune surveillance hypothesis has been that while immunosuppressed and genetically immunodeficient animals and people have an increased tumor incidence, most of these excess neoplasms are lymphoreticular; tumors of many other cell types are not increased in frequency. Nevertheless, immune responses to antigens on spontaneous tumors certainly occur. It is currently felt that specific cytotoxic T lymphocytes, together with non-specific "natural killer" cells and activated macrophages may have important controlling effects. The immune response to tumor (and other) antigens is extremely complex, and may involve not only these non-specific elements and specific effector cells but also suppressor T cells and antibodies with various kinds of relationship to the tumor - e.g., blocking, unblocking and anti-idiotype antibodies.

Patterns of cancer growth furnish another line of evidence which points strongly to fluctuating control by the body. Devitt (1979) and Stoll (1979) have recently summarized this work:

(1) Precancerous lesions, e.g., in prostate, are quite common in normal people.

(2)  It is unlikely that any treatment kills every cancer cell, yet cures are achieved, implying that the remaining cells are controlled; for example, incompletely excised tumors may fail to recur; metastases of breast cancer in lymph nodes may fail to grow beyond a certain size.

(3)  Recurrence of a tumor (after treatment of the primary) may be delayed a long time, sometimes more than 20 years, and yet growth subsequent to its reappearance may be very rapid.  Breast cancer fits into this last pattern, with a variable and sometimes long dormancy often followed by a "shower" of metastases and rapid growth.

(4)  The most dramatic example of putative control of cancer by the body is, of course, the rare spontaneous regression without treatment or with apparently inadequate treatment (Everson and Cole, 1966; Boyd, 1966; Lewison, 1976).  Where all lesions of a multifocal tumor regress simultaneously it is very difficult to argue that some local chance event, like blockage of a blood vessel or exhaustion of cell proliferative capacity, is responsible.  Instead, a reassertion of systemic control seems to have occurred.  All of the above patterns of tumor growth could be accounted for by making special assumptions about behaviour intrinsic to the cells, but taken together they seem much more compatible with the idea that tumor cells are normally under some control, and that this control varies with time and is influenced by currently unrecognized factors.

## 4. RESEARCH EVIDENCE FOR AN ASSOCIATION BETWEEN MENTAL STATE AND CANCER

We can identify 3 main areas of research under this heading; attempts (mostly with animals) to relate stress to cancer growth and dissect out relevant neural and hormonal mechanisms; studies with human patients comparing mental attributes of people with or without cancer; and correlations, within cancer patient groups between mental attributes and the course of the disease.

(1)  The effects of  stress, and mechanistic studies

The most common type of animal experiment has been to attempt to alter the course of tumor growth by stress of various kinds, and then, in some cases, to study possible mechanisms responsible for the change.

Diverse effects of stress have been reported: e.g., according to the review by LaBarba (1970) tumor growth may be enhanced or diminished by handling or early weaning; it is enhanced by isolating animals or inducing neuroses experimentally, and tends to be diminished by chronic stress.  Riley (1975) found that the development of mammary tumors in C3H/He strain mice (carrying the Bittner oncogenic virus) was considerably increased by chronic stress.  At 400 days of age, incidence ranged from 92% under stress to 7% in a protected environment. Sklar and Anisman (1979; 1981) discerned a pattern in response to stress, elucidated by their own very interesting work. Acute stress appears to enhance tumors, chronic to depress them. The effect of acute stress is possibly mediated by the influence of hormones, notably corticosterone, on the immune system. The existence of coping mechanisms, such as fighting, or learning how to turn off a stressful, regular shock prevented the increase in tumor growth which would otherwise have been seen, and was correlated with lower plasma corticosterone levels. A further dimension of complexity is added by the observation that the animals' previous history influences the effects a stressor will have (Ader and Friedman, 1964). For example, isolating mice increases tumor growth only if the individuals had previously been housed in groups (Sklar and Anisman, 1979).

The mechanisms by which stress might affect tumor growth has been the subject of several recent reviews (Gisler, 1974; Amkraut and Solomon, 1975; Rogers et al., 1979). While effects on tissue-specific homeostasis and tumor angiogenesis have been mentioned, the great majority of the work reviewed concerns the immune system. Acute stress or ACTH tend to depress immune responses, probably mainly through effects on B cells and macrophages, and on circulating T cells. Thymus involution also occurs in stressful situations and T cells migrate to the bone marrow. Lymphocytes may be direct targets for many hormones as they have $\alpha$ and $\beta$ adrenergic receptors and receptors for corticosteroids, somatrophic hormone, insulin and histamine.

(2) Comparing personality attributes of people with and without cancer

A different approach to establishing a relationship between mind and cancer is to bypass mechanisms and look directly for a correlation between mental characteristics and liability to the disease. The dominant kind of study has been a retrospective comparison between people who already have the disease, and otherwise comparable normal individuals. Several hundred such papers exist (see reviews by Fox, 1978; Scurry and Levin, 1978; Greer, 1979). Although many characteristics have been considered, it has proved extremely difficult to draw unequivocal conclusions. However, two fairly definite correlations seem to emerge.

(a) Cancer is often associated with a relative inability to express emotion, particularly anger. This would fit with the idea (e.g., Bahnson, 1969) that if conflict is not resolved by interpersonal expression or mental derangement it is liable to break out as somatic pathology.

(b) Cancer patients, more often than normal individuals, have a feeling of lack of control over events (the "helpless/hopeless" syndrome), and have frequently suffered the loss of an important relationship prior to getting the disease. Other points raised by various authors are: the importance of social support, a sense of belonging, will to live and meaningfulness of existence in preventing cancer onset; the need for a sense of control and coping ability in avoiding the disease; existence of "general emotional lability" in cancer patients, some correlation with anal character traits among cancer patients; the importance of social stress.

Many difficulties beset this kind of study. Human personality attributes are clearly complex, subtle and variable, which may lead to low reliability of psychosomatic tests. Amongst groups with high or low incidence of disease mental attributes may be confounded with other variables: for example, Fox (1978) points out that the low incidence of certain kinds of cancer among Seventh Day Adventists could be caused by genetic or dietary factors, strong family and social support structures, strong religious feeling, low stress, not smoking, low promiscuity, or a tendency to work in particular occupations. A common criticism of retrospective studies is that having the disease may change personality, so that any correlations are not causative. Prospective studies are obviously much more difficult, but several have now been reported, demonstrating a number of characteristics common to individuals who later developed cancer: repressive tendencies (Dattore et al., 1980; Grossarth-Maticek, 1980); lack of closeness to parents (Beddell-Thomas, 1974); depression (Hagnell, 1966; Bieliauskas, 1979); and oral-dependent traits (Greenberg and Dattore, 1981).

Overall, while measured psychological attributes have very weak predictive power there is a fair consensus that certain personality traits may be associated with increased likelihood of developing cancer. It seems that the mind may, indeed, have some influence on this disease.

(3)  Correlating mental attributes with outcome in patients who already have cancer

In this approach, correlations are made between different mental attributes and the progress of cancer among groups of patients all of whom have the disease. It has been used much less than the retrospective study design just discussed - there are about 10-20 published reports. Results from this kind of study seem similar to those of retrospective comparisons: relatively good outcome is associated with ability to express hostility, and with a sense of control over events in life. For example, Blumberg et al., (1954), using the M.M.P.I. (Minnesota Multiphasic Personality Inventory), found that people in whom  disease progressed fast were lacking in ability to reduce excessive emotional stress and were "over-nice, cooperative, serious, painful". Stavraky (1968) found no great abnormality among patients with poor outcome, (using the M.M.P.I., Wechsler verbal IQ test, and a projective personality assessment), but noted that favourable outcome was associated with expression of hostility and high IQ. Derogatis et al., (1979) similarly observed a correlation between expression of hostility and longer survival. The recent paper of Greer et al., (1979) sparked an exchange of views in the columns of Lancet in which some difficulties of interpretation were pointed out, for example, that denial of the importance or likelihood of disease could be correlated with a slower-growing and so less threatening tumor.

A most interesting study has recently been published by Achterberg and Lawlis (1978). Patients were asked to draw the way they saw their cancer cells and their defense mechanisms. Many chose symbolic modes, e.g., cancer cells were meat eaten by dogs representing phagocytic cells. The drawings were assessed by independent workers according to several criteria, the main aim being to arrive at a number representing the relative strength of defense mechanisms and cancer cells as perceived by the patient. People who scored well in this test had a better outcome, on average, than those who scored badly. This fascinating result offers the possibility of objective diagnosis from material produced by the patient's psyche. It may reflect the same processes that persuaded earlier workers (Booth, 1969; Mezei and Nemeth, (1969) that cancer patients given Rorshach tests had anal characteristics and a poor ability to recognize anatomical parts on the blots. The logical next step is obviously to try to change outcome by teaching "strong" imagery, and we turn now to a brief consideration of this type of work.

## 5. CLINICAL SUPPORT FOR A POTENTIAL THERAPEUTIC EFFECT OF MIND

There is growing interest in teaching patients to attempt to control their cancer by visualizing the treatment and their own body defenses as having a powerful healing effect. This is a way of mobilizing expectation of cure which derives from the early practice of medicine in many cultures. It has been revived and extensively used for about the last 10 years, in conjunction with other modes of psychotherapy by the Simontons (1978), who have taught the techniques to many other therapists. They report an approximately two-fold average prolongation of life-span in patients with a variety of types of cancer who received this kind of psychotherapy (Simonton et al., 1980). These results are not conclusive, since the life-span comparison has been made against the median national (U.S.A.) survival time, and it is clear that the

Simontons' patients were a highly self-selected group. Nevertheless, this approach is extremely interesting and deserves investigation now in trials with randomized controls.

The other body of published work describing systematic use of a form of psychological intervention as therapy for cancer comes from an Australian psychiatrist, A. Meares (1980) who uses intensive meditation. Of 73 patients he reports that 5 made "what appears to have been a complete regression of their growth in the absence of any organic treatment which could possibly account for it". Five others, at the time of publication, appeared to be "well on the way to similar regressions". Many more enjoyed significant psychological benefits. Again in the absence of controls and of details about the medical conditions of the patients (most were said to be advanced), it is difficult for an outsider to assess this work, although no doubt it is extremely convincing to the therapist himself, since he is able to observe small fluctuations in the medical state of individual patients and to correlate these with mental changes.

In addition to the work of Meares and of the Simontons and their colleagues there exist anecdotal clinical reports on small numbers of patients. A particularly dramatic case was reported by Klopfer (1957): a patient with multiple large lymphosarcoma tumors, apparently moribund, was restored to good health within a few days by injection of "Krebiozin", touted as a miracle drug. He relapsed, two months later, after reading reports that this drug was ineffective, but was again put into rapid remission by a reassurance that those reports were untrue and by an injection of what was described a "double-strength super-refined product" (in fact water was injected!), only to relapse again and die when he saw an AMA announcement that Krebiozin was worthless. Such a course seems almost impossible to attribute to coincidence; it appears instead to attest to the remarkable power that expecting to be healed may have over some tumors. Ikemi et al., (1975) similarly describe 5 cases of spontaneous recovery from cancer associated with dramatic changes in the patients' outlook on life, in particular with development or reaffirmation of religious faith. Among non-malignant tumors, there are a number of studies, some well-controlled, some not demonstrating the removal of warts by suggestion/ expectancy (Ullman, 1959).

## 6. LEVELS AT WHICH EFFECTS OF MIND ON BODY AND ON CANCER MAY BE STUDIED

Figure 2 shows some of the events that may occur between the perception
of a stimulus by the mind and its ultimate effect in the body. Many more
could be added. Most research involves examining the events within one "box"
or correlating effects in two, rarely more. For example, classical psychology
compares (1) and (10); study of the immunology of infectious disease - (8) and
(9); endocrine control of immune responses - (5) or (6) and (8); psychological
conditioning of immune responses (Ader et al., 1975) (2) or (3) and (8).

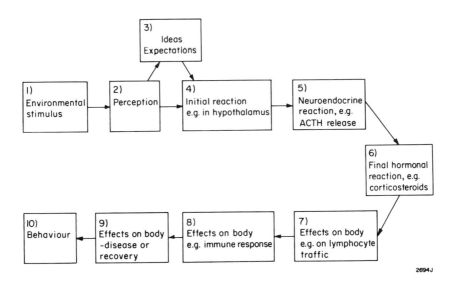

Fig. 2. Some events in the pathway mental perception - body response.

We need to ask ourselves: What does it mean to try to "understand" the
effects mind may have on cancer? The reductionist answer is that we need to
know details of all intermediate mechanisms. This is a laudable aim, but one
which may take many decades to even begin to fulfill. A review of the recent
book Psychoneuroimmunology (Ader, 1981) from which Figure 2 is taken
(Cunningham, 1981) shows the enormous complexity of interactions between

94

nervous, endocrine and immune systems, each of which is complex enough in
its own right. It is unfortunate that "explanation" of a phenomenon is
often equated with gaining a knowledge of the mechanisms involved. But this
is not the only way - and may be not the best way - to proceed when faced
with a problem like understanding the impact of mind on cancer. Scientific
hypotheses can be framed at any level, then tested by experiment, and it can
be argued that the most efficient level at which to formulate hypotheses in
this area is the psychological one, that is, comparing events in boxes (1)
to (3) with (9). The correlations between personality and cancer
susceptibility discussed in section 4 are examples of testing such hypotheses.
Knowledge of intervening mechanisms, while desirable, is not essential in
tackling the practical problem of using the mind therapeutically.

However, we do need some kind of theoretical structure within which to
formulate our theories. I suggest that, rather than concentrating
exclusively on the material interactions that accompany an influence of
mind on body, we also consider the informational aspects of these processes.
The human brain, with about $10^{11}$ neurones (all different) and $10^{14}$ synapses
(Hubel, 1979) is the most complex structure known. It serves as a computational
network, an information processor, evolved to coordinate the body's activities
and its interactions with the environment. "Mind", we may consider as an
emergent property of brain (some philosophers would disagree). An "idea" is
a way of conceptualizing an activity of the brain - it corresponds to a
particular pattern of neuronal activity, to a change in form. This alteration
may extend into the body, as, for example, when an emotion causes a blush. In
fact, there is no real separation between mind and body. Information about the
environment is recorded not only in the mind but in the body also, as adaptive
changes in form, although because of its much greater complexity the mind is
able to store a great deal more information than the body. Disease can be
viewed as a distortion of the form of the mind-body complex outside the limits
of normal healthy function.

While there is no space to develop these ideas here, a diagram (Fig. 3)
comparing the informational aspects of an asthmatic attack provoked either
psychogenically or allergically may show the usefulness of this kind of
analysis in bringing together phenomena that might otherwise seem very
different.

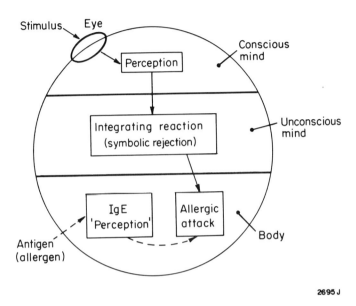

Fig. 3.  Similarities between allergic and psychogenic induction of allergy.

## 7. DESIGNING PSYCHOTHERAPY FOR CANCER

The remainder of this paper will consist of speculations on what kinds of
psychological technique might prove useful against cancer.  Our aim, as in all
psychotherapy, is to transfer information to the patient in a form that he can
accept (that bypasses resistance).  But instead of attempting to induce a
behavioural change we are interested to have this information "translated" into
a useful change in body form.  The mind contains "programs" for healthy
function, i.e., it has the potential for certain patterns of nerve action that
promote health; this is simply a way of restating the experimental observations
that mind influences disease, including cancer.  We would like to know, then,
how these programs can be activated or reinforced.  They are likely to be largely
unconscious: is there some way we can make them available for cognitive
inspection and manipulation?  Clearly, such "programs for health" will need to
be conceptualized in psychological rather than neurophysiological or electro-
chemical terms: there is nowhere near enough information available for the

latter kinds of description.

Perhaps the most useful way to think of these programs is as images of health coupled with strong affect and expectancy that the imagined changes can come about. An image is a neurological firing pattern in the brain that can occur in any sensory mode, has cognitive emotional and somatic associations, and embodies a vast amount of information (Sheikh and Panagiotou, 1975). There is evidence from biofeedback research and elsewhere that imagining some kinds of body response tends to bring them about (Lang, 1979): to paraphrase McLuan, "the image is the message"; it connects stimulus and response. Most ways of influencing the body through the mind, e.g., via placebo effect, hypnosis, psychological conditioning or faith-healing, may involve the formation of an intermediate image of the desired effect associated with a strong expectancy that it can and will occur (Fig. 4).

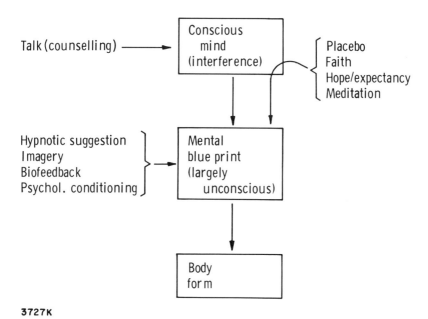

**3727K**

Fig. 4. Influence on body of various kinds of psychotherapy.

This all provides a post hoc rationalization for the widespread use of imagery therapy for cancer both in our culture and in earlier times. What is not clear is whether the attempts by the patient to "see" his white cells gobbling up cancer cells or to visualize other specific changes in tissues makes sense. The closest one can come to justifying this is to point to biofeedback work training individuals in controlling blood flow to certain areas. It may be that worthwhile effects are produced at higher "levels", e.g., imagining the specific tissues as restored to health, or, higher still, imagining (and strongly desiring) the return of the whole body to health, leaving the details of how this is accomplished to the unconscious mind. Modern clinical hypnosis favors such an approach where the desired end result is suggested rather than detailed instructions on body changes being given. It may, however, be important for the patient to have a concrete image to focus his attention on, either a quasi-realistic impression of cells interacting or a symbolic representation like large dogs as host defenses eating piles of meat, the cancer cells (Simonton et al., 1978).

In addition to having patients provide themselves with images of somatic change it is clearly important to have their minds as receptive as possible to the new suggestions. Relaxation, meditation and light hypnotic trances are useful techniques for this preparation. Counselling can help remove resistance to change and here we can be guided by the literature in psychosocial medicine: identifying strong goals in life, developing a sense of control over events and learning to give and accept love and support from others are all likely to promote a state of mind favourable to health. Teaching patients to express emotion rather than bottle it up (and thus somatise its expression?) also seems valuable. Speculating more wildly still, it may turn out that the increasing prevalence of cancer in our society reflects an absence of meaning in our lives; that a neoplasm is a kind of representation of the perceived lack of general order and control "written" into our body, much as an attitude of despair may be written into the mind by repeated demoralizing experiences. If this is true, attempts to assist in cure of cancer by psychotherapy may involve some very deep existential questions.

In fairness to the Simontons and others, it should be said that they have been doing for some time what I have tried to represent as logical approaches to psychotherapy for cancer. The overwhelming need now is for controlled clinical trials of this approach. It would seem sensible to use, at first, an intensive program including many different techniques, to try and get evidence for some physical effect, after which the significant parts of the program could be dissected out. Getting this evidence will not be easy, and the methods will probably be suitable at first for only a small proportion of patients. Nevertheless, extremely important issues are at stake: not only relief for victims of a devastating disease, but also the possibility of contributing to a new and broader biomedical paradigm which will include consideration of the impact of mind on disease generally.

SUMMARY

This paper suggests that it is time for properly controlled studies on the efficacy of psychological techniques as adjunctive therapy against cancer. The reasons for saying this are set out in the following chain of arguments.

(1) The mind has a profound controlling effect on the body as shown by research in hypnosis, placebo effect, psychosomatic disease, psychological conditioning, biofeedback, and other areas.

(2) There is also considerable evidence that mental states can contribute to many kinds of physical disease; for example, the association between type A personality and cardiovascular disease is well established.

(3) Tumors are not autonomous, but are subject to some regulation by the body. This can be inferred from cancer growth patterns and from knowledge of the effects of hormonal and immune mechanisms on at least some tumors. The brain, as ultimate controller of events in the body, is thus likely to exert an indirect effect on such tumors.

(4) There is now a body of evidence for some association between certain mental states and predisposition to cancer. This includes several prospective trials.

(5) There are anecdotal clinical reports describing beneficial effects of psychotherapy with certain cancer patients.

Some suggestions have been offered as to how the effect of mind on cancer might best be studied. It is argued that the immensely complex mechanisms connecting psyche and soma will take many decades to elucidate. It may be more immediately rewarding to consider informational (rather than material/ energetic) aspects of these interactions, framing hypotheses at the psychological level and testing directly for outcome on cancer. There is a rational basis for teaching patients to use images of healing coupled with strong desire for and expectancy of recovery. This needs to be validated by controlled scientific investigation.

REFERENCES

Achterberg, L. and Lawlis, G.F. (1978) Imagery of Cancer, Institute for Personality and Ability Testing, Illinois.
Ader, R. ed. (1981) Psychoneuroimmunology, Academic Press, New York.
Ader, R. and Cohen, N. (1975) Psychosom. Med. 37, 333.
Ader, R. and Friedman, S.B. (1964) in Medical Aspects of Stress in the Military Climate, Walter Reed Army Institute of Research, p. 457.
Alexander, F. (1950) Psychosomatic Medicine, Norton and Co., New York.
Amkraut, A. and Solomon, G.E. (1975) Int'l. J. Psychiatry in Medicine 5, 541.
Antonovsky, A. (1979) Health, Stress and Coping. Jossey-Bass, San Francisco.
Bahnson, C.B. (1969) Anns. N.Y. Acad. Sci. 164, (art. 2), 319.
Bartrop, R.W., Lazarus, L., Luckhurst, E., Kiloh, L.G. and Penny, R. (1977) Lancet i, 834.
Basmajian, J.V. ed. (1979) Biofeedback Principles and Practice for Clinicians. Williams and Wilkins, Baltimore.
Beddell-Thomas, C. and Duszynski, K.R. (1974) Hopkins Med. J. 134, 251.
Bieliauskas, L.A., et al., cited by Bahnson, C.B. (1980) Psychosomatics 21, 975.
Benson, H. and Epstein, M.D. (1975) J. Amer. Med. Assoc. 232, 1225.
Blumberg, E.M., West, P.M. and Ellis, F.W. (1954) Psychosomatic Medicine 16, 277.
Booth, G. (1969) Ann. N.Y. Acad. Sci. 164, (art. 2), 568.
Bowers, K.S. (1979) Aust. J. Clin. Exp. Hypnosis 7, 261.
Boyd, W. (1966) Spontaneous Regression of Cancer. Thomas, Springfield, Ill.
Brody, H. (1980) Placebos and the Philosophy of Medicine, University Chicago Press, Chicago.
Burnet, F.M. (1970) Immunological Surveillance. Pergamon Press, Australia.
Cassel, J. (1979) Stress and Survival. The Emotional Realities of Life-Threatening Illness. Garfield, C.A., ed., C.V. Nosby, St. Louis.
Chesney, M.A., Eagelston, J.R. and Rosenman, R.M. (1981) in Medical Psychology, Contributions to Behavioural Medicine, Prokop, C.K. and Bradley, L.A. eds., Academic Press, N.Y., p. 19.
Cunningham, A.J. (1981) in Psychoneuroimmunology, Ader, R., ed., Acad. Press, N.Y., p. 609.
Dattore, P.J., Shontz, F.C. and Coyne, L. (1980) J. Consult. Clin. Psychol. 48, 388.
Derogatis, L.R., Abeloff, M.D. and Melisaratos, N. (1979) J.A.M.A. 242, 1504.
Deutsch, F. (1953) The Psychosomatic Concept in Psychoanalysis. Internat. Universities Press, New York.
Devitt, J.E. (1979) in Mind and Cancer Prognosis, Stoll, B.A., ed., John Wiley, p. 9.
Dunbar, H.F. (1943) Psychosomatic Diagnosis. Hoeber, New York
Engel, G.A. (1967) Proc. R. Soc. Med. 60, 553.
Everson, T.C. and Cole, W.H. (1966) in Spontaneous Regression of Cancer, Saunders, Philadelphia/London.
Fox, B.H. (1978) J. Behav. Med. 1, 45.
Fox, B.H. (1981) in Psychoneuroimmunology, Ader, R., ed., Academic Press, N.Y. p. 103.
Gisler, R.M. (1974) Psychosom. 23, 197.
Grace, W.J. and Graham, D.T. (1952) Psychosom. Med. 14, 243.
Greer, S. (1979) Psychological Medicine 9, 81.
Greer, S., Morris, T. and Pettingale, K.W. (1979) Lancet ii, 785.
Grossarth-Maticek, R. (1980) Psychother. Psychosom. 33, 122.
Hagnell, O. (1966) Anns. N.Y. Acad. Sci. 125, 846.
Holmes, T.H. and Rahe, R.H. (1967) J. Psychosom. Res. 11, 213.
Hubel, D.H. (1979) Sci. American 241, 45.
Huggins, C. (1967) Science 156, 1050.
Ikemi, Y., Nakagawa, S., Nakagawa, T. and Sugita, M. (1975) Dynamische Psychiatrie 8, 77.

Klopfer, B. (1957) J. Projective Techniques 21, 331.
LaBarba, R.C. (1970) Psychosom. Med. 32, 259.
Lang, P.F. (1979) Psychophysiology 16, 495.
Lewison, E.F., ed., (1976) in Conference on Spontaneous Regression of Cancer, NCI Monograph.
Llynch, J.L. (1977) The Broken Heart, The Medical Consequences of Loneliness. N.T. Basic Books.
Meares, A. (1980) Aust. Family Physician 9, 332.
Mezei, A. and Nemeth, G. (1969) Anns. N.Y. Acad. Sci. 164, 560.
Razran, G. (1961) Psychol. Rev. 68, 81.
Riley, V. (1975) Science 189, 465.
Rogers, M.P., Dubey, D., Reich, P. (1979) Psychosom. Med. 41, 147.
Ruesch, J. (1948) Psychosom. Med. 10, 134.
Scurry, M.T. and Levin, E.M. (1978) Int'l. J. Psychiatry in Medicine 9, 159.
Shapiro, A.K. (1968) in Modern Perspectives in World Psychiatry, Howells, J.G. ed., Oliver and Boyd, Edinburgh, p. 596.
Sheikh, A.A. and Panagiotou, N.C. (1975) Percept. Motor Skills 41, 555.
Simonton, O.C., Mathews-Simonton, S. and Creighton, J. (1978)   Getting Well Again. J.P. Tarcher, Los Angeles.
Simonton, O.C., Mathews-Simonton, S. and Sparks, T.F. (1980) Psychosomatics 21, 226.
Sklar, L.S. and Anisman, H. (1979) Science 205, 513.
Sklar, L.S. and Anisman, H. (1981) Psychol. Bull. 89, 369.
Stavraky, K.M. (1968) J. Psychosomatic Res. 12, 251.
Stoll, B.A. (1979) in Mind and Cancer Prognosis, Stoll, B.A., ed., John Wiley, p. 19.
Ullman, M. (1959) Psychosom. Med. 21, 473.

## DISCUSSION

DR. VERNON RILEY: On the positive side, perhaps, I've seen the epidemiological data on the Mormons and the Seventh Day Adventists. Here it looks as though this group as a whole is protected in some way in that the incidence of cancer among the Mormons is significantly lower than the general population.

The smoking-non-smoking, non-drinking, would have something to do with some of the obvious sites, but the intriguing thing here is that apparently there is a protection against cancer for sites that as far as we know have nothing to do with smoking and drinking. I think we do know that these people have a rather special lifestyle in that they have internal support within their group; they have a year's supply of food under the bed; they help each other on employment problems, and there may be other aspects to their security. Is there something about that we should learn? Are they--do they know something about a lifestyle that has protective effects?

DR. BORYSENKO: They're protected in other ways too, against hypertension. Even churchgoers are protected against hypertension compared to the population as a whole. And I'm always thinking about the mechanisms. I'm sorry, Dr. Cunningham. But one possible thing that comes up is that in both groups these people are probably eliciting what one would refer to as a relaxation response, which seems to be an antedote, if you will, for sympathetic arousal. Most of the physiological effects of this response lead to decreased arousal of the sympathetic nervous system. And perhaps there is something in that mechanism that might have some intervening effect on the diseases in question.

DR. CUNNINGHAM: There's a difficulty, and Dr. Fox has written a couple of lovely reviews to point out some of these difficulties. In looking at a mass of data like that, you always have the chicken and egg problem. It seems to me that the time is ripe now for intervention studies rather than simply correlative studies. We'll only get over that problem of the chicken and the egg when we start using psychotherapy in a controlled way and observing whether it makes a difference.

I'd like to hear your comments on it.

DR. FOX: Yes. There is a little difficulty. First, with respect to the Mormon and Seventh Day Adventist data, a substantial amount of this has been attributed by epidemiologists to dietary differences. The only finding which is a puzzle, and which is contrary to the general picture, is that Mormons do not, in fact, have a lesser meat consumption than the public at large. But in most other dietary habits, they and the Seventh Day Adventists, have a more meager diet, and a healthier diet overall. This fact would at least seem to be a contributor to the lower incidence of cancer. Whether it is sufficient to account for all of it, I'm not sure.

One of the things that they did not control for very will was occupation and exposure to external carcinogens. Also the geographic region in which they live seems to be enviromentally more healthy. Nevertheless, there are enough questions to be asked in that whole picture that would make further investigation of this very important.

So far as the application of the study method that you're suggesting, Dr. Cunningham, I would be very worried about embarking on such a thing without instituting necessary controls, namely controlling for the variables that we already know are precursors to cancer. And unless you do that, you always have the danger that these uncontrolled factors could have been the reasons for differences found.

Now the problem is that in epidemiological investigations researchers are at a very primitive level in defining the precursors, the causative precursors. They only have associative precursors, to some degree (for example, socioeconomic level, which is not a causitive precursor). For that reason it becomes very difficult to control for the true causes if indeed they are the ones that are active in the mind/cancer paradigm. So this is not a rejection of the idea that you propose; I think it is a very good idea. But I think that in doing such an intervention study, one should proceed with great caution and circumspection.

DR. CUNNINGHAM: In an intervention trial would it not be possible to randomize out those other factors?

DR. FOX: No. One of the most difficult ones of all which has never been controlled, and probably right at this time cannot be controlled, is the prior rate of growth of a cancer. If you have a lognormal distribution of the rate of growth of cancer and you start with a person whose rate of growth is unknown, you don't know where they lie on the curve. And in order to decide whether there is a difference, you have to make sure that these rates of growth are not related to things that are parts of your experimental design. And to do that, I think, right now is impossible.

DR. CUNNINGHAM: You'd have to randomize the groups, wouldn't you?

DR. FOX: Well, it's true. You could do it that way. But in order to do it that way, because of the breadth of the distribution, you need a very large number of cases. You can do it but that only controls for that one confounding factor of growth rate.

DR. CUNNINGHAM: Right. I picked that up from your paper. There would be advantages of selecting a much more restricted group.

DR. FOX: Yes. If you do that then you eliminate a lot of variability associated with diversity of tumor behavior. But you still would have many potentially confounding variables. I think it is possible to do a study of that kind, but you have to do it with great control. I think a large number is absolutely necessary; and if you don't have a large number, one really can't have terribly much confidence in the results.

DR. LOCKE: What's a large number?

DR. FOX: Well, for a progression experiment, that is, examining what might change the progress of cancer, I would guess you would need something on the order of 150-200 per group of experimental and control subjects. For precursor and cause, you would need something on the order of 5,000-10,000 in such a group, and even then you're not sure.

DR. LOCKE: The progression numbers aren't overwhelming. That could be done, if it was done as a collaborative, multi-institutional study, which is of course the way the chemotherapy protocols are done.

DR. LEVY: You could do a randomized clinical trail of intervention modalities.

DR. LOCKE: Yes.

DR. LEVY: Okay, Dr. Cunningham, I just had a quick note. Looking at your Figure I, it struck me that you really have a closed-loop in the sense that behavioral response can not only be altered by feedback (how one perceives the environment, the perceptional interpretation) but the behavioral responses, broadly defined (in the sense of fight or flight, or whatever) certainly directly affect the rest of the chain.

DR CUNNINGHAM: That's a good point. Thank you.

DR. LOCKE: I just wanted to comment briefly, Dr Cunningham, on your hierarchy which is out of systems theory. You already referred to the fact that most of our treatment interventions for cancer are oriented at the local tissue control area or the cellular mechanism control level, and certainly chemotherapy is targeted specifically at the cellular mechanism level, at least in theory. But in reality, what we may have is a very important placebo effect which may be a component of the chemotherapy process because of the strong belief that doctors have that the treatment is going to work. Anecdotal observations, at least, would suggest that the doctor's belief in the treatment efficacy may affect the patient's clinical course. There may in fact be a misinterpretation by many researchers investigating the treatment of cancer because they ignore the whole top half of the pyramid. The point that I tried to make was that we really have an ethical dilemma which is hamstringing us in our ability to study the importance of that factor. It is very difficult to tease out what may be happening in clinical treatment which is in fact occurring at a much higher level than the cellular level and is a function of the person's belief in the treatment.

DR. VERNON RILEY: There is also the sabertooth concept of stress, in that evolutionary biologists are puzzled by the development in the animal organism of a physiological mechanism that seems to be only a handicap in terms of response. You would think that from an evolutionary standpoint that that would not be a possibility.

However, and as some of these papers have indicated, the timing is the critical thing. It can be demonstrated that the very same stressor will cause first an immunological impairment, and then that will be followed by an immunological enhancement at various times in the future.

Now, if a person was injured and the immune system was activated-even though it was originally impaired-if 14 days later when it really needed to face an immunological crisis due to infection or something, the immune system might actually be benefited. So that the paradox perhaps is not a paradox after all, except in terms of timing. An article of Monjan and Collector's that appeared a couple of years ago in Science demonstrated that when they stressed animals by noise, at first they had an immunological impairment. This was expressed by an elevation in corticosterone followed by a decrease in the number of white cells. Both B-cells and T-cells were diminished. Then there was a recovery, but there was an overshoot, and it was during the overshoot period that they demonstrated an enhancement. And this certainly would explain a lot of the apparent contradictions in the literature. One laboratory will say, "Stress impairs immunity and causes the tumor to grow faster," and other laboratories (like Newberry's at Ohio University) have found tumor enhancement. It could be a simple matter of the timing.

DR. ADER: I was going to make a plea. We see it so much in the literature, futile arguments about who's right and who's wrong, as opposed to an analysis of why you get another effect under another set of conditions. I consider the latter analysis a far more fruitful way to approach the problems.

DR. LOCKE: I'd like to return to the jungle with you in this notion of the sabertoothed tiger and the selective advantage of possible inhibition of the immune system in the face of stressful circumstances. In the acute situation of danger, where tissue damage is imminent, the selective value may be to prevent autoinnoculation with autoantigen and to contain the response to a local area to prevent systemic spread. Later, due to the nature of virus and bacteria reproduction, the host defenses against the spread of those pathogens may occur somewhat later in time. I don't know whether the immunologists would support that notion as having any potential validity, but it is a possible explanation.

DR. FOX: I have two or three things to remark on, but I'll bring them out in the order in which I think they're important. I have seen some references in these papers to the findings on anger suppression and expression. That seems to be a very potent variable in the minds of prospective researchers. Dr. Levy is doing her work essentially on that as its mainstay. Now I asked myself the prior question: Shouldn't we look at the mechanisms for any of the psychological precursors? And I asked, what about that kind of response? Could it explain a possible change in progress? And I came up with two possible variables which I think now should be controlled in any experimentation that is done with that as a variable, as the main variable.

One of these has to do with the fact that it is well-known that people in low socioeconomic levels have a much lower survival rate. That is, the average time of death following discovery of cancer is earlier in those with low socioeconomic level than in high. One can speculate as to the reasons for this, but SES should be controlled, because it may contribute to the reason why you get differences. And one has to ask, is there a difference in the degree to which anger is expressed or suppressed in low and high socioeconomic levels? Now it turns out this is not only true but it can be demonstrated very clearly. Those who are at the low socioeconomic level are likely not to express their anger and to suppress it because of the total environment in which they live. Other people who are more familar with the sociology of it can develop this further, but that's the basic idea.

Now, there's a second issue in that whole affect and progression area. What is the actual measure? The measure is how long does it take for a recurrence of the tumor, which in turn is related to how long does it take to die, so that usually the two are correlated although not all that well. So one has to ask, why should a tumor recur? And the usual explanation is not that the same tumor recurs, especially in a mastectomized situation, but metastases occur. And because we know something about the rate of growth in metastases, usually these are already present at the time of the diagnosis.

If that's the case, one has to ask, how long has it been between the time of the first symptomatology and the time of diagnosis? How long has it been from the time of diagnosis to whatever treatment, et cetera? Now, it also turns out that those with low socioeconomic levels delay much longer. And even when one has equated the stage, it turns out that those with low SES have a shorter survival time. And the reason they have found is that within stage they will report a symptom later than those at high SES.

So what you have is that the tumor has been allowed to sit in the body for a longer time before it's exposed to the doctor. And if you take the whole length of time for survival from the first cell to the last, then it looks as if you have delayed by several months, or whatever it is, the time at which it came to the attention of the doctor. And therefore this whole business can be displaced to the time of death. And usually time of death, on average, is only a matter of months in the two groups, not a matter of years.

Now, if that's the case, then that phenomenon should be examined in the patients, because if you don't control for that, you may get a spurious difference.

Now this was examined in the study which I was involved in, with Rogentine, and part of the reason--Well, no relationship was found. But I am certain that part of the reason was that we had such a small number of cases. We only had 64, overall. And the phenomenon is a rather weak one and you can't really expect to find that kind of difference with only a small number of cases because survival itself happens to have a negative exponential distribution.

DR. VERNON RILEY: Dr. Fox, I probably missed the point, but how does this relate to the problems of stress and the immune system? Is there some connection that I don't realize?

DR. FOX: Well, I was talking about the studies in which people are using psychological characteristics as a predictor of survival. Now I think that there may be a connection with stress, theoretically, but in terms of research, this is a different class of experiment entirely and does not belong to the class of stress studies that you've been talking about.

DR. MILLER: He's saying that psychological characteristics may be a function of the socioeconomic status, or highly correlated with that, and that may be highly correlated with an aspect of medical care like how soon you go to see the doctor.

DR. FOX: Right. This is a suggestion for two other controls that should be put in because of their possible effect on the outcome.

DR. LEVY: Of course, even if you found a relationship between style of anger expression and social class, it doesn't necessarily then negate the possibility that there are hormonal differences or that there are mediating pathways that can have an effect?

DR. FOX: Not at all. But surely if you control for it, then you have removed that as a possibility.

DR. MILLER: I'm a little surprised by your saying that the lower socioeconomic class has less expression of anger because early studies seemed to show exactly the opposite. There does seem to be more, say, in Harlem than it is in--

DR. FOX: Well, it turns out that it is a circumstantial thing. In the environment of these doctors whose magic is presented to you, and when you have this terrible disease, and all the people around you have major control over you and you are in no way in control of your own life, you sit back and become very passive. And this has been observed among the various classes of patients.

DR. BORYSENKO: I wanted to discuss some things about running clinical trials that have come up. I think it's very important when you say, "It would be good to study an intervention," and I think that it is also in that context that you have the capability of looking at the intermediary mechanisms. I don't think that the extreme right and left need rule each other out, but that hopefully when you design a study you will both take the leap forward into behavioral interventions and look back and see what change your intervention promoted in various intervening biological mechanisms.

In the design of a study like this, Dr. Fox has made the very relevant point that you have to define your patient population. There are a limited number of things you want to stratify within a modest clinical trial. It turns out that it's darned hard to scrape together an appropriate clinical population, and I addressed that briefly in my paper. If you take something like colo-rectal cancer, where you've got a lot of patients who are coming in and you have the best chance of getting enough of them with several hospitals combined, you still have the very real problem of accrueing enough patients to make it meaningful. You make the estimate that if you do a behavioral intervention maybe you'll get a 15 percent difference in time to recurrence. It will take 210 patients in the case of colo-rectal cancer patients to test that assumption. If you are talking about a smaller effect, then exponentially the number of patients you need increases.

Now if you're saying it would be nice to compare several different behavioral interventions, there is a real can of worms that you're opening. First of all, if you're going to compare several different interventions, the number of patients you need goes way up. Futhermore, the old, ugly question rears its head: Is it the intervention or is it the therapist that produces the effect? So that ideally, if you were going to compare a number of interventions there would be two therapists to provide each intervention so that you would at least have some control over whether it's the therapist or whether it's the intervention. By this time we need about 10 to the 10th patients and that's a very difficult logistical problem. That is going to somewhat limit our ability to run a single prospective study that is going to look at all of these things, and it's something very real that needs to be taken into consideration.

DR. ANISMAN: Every year or so I feel inspired to do a human study. This feeling lasts about a week; it goes away and I feel normal again. I see no way of doing a study without having a thousand confounds in it. I started a study last summer. This was going to be with stress and depression. And the first thing I ran into was that the stresses I was looking for were all the wrong stressors. Here was a--In this particular case, my first subject, was a lady who had been chronically depressed, and I was looking for all sorts of major stresses. It turns out she was very relaxed and laid back. Her husband was a Type A and he was essentially a stress giver. Okay? Pushing her and things like this. That was one source of stress I hadn't even considered. It came out after all my little scales and questionnaires and things like this. I was looking in the wrong place entirely. It also turned out that for her, vacation was a trauma. Again, this was a second stressor that I hadn't even considered. She would go into her cottage which was a terrible event for her. Whether now the affective state was being affected by the stress, or whether the stress was actually related in some other way to the affective state, I don't know.

You can go on with a dozen examples of this nature. To put that now in the context of the cancer work, you have all the other factors that were already mentioned, such as diet, culture and so forth. You can't possibly design a study that is going to account for any great degree of the varience.

DR. LOCKE: We seem to be focusing somewhat on some of the methodological problems in doing this kind of research. One additional comment that your point suggested to me is the problem of differences in designing intervention-oriented studies. Differences in attitudes of the person applying the intervention may account for observed outcomes. If the person who is actually controlling the experiment and designed the experiment isn't removed in some fashion from the application of the treatment, the involvement with the patients will be such as to have a significant influence on the outcome. The example of this that's quite clear is in the biofeedback literature. People who believe that they can train people to warm their hands easily train people to warm their hands with biofeedback. Practitioners who take a purely scientific attitude and who state that they have no vested interest in whether the person warms or cools, have tremendous difficulty achieving an effect.

Studies that involve behavioral interventions in treating cancer patients are going to have to be run by people who are not actually themselves applying the treatments or any outcome is going to be confounded. Whatever your comparisons are--for example if you're comparing two treatments--those therapists both have to believe very strongly that they are going to help, whether it be chemotherapy versus a behavioral intervention or some combination of them.

DR. MILLER: That's true if you're trying to compare treatments. If you took the simpler problem of taking a sort of grab bag of behavioral treatments, all of which you think might be good, for logical reasons, and which wouldn't conflict with each other, and ask--do you get any effect there versus doing nothing. Then you wouldn't have quite those problems. And then, if that doesn't produce anything, you wouldn't want to be going after little things piecemeal to see if "A" is more effective than "B". I'm not saying that's necessarily the strategy, because, you know, there are problems with that. But certainly one possible way to react to this situation we've been describing is to see if there's any effect there at all.

DR. LOCKE: Really load it in favor of demonstrating an effect?

DR. MILLER: Yes. But be very careful. Well, you can supposedly do that if you randomize patients right so that you don't load it in favor of any of the biasing factors that Dr. Fox has been pointing out so clearly and so usefully.

When I was suggesting the grab bag thing, of course I would assume that Dr. Borysenko's point would be included. When you were doing that you would be measuring as many of these intervening hormonal variables and other factors as you could and as many direct measures of effects on the immune system as you could. You wouldn't just be jumping across from one side to the other, but would be putting as much in the biological middle as possible.

DR. CUNNINGHAM: How would you feel about a grant proposal which failed to contain those intermediate variables.

DR. MILLER: I think I would feel a little negative towards it for this reason, that your are investing considerable effort. I mean, even if you simplify it the very best you can, you're investing an effort in it and once you have that effort invested, perhaps you should invest a bit more to get some of these other things in.

Now, maybe when I say "a bit more," I'm just betraying my gross ignorance of what it takes to get those other measures.

DR. CUNNINGHAM: That's the difficulty, isn't it? I agree with you. In an ideal world, measure everything. But the problem is that is does take a lot, from my experience, to measure one or two simple physiological parameters.

DR. ADER: Even so, Dr. Miller, let me put a different label on the same study--

DR. MILLER: Okay.

DR. ADER: --and I don't mean to denegrate it, because I think that's the level that we are at now, but I think the response you're going to get back from that application is, "This is a fishing expedition."

Now at certain levels of science, I don't see anything wrong with fishing expeditions, provided you label them as fishing expeditions. But given that you did that, I'd give you odds that's the response you're going to get. Unless you can tell me why you're measuring this in relation to something else, you're doing a fishing expedition and we don't want any part of it. That's where we are.

DR. MILLER: I agree. That's the way Study Sections are. But I think at certain stages--Now, I don't want to push this thing too hard because I'm certainly not an expert in this field. I just want to have it considered as one of the possibilities. But I think that's one of the problems of Study Sections too, that they will label certain things fishing expeditions, and if they do it's utterly damning. But, you know, if you have a good fisherman fishing in an appropriate spot, you can catch quite a few fish.

II


BIOLOGICAL MEDIATORS OF BEHAVIOR AND NEOPLASIA :

ANIMAL MODELS

SOME BEHAVIORAL FACTORS RELEVANT TO CANCER

NEAL E. MILLER
The Rockefeller University, New York, NY 10021, USA

DIRECT EFFECTS OF "STRESS" ON IMMUNE SYSTEM

One thing that comes out very clearly from many experiments on animals and some on people is that conditions that may be described loosely as stressful can have an effect on the immune system that is relevant to malignancy and to infections by viruses that may play a role in malignancy. But another thing that comes out clearly is that the effects of behavioral factors on the immune system are complex, so that a large amount of research that is more systematic is needed to sort out the variables. Many experiments have shown that stress can interfere with the effectiveness of the immune system and can increase the susceptibility to experimental transplants of malignant tissues and to experimental inoculations of viruses that can produce malignancy. On the other hand, there are a number of published, and without doubt a larger number of unpublished, studies that have failed to show such effects. Furthermore, a significant minority of apparently equally good experiments have produced opposite results: increased effectiveness of the immune system or a reduced susceptibility to implanted tumors or experimental injections. In some cases, the paradoxical results can be explained by the fact that the implanted tumor was derived from a tissue (e.g., lymphatic) that is inhibited by the corticosteroids; in other cases, this explanation does not appear to be possible (LaBarba, 1970; McClelland et al., 1980; Miller, 1980a; Newberry, 1981; Rasmussen, 1969; Riley, 1981a,b; Stein et al., 1976).

That there should be effects of emotional factors, such as stress, on malignancies is to be expected from the facts that lymphatic and other relevant tissues are innervated by the autonomic nervous system and that, as other chapters in this book will show, receptors for a variety of hormones that are affected by emotional factors are to be found on different cellular components of the immune system. These effects may be expected to be complex because different hormones have different time courses and are beginning to be found to have different, sometimes opposite, effects on different components of the immune system (see papers by Wunderlich, Herberman, this volume).

Unfortunately, most of the studies to date have involved comparing only two groups, one subjected to supposedly normal conditions and the other to an elevated level of "stress." But if, as a few studies (e.g., Jensen, 1969) suggest,

the dose-response curve should be a non-monotonic one -- for example, an in-
verted J-shaped one -- then the comparison between the two groups would be expected to show either an effect in one direction, no effect, or an effect in the
opposite direction, depending on where these two points were located on such a
curve. Thus, we need dose-response studies involving multiple points on a curve
that extends through a considerable range. Riley's (1981a, and chapter 7 in
this volume) studies are a laudable step in this direction, but in his commend-
able interest in avoiding possibly confounding effects of tissue damage, he has
confined himself to comparatively low levels of stress. That under appropriate-
ly chosen and carefully controlled conditions these relatively low levels of
stress can produce such significant results indicates the potential fruitfulness
of research in this area. In addition to dose-response studies, we need time-
course studies, studies of rebound effects after the termination of stress, and
studies of closely-spaced versus more widely-distributed stresses. Ideally, such
studies should involve direct measurements of effects on different components of
the immune system (e.g., Keller et al., 1981) and ideally also include measurements of some of the relevant hormones.

The problem is complicated additionally by the fact that we do not know which
elements of the immune system have what effects on possible carcinogenic viruses
and on the development or spread of cancer (Holland and Rowland, 1981). Therefore at the most analytic level additional information is needed at four points:
effects of stress on the immune system that are mediated by direct neural con-
nections; effects of stress on various hormones; effects of various hormones on
different components of the immune system; and effects of different components
of the immune system on different aspects of the development or progression of
cancer. Because of the complexities of the most highly analytical approach, it
will be worthwhile to secure more systematic information also on the effects of
stress on the immune system, on the effects of hormones on cancer, and on the
effects of stress on cancer. The evidence that we already have on the effects
of stress on implanted and virus-induced tumors (Riley, 1981a,b and chapter 7
in this book), along with the accumulating evidence on some of the intervening
links that is described in this book, indicates that all of the foregoing lines
of investigation are likely to be fruitful.

If the work to be done seems formidable, we should remember "how many generations of talented scientists, beginning with Pasteur, worked out their lives on
the problems of infection before the stage was set for the era of antibiotics"
(Thomas, 1976, p. 6). Furthermore, more data from systematic studies may allow
us to reorient our perspective and perceive a pattern that is much simpler,

analogous to the great simplification when the complex cycles and epicycles of
the earth-centered Ptolemaic view of the solar system was supplanted by the
heliocentric Copernican one, and to the additional great simplification that was
introduced by Newton's laws of gravitation and motion.

## EFFECTS OF POSITIVE EMOTIONS ON IMMUNE SYSTEM

The work that has just been described has involved situations that might be
expected to arouse negative or unpleasant emotions, such as fear.  To my knowledge, there has been little or no work on the effect of a situation that might
be expected to elicit positive or pleasant emotions, such as joy, love, or hope.
Yet there is evidence to suggest that an investigation of these neglected emotional responses might be scientifically interesting and therapeutically significant.  Norman Cousins (1979) has suggested that laughter may be therapeutic.
There is experimental evidence that a positive situation can counteract stress.
Pavlov (1927) reports that physiological reactions to pain can be inhibited by
making it the signal for a strongly rewarding stimulus, such as the presentation
of food to a very hungry animal.  He says:

> "Subjected to the very closest scrutiny, not even the tiniest
> and most subtle objective phenomenon usually exhibited by
> animals under the influence of strong injurious stimuli can be
> observed in these dogs.  No appreciable changes in the pulse or
> in the respiration occur in these animals, whereas such changes
> are always most prominent when the nocuous stimulus has not been
> converted into an alimentary-conditioned stimulus." (p. 30)

He called this phenomenon counterconditioning.  We have verified it with one
dog (Miller, 1980a).  Ball (1967) has shown that stimulating rewarding areas of
the rat's brain inhibits evoked potentials in the trigeminal nucleus to presumably painful stimulation of the face.  Similarly, Beecher (1956) found that sol-
diers for whom a severe wound means being sent home from harrowing combat may
show astonishingly little sign of pain and not request any pain-relieving drugs.
But, in spite of the extensive theoretical use made of the concept of counterconditioning by behavior therapists, it has not been investigated by modern
physiological techniques.

Another suggestive fact comes from a study in which Goldman et al. (1973)
found that opposite shifts in schedules of reinforcement can change levels of
plasma corticosterone in opposite directions.  Shifts to schedules of reinforcement that delivered fewer or no rewards produced elevations of plasma

corticosteroids, and shifts to schedules of reinforcement that delivered more rewards produced reductions in the level of plasma corticosteroids. Hennessy and Levine (1979) summarize additional data indicating that performing a variety of consummatory responses (i.e., achieving a variety of goals) can reduce the level of plasma corticosteroids.

We must not jump to the conclusion, however, that pleasant and unpleasant situations are simple opposites. Frankenhaeuser (1976) found that a Bingo game rigged so that everyone was winning caused the subjects to be happily excited but produced as great an elevation in urine metabolites of epinephrine and nor-epinephrine as the aversive situations that she had studied earlier.

As far as I know, no one has studied the effects on the immune system or on cancer of pleasant emotions, of possessing a sense of humor, or of achieving important goals. I believe that it will be profitable to investigate this neglected area.

## EXPRESSION OF AGGRESSION

There is some suggestive evidence that, in a situation that would be expected to arouse strong anger, being able to express aggression relieves stress in the same way as does performing a consummatory or other goal response. Conner et al. (1971) have shown that rats shocked in pairs so that they can attack each other have less ACTH secretion than those individually shocked without any opportunity to attack. Similarly, Weiss et al. (1976) have used fixed electrodes on the tails of rats, to be sure to control the strength of electric shock, and shown that being able to attack another rat in this situation reduces the amount of stomach lesions. Pettingale et al. (1977) have linked the mode in which anger is expressed to an immunological parameter, and Sklar and Anisman (1981; see also chapter 5 in this volume) have found slower growth of tumors in animals that are transferred from isolation to a group cage, if such animals fight their cage-mates.

## INDIRECT EFFECTS OF "STRESS"

In addition to the effects of stress on the immune system, there are other effects that may be relevant to cancer. For example, stress may produce stomach lesions (Weiss, 1977); it also affects gastrointestinal motility (Miller, 1977). It is conceivable that it might affect the detoxification and elimination of carcinogens by the liver and the kidneys. There are many new avenues to be investigated.

Furthermore, stress can lead to behavioral changes which, in turn, can affect carcinogenesis. For example, some people respond to stress by increased smoking, drinking, or overeating. Indeed, the same stressful factors that show up in both epidemiological studies and experiments on animals as producing effects on the immune system also produce many psychological symptoms (Miller, 1980a). One of these effects is the symptom of depression. Being depressed can lead to a lack of following good rules of personal hygiene, a failure to note and report suspicious symptoms, delay in securing medical care, and poor compliance with medical procedures such as Pap smears, breast examinations, and reporting danger signals such as bleeding. Depression can cause people to fail to avoid risks such as obesity and exposure to carcinogens such as cigarette smoke, or excessive exposure to the sun and industrial hazards. Conversely, positive factors such as hope can help in preventive hygiene and in compliance with therapeutic regimes. Furthermore, habituation to stress and learning various coping responses can greatly reduce the effects of a given stressor (Miller, 1980a; Weiss et al., 1975).

ADDITIONAL BEHAVIORAL FACTORS

An important behavioral principle involved in prevention and compliance is the Gradient of Reinforcement, namely, the fact that immediate rewards and punishments are much more effective than delayed ones. Thus, the person tends to respond to the pleasure or convenience of the moment and to ignore long-range consequences. Programs to promote healthier behavior must try to discover and to utilize immediate reinforcements. In my opinion, some of the effects of the Surgeon-General's report have been to change smoking in certain circles from being the thing to do, providing some immediate reward of being "in," to being the thing not to do, so that at least some smokers immediately feel a bit conspicuous and some social disapproval when they light up. If the person conceptualizes his inability to quit as a sign of weakness, this provides an immediate deterrent. Another effect has been to give non-smokers a licence to complain, which supplies some immediate negative reinforcement for the smoker when he starts to light up. Along this line, campaigns capitalizing on the offensive odor of tobacco to the nonsmoker might be effective. There have been psychologically sophisticated programs of trying to immunize the teenager against peer pressure to take up smoking (Evans et al., 1981).

Another behavioral principle relevant to the problem of encouraging healthy and discouraging unhealthy behavior is that any response that reduces fear (or anxiety, as it frequently is called) is immediately reinforced (Miller, 1948). Thus, there is a tendency to learn to escape from and to avoid fear-inducing

stimuli and thoughts (Dollard and Miller, 1950; Miller, 1980b). This tendency
is called <u>suppression</u> when it is mild and <u>repression</u> or <u>denial</u> when it is
stronger. This means that the messages in campaigns against unhealthy behavior
that are based primarily on fear, especially those based on strong fear, run a
risk of being ignored or quickly forgotten unless some relatively easy course of
action is immediately available to reduce the danger eliciting the fear. Wher-
ever possible, it probably is much better to concentrate on the immediate rewards for healthy behavior. Evidence relevant to the problem of denial is discussed in chapter 8 of Janis et al. (1969).

In certain people, emotions such as fear, anger, or forms of stress tend to
motivate behaviors such as smoking, consuming alcohol, or the use of drugs, all
of which can have apparently calming or distracting effects. They also are risk
factors for malignancies. A person who has given up one of these unhealthy
habits is more likely to relapse under stress. Furthermore, strong emotions may
narrow the range of the attention; the strong response that they motivate can
conflict with other types of behavior and cause the person to neglect personal
hygiene; for example, be less likely in the work place to take special measures
to avoid carcinogens.

RELIEVING STRESSFUL EFFECTS OF DIAGNOSIS AND TREATMENT

It is obvious that the diagnosis of cancer and some of its treatments can
serve as strong stressors. As an extreme example, there are some patients who,
when told that they have inoperable cancer, will give up, turn their face to the
wall, and die within a few days from no obvious physical cause (Lewis Thomas,
personal communication). It should be profitable to give half of some suitably
selected group of patients, approximately half of whom are likely to go five
years without recurrence, a total-push program with a variety of components
ranging from training in relaxation through training in coping responses to
maximizing affection and social support -- all aimed at counteracting the
stress. With a moderately high-risk group, suitable follow-up measures will
yield meaningful positive or negative results in a reasonably short time. If
an overall package appears to be promising, additional, more analytical, studies
can be carried out to determine the effects of different components and to opti-
mize the procedures. In designing such a study, one should give thought to the
possibility that the different components of the procedure may interact with
each other and with the personality of the patient. Thus, an alternative approach could be a factorially designed study of the type conducted by Cromwell
et al. (1977) on the effects of different types of care after myocardial
infarction.

In short, in studying the role of biobehavioral factors in cancer, there is room for highly analytical studies investigating the effects of specific hormones and specific components of the immune system, for total-push studies determining the effects of a combination of hopefully favorable inputs on outcome, and for various combinations of these approaches. Further ideas for behavioral interventions along with cautions are presented by Holland and Rowland (1981).

COUNTERACTING THE GARCIA EFFECT

If an animal or a person has tasted a distinctive flavor and subsequently been nauseated by chemical poisoning or by X-ray radiation, the aversion to the nausea will become conditioned to the flavor in spite of a considerable lapse of time between the two exposures (Garcia and Koelling, 1966; Garcia et al., 1966). This type of aversion appears to be a problem for patients undergoing certain types of treatment for cancer. Therefore, it should be worthwhile to test the effectiveness of one procedure that has been found in experiments on rats to reduce the effects of such aversion. This is to interpose a very distinctive and novel flavor between the meal and the nausea-inducing event. Then the nausea will tend to become conditioned to that flavor instead of to the flavors of the meal. In extreme cases, another approach might be to try biofeedback training to teach the patient to counteract each of the specific symptoms in the nausea complex. Cowings et al. (1977) have reported success in using such procedures in warding off the symptoms involved in motion sickness.

SPECIAL PROBLEM OF SUPPORT FOR INTERDISCIPLINARY RESEARCH

Much of the research in the new area of the behavioral biology of cancer by its very nature will be interdisciplinary; it will involve links between the behavioral and other biological sciences. From a lifetime of experience with interdisciplinary work, I can point out certain hazards that must be overcome if such work is to flourish. One of these is the "Stephen Leacock phenomenon." Its name is derived from a quotation in which he said, "Among humorists I am known as a political scientist whereas among the political scientists I am known as a humorist." Similarly, a new area of interdisciplinary research habitually suffers from a lack of understanding by the various disciplines involved. In universities, each academic department tends to breed true and to be reluctant to waste its precious positions on people on the borders of the discipline whose work seems a bit strange. Sometimes, each department is willing to cooperate provided the appointment is charged to the budget of the other one.

The foregoing tendency is exaggerated in times when budgets are being cut or

120

there is even the threat of cuts. Then each discipline tends to retreat toward
its heartland and to be even more reluctant to waste scarce funds on its own
members who have strayed from the fold across the border into a different area
or, worse still, on those rash intruders who are trying to crash in from some
alien field.

The problem affects not only academic departments but also the specialists
who evaluate applications for research grants. It is not solved by assembling
an ad hoc group with conventional experts from the two or more fields involved.
In the case of the behavioral biology of cancer, the traditional molecular bio-
logist is likely to feel that, ingenious or interesting as the work may be, it
is beside the point in that it is not advancing the fundamental knowledge of the
molecular biology of the genome that will provide the eventual solution to the
problem. Similarly, the traditional experimental psychologist is likely to believe that research funds can be concentrated much more profitably in some central area of his field such as the mechanism of information processing involved
in transfer from short-term to long-term memory and in retrieval. Furthermore,
the technical specialists in each field are likely to look askance at the com-
promises that often are required in order to adapt the procedures that have
evolved in their field to the difficulties involved in working on the border of
some different field.

Under present circumstances, it requires only a few less than highly enthu-
siastic ratings to derail a promotion or to put a grant proposal into the "ap-
proved but not funded" category. In short, the promotions of interdisciplinary
investigators and the funding of interdisciplinary research projects must be
judged by people who have experience with the particular problems and the prom-
ise involved in that type of interdisciplinary work. For peer review of an
interdisciplinary project, the only appropriate peer is another interdisciplinary investigator. Failure to recognize this fact and to provide appropriate
review groups inevitably will impede desirable progress in the field of the
behavioral biology of cancer.

REFERENCES
Ball GG (1967) Electrical self-stimulation of the brain and sensory inhibition.
    Psychon Sci 8: 489-490.
Beecher HK (1956) Relationship of significance of wound to pain experienced.
    J Amer Med Assoc 61: 1609-1613.
Conner RL, Vernikos-Danellis J, Levine S (1971) Stress, fighting and neuroendo-
    crine function. Nature 234: 564-566.
Cousins N (1979) Anatomy of an Illness. New York: Norton.

Cowings PS, Billingham J, Toscano BW (1977) Learned control of multiple autonomic responses to compensate for the debilitating effects of motion sickness. Theory in Psychosom Med 4: 318-323.

Cromwell RL, Butterfield EC, Brayfield FM, Curry JC (1977) Acute Myocardial Infarction: Reaction and Recovery. St. Louis, Mo.: CV Mosby.

Dollard J, Miller NE (1950) Personality and Psychotherapy. New York: McGraw-Hill

Evans RI, Hill PC, Raines BE, Henderson AH (1981) Current behavioral, social, and educational programs in control of smoking: a selective, critical review. In Weiss SM, Herd JA, Fox BH (eds). Perspectives on Behavioral Medicine. New York: Academic Press.

Frankenhaeuser M (1976) The role of peripheral catecholamines in adaptation to understimulation and overstimulation. In Serban G (ed). Psychopathology of Human Adaptation. New York: Plenum Press.

Garcia J, Koelling RA (1966) Relation of cue to consequence in avoidance learning. Psychon Sci 4: 123-124.

Garcia J, Ervin FR, Koelling RA (1966) Learning with prolonged delay of reinforcement. Psychon Sci 5: 121-122.

Goldman L, Coover GD, Levine S (1973) Bidirectional effects of reinforcement shifts on pituitary-adrenal activity. Physiol Behav 10: 209-214.

Hennessy JW, Levine S (1979) Stress, arousal, and the pituitary-adrenal system: a psychoendocrine hypothesis. Progr Psychobiol Physiol Psychol 8: 133-178.

Holland JC, Rowland JH (1981) Psychiatric, psychosocial, and behavioral interventions in the treatment of cancer: an historical review. In Weiss SM, Herd JA, Fox BH (eds). Perspectives on Behavioral Medicine. New York: Academic Press.

Janis IL, Mahl GF, Kagan J, Holt RR (1969) Personality: Dynamics, Development, and Assessment. New York: Harcourt, Brace, and World.

Jensen MM (1969) The influence of vasoactive amines on interferon production in mice. Proc Soc Exp Biol Med 130: 34-39.

Keller SE, Weiss JM, Schleifer SJ, Miller NE, Stein M (1981) Suppression of immunity by stress: effect of a graded series of stressors on lymphocyte stimulation in the rat. Science 213: 1397-1399.

LaBarba RC (1970) Experiential and environmental factors in cancer: a review of research with animals. Psychosom Med 32: 259-276.

McClelland DC, Floor E, Davidson RJ, Saron C (1980) Stressed power motivation, sympathetic activation, immune function, and illness. J Human Stress June 11-19.

Miller NE (1948) Studies of fear as an acquirable drive: I. Fear as motivation and fear reduction as reinforcement in the learning of new responses. J Exp Psychol 38: 89-101.

Miller NE (1977) Effect of learning on gastrointestinal functions. Clinics in Gastroenterology 6: 533-546.

Miller NE (1980a) A perspective on the effects of stress and coping on disease and health. In Levine S, Ursin H(eds). Coping and Health. NATO Conference Series. New York: Plenum Press.

Miller NE (1980b) Application of learning and biofeedback to psychiatry and medicine. In Kaplan HI, Freedman AM, Sadock BJ (eds). Comprehensive Textbook of Psychiatry, 3ed edition. Baltimore: Williams & Wilkins.

Newberry BH (1981) Effects of presumably stressful stimulation (PSS) on the development of animal tumors: some issues. In Weiss SM, Herd JA, Fox BH (eds) Perspectives on Behavioral Medicine. New York: Academic Press.

Pavlov IP (1927) Conditioned Reflexes (Anrep G, translator) London: Oxford University Press.

Pettingale K, Greer S, Tee D (1977) Serum IGA and emotional expression in breast cancer patients. J Psychosom Res 21: 395-399.

Rasmussen AF Jr (1969) Emotions and immunity. Ann NY Acad Sci 164: 458-461.

Riley V (1981a) Psychoneuroendocrine influences on immunocompetence and neoplasia. Science 212: 1100-1109.

Riley V (1981b) Biobehavioral factors in animal work on tumorigenesis. In Weiss SM, Herd JA, Fox BH (eds). Perspectives on Behavioral Medicine. New York: Academic Press.

Sklar L, Anisman H (1981) Stress and cancer. Psychol Bull 89: 369-406.

Stein M, Schiavi RC, Camerino M (1976) Influence of brain and behavior on the immune system. Science 191: 435-440.

Thomas L (1976) The place of biomedical science in medicine. Report of the Overview Cluster In Report of the President's Biomedical Research Panel, Appendix A, The Place of Biomedical Science in Medicine and the State of the Science. Washington, DC: DHEW Publ No (05)76-501.

Weiss JM (1977) Psychological and behavioral influences on gastrointestinal lesions in animal models. In Maser JD, Seligman MEP (eds). Psychopathology: Experimental Models. San Francisco: Freeman.

Weiss JM, Glazer HI, Pohorecky LA, Brick J, Miller NE (1975) Effects of chronic exposure to stressors on avoidance-escape behavior and on brain norepinephrine. Psychosom Med 37: 522-534.

Weiss JM, Pohorecky LA, Salman S, Gruenthal M (1976) Attenuation of gastric lesions by psychological aspects of aggression in rats. J Comp Physiol Psychol 90: 252-259.

# STRESS PROVOKED NEUROCHEMICAL CHANGES IN RELATION TO NEOPLASIA

HYMIE ANISMAN[+] AND LAWRENCE S. SKLAR[++]
[+]Department of Psychology, Carleton University, Ottawa, Ontario, Canada;
[++]School of Medicine, University of Toronto, Toronto, Ontario, Canada

## INTRODUCTION

Considerable attention has been devoted to the analysis of the relationship between stressful life events and neoplastic disease. Numerous studies involving retrospective, prospective and prognostic analyses in human populations indicated that physical and psychological stressors are associated with several forms of neoplasia. Furthermore, the pathological consequences of aversive experiences appear to be related to the effectiveness of psychological or behavioral coping mechanisms (see for example, Fox, 1978; Schmale & Iker, 1966; Thomas & Duszynski, 1974; Thomas, Duszynski & Shaffer, 1979). Unfortunately, in many instances the experimental paradigms are flawed (see Fox, 1978; Sklar & Anisman, 1981; for a fuller discussion of this issue) and thus conclusions derived from these human experiments must be considered provisionally. Nevertheless, studies involving infrahuman subjects also revealed that environmental and social stressors will either exacerbate or inhibit tumor development, depending on variables such as stress chronicity and type, the availability of coping responses, the organism's premorbid stressful experiences, and the environmental context in which the stressor is applied (see reviews in Riley, 1981; Sklar & Anisman, 1981).

Although the involvement of immunological and hormonal mechanisms in the oncogenic process has been extensively examined, less attention has focussed on the contribution of central neurotransmitters. Yet, a large body of evidence indicates that central neurochemical events may influence hormonal functioning, and directly or indirectly affect immunocompetence as well (see reviews in Riley, 1981; Sklar & Anisman, 1981; Stein, Schiavi & Camerino, 1976). Interestingly, the alterations in tumorigenicity associated with aversive events are paralleled by predictable changes in central neuronal activity. Although the final mechanisms directly subserving the stress-related neoplastic changes might be hormonal, immunological, or metabolic, it seems likely that these variations are influenced by the initial neurochemical alterations provoked by a stressor.

*Supported by Natural Sciences and Engineering Research Council of Canada Grant A9845 and by Medical Research Council of Canada Grant MA6486.

The present review will delinate some of the conditions under which stressors will influence neurochemical activity, as well as describe some of the organismic and experiential variables that increase vulnerability to the neurochemical alterations. As will be seen, a remarkable congruency exists between the effects of stressors on central nervous system functioning and on tumor development. Although the mechanisms ultimately responsible for the effects of aversive events on tumorigenicity have not been deduced, some provisional hypotheses will be offered.

## PHYSIOLOGICAL CONSEQUENCES OF STRESS

### Neurochemical alterations

Exposure to aversive stimulation results in profound physiological alterations, which probably have adaptive value in that they may be essential for the organism to meet the demands placed upon it. However, these physiological changes may also be detrimental, since they appear to render the organism more susceptible to various pathologies such as depression, ulceration and heart disease (Akiskal & McKinney, 1973; Galosy & Gaebelein, 1975; Seligman, 1975; Weiss, 1971). The central nervous system response to a stressor is fairly extensive. In considering norepinephrine (NE), it appears that upon stress inception (e.g., electric shock, restraint, cold, shaking, etc.) the utilization and synthesis of this amine is increased (Kvetnansky et al., 1976; Thierry, Fekete & Glowinski, 1968; Weiss, Glazer, Pohorecky, Brick & Miller, 1975; see also reviews in Anisman, Kokkinidis & Sklar, 1981; Stone, 1975). Indeed, levels of NE may actually rise initially, possibly owing to a transient inhibition of monoamine oxidase (Modigh, 1976; Welch & Welch, 1970). When behavioral methods of coping are available (i.e., escape from the aversive stimulus) NE synthesis will keep pace with utilization resulting in fairly stable levels of the transmitter (Weiss, Glazer & Pohorecky, 1975; Weiss, Stone & Harrell, 1970). However, if behavioral control is not possible (or perceived as not being possible) then the burden of coping is placed more fully on endogenous systems. Under such conditions the rate of NE utilization increases, eventually exceeding synthesis, hence resulting in a net amine reduction (Anisman, Pizzino & Sklar, 1980; Weiss et al., 1970, 1976). This in turn will result in various behavioral effects, and also in serial alterations of other neurotransmitters and hormones (see reviews in Anisman, 1978; Anisman et al., 1981; Sklar & Anisman, 1981).

The effects of aversive stimulation on brain dopamine (DA), while similar to NE, are much less extensive and occur for the most part in discrete brain regions, such as the arcuate nucleus, frontal mesocortical neurons and the nucleus accumbens. As in the case of NE, stress inception results in increased synthesis and utilization of central dopamine. If the stress is protracted, then the utilization of DA will exceed its synthesis resulting in a relative depletion of this transmitter in some of these areas (Blanc et al., 1980; Kvetnansky et al., 1976, 1977; Kabayashi et al., 1976; Thierry et al., 1976).

While the effects of coping on DA levels have not been examined in these particular regions, it has been observed that coping behaviorally with stress may influence DA receptor binding. Relative to rats that received four sessions of escapable shock, binding to low affinity DA receptors increased in the frontal mesolimbic cortex of rats that had received an identical amount of yoked inescapable shock. In other brain regions such as striatum, hippocampus and diencephalon, decreased DA receptor binding occurred following yoked inescapable shock (Cherek et al., 1980). It is possible that the alterations of DA receptor binding as a function of coping factors are related to the alterations in turnover and levels of this transmitter.

Catecholamines are not the only central transmitters influenced by stress. Acute uncontrollable stress in the form of shock, cold or restraint increased both the synthesis and release of serotonin (5-HT) in several brain regions (Palkovits et al., 1976; Telegdy & Vermes, 1976; Thierry et al., 1968; see also Anisman et al., 1981). Moreover, these increases occurred in direct proportion to the severity of the stress (see Thierry, 1973). With sufficiently severe stress utilization of 5-HT exceeded synthesis in the hypothalamus resulting in reduced 5-HT levels in this brain region (Telegdy & Vermes, 1976). In general, as in the case of NE, the 5-HT depletion is fairly transient, and depending on stress parameters, the initial depletion may be followed by an increase in the levels of this transmitter (Palkovits et al., 1976). More severe stress is necessary to produce the 5-HT changes than is needed to produce comparable changes in NE or DA (Thierry, 1973).

It has been reported that stress will influence central acetylcholine (ACh) activity as well. Stressors such as restraint plus cold were found to reduce turnover of ACh in frontal cortex and in the hypothalamus (Costa et al., 1980). Moreover, several forms of stress were found to increase levels of brain ACh (Saito et al., 1976; Zajaczkowska, 1975); however, the latter effect was observed at least 1 hr after stress termination (Zajaczkowska, 1975), suggesting that the ACh increases might be secondary to the rapid catecholaminergic effects (Costa et al., 1980). It is interesting that some of the ACh alterations induced by stressors also seemed to be dependent upon the controllability of the aversive stimulus. In one study using escapable stress, Karczmar, Scudder and Richardson (1973) found that ACh levels were not appreciably influenced, but increased ACh levels were noted in a second study using uncontrollable stress. Furthermore, Cherek et al. (1980) found that relative to escapable stress, exposure to an equivalent amount of uncontrollable stress increased central muscarinic ACh receptor binding.

It has been our contention that the failure to cope with stress, rather than the stress per se, represents the fundamental variable responsible for amine changes and for some forms of pathology. This should not, however, be taken to imply that other adaptive changes, unrelated to behavioral control, will not modify neurochemical activity. For example, in contrast to the NE and DA depletions seen after acute exposure to uncontrollable stress, basal levels of these amines are seen after a chronic regimen of uncontrollable stress (Kvetnansky et al., 1976; Weiss et al., 1975). Evidently, the activity of the synthetic enzymes, tyrosine hydroxylase, and dopamine-β-hydroxylase are increased appreciably with chronic stress, thus resulting in increased amine levels (Kobayashi et al., 1976; Kvetnansky, 1980; Weiss et al., 1976). In addition, with chronic stress catecholamine degradation is inhibited owing to reductions in the activity of catechol-o-methyl transferase and monoamine oxidase (Kvetnansky, 1980). Not only are amine levels increased, but reuptake of catecholamines is blocked, thereby maximizing the effectiveness of the released-transmitters (Weiss et al., 1976). Finally, the excessive neuronal activity provoked by chronic exposure to a stressor appears to be moderated by the subsequent development of receptor subsensitivity (Stone, 1979).

The effects of stress on neurochemical change are dependent on a variety of other experiential, environmental and organismic factors as well. For example, it has been shown that social isolation will reduce the turnover of NE in several brain regions (Modigh, 1976; Thoa, Tizabi & Jacobowitz, 1977; Welch & Welch, 1970). Unlike physical stressors, amine levels are not affected by isolation, and adaptation to the effects of isolation are not evident, although we have noted that the greatest effects of isolation occur within the first few hours of separating mice from their cage mates. Furthermore, the response to physical stressors varies as a function of housing condition. For example, footshock was shown to have more profound effects on central DA and NE activity in animals housed individually than in group housed animals (Anisman & Sklar, 1981; Blanc et al., 1980).

In addition to social factors, the effects of stress on neurochemical change vary as a function of age. Ordinarily, turnover of brain NE is more rapid in younger rats (3 months) than in older animals (8 months). Upon exposure to stress of cold water immersion or footshock a more rapid and pronounced depletion of NE, with a slower recovery rate, was seen in the older animals (Ritter & Pelzer, 1978, 1980).

Finally, it should be considered that species specific defense behaviors may influence the effects of stress on neurochemical functioning. Specifically, if rats were permitted to fight during shock, the NE depletion normally observed was diminished. Furthermore, the magnitude of this protective effect was directly proportional to the number of fighting bouts in which rats engaged (Stolk et al., 1974). Fighting, it seems, may act as a behavioral coping response much in the same way that escape from an aversive stimulus does.

Although the neurochemical consequences of stress are fairly transient, they can readily be re-induced if animals are subsequently exposed to even mild stressors that would ordinarily have no substantial consequences in naive subjects. For example, we found that re-exposure to just 10 footshocks, a treatment that has little effect on its own, elicited significant hypothalamic NE depletions in mice previously exposed to more severe stress (Anisman & Sklar, 1979). Similarly, a CS that had been paired with shock was found to subsequently enhance the utilization of both NE (Cassens et al., 1980), and the endogenous opioid, leuenkephalin (Chance et al., 1978), as well as increase brain levels of acetylcholine (Hingten et al., 1976).

While cues associated with a stressor or re-exposure to a mild stressor may come to elicit the neurochemical changes ordinarily provoked by more severe trauma, previous encounters with controllable stress can protect the organism from the neuronal consequences of subsequent uncontrollable stress. Specifically, if mice were first exposed to escapable shock, subsequent exposure to inescapable shock no longer produced the reduction of NE levels ordinarily observed in the hippocampus, and provoked only relatively small depletions in hypothalamus (Anisman et al., 1980). It seems that traumatic stress experiences sensitize the organisms to later stressors or cues associated with a stressor, thereby maximizing neurochemical change, and experience with controllable stress events protected the organism from later uncontrollable trauma.

## Hormonal change

In view of the fact that the hypothalamic factors which initiate or inhibit pituitary function are controlled by neurochemical activity (see reviews in Ganong, 1980; Guillemin, 1978; Terry & Martin, 1978), it seems likely that the hormonal consequences of aversive stimulation are provoked by the initial neurochemical alterations (Sklar & Anisman, 1981). The hypothalamic NE and DA depletions or the ACh and 5-HT increases induced by acute uncontrollable physical stress result in increased corticotropin releasing hormone (CRF) and adrenocorticotropic hormone (ACTH) secretion. The ACTH secretion in turn promotes synthesis and release of adrenal corticosteroids (for details see review in Terry & Martin, 1978). In addition, since endorphins and ACTH are present in the same secretory granules of the pituitary (Weber, Voigt & Martin, 1978), the stress-provoked endorphin release (Rossier et al., 1977) may be mediated by the same mechanisms. Predictably, coping factors influence the corticosteroid activation. Escapable shock increases plasma corticosterone to a much smaller extent than does yoked inescapable shock (Weiss et al., 1971). Thus again it seems that the ability to cope with stress is a fundamental determinant of the ultimate physiological consequence.

Similarly, the stress-induced DA depletions and possibly the stress-induced 5-HT and histamine increases (Mazurkiewicz-Kwilecki & Taub, 1978) appear to mediate the stress-provoked increased prolactin secretion (see review in Terry & Martin, 1978). Indeed, since DA is considered to be prolactin inhibiting factor, it is likely that arcuate and tuberoinfundibular DA depletion following acute uncontrollable physical stress disinhibits the pituitary and causes enhanced prolactin release. Central nervous system alterations are probably also responsible for the transient growth hormone variations induced by stress. The initial enhancement of catecholamine release is probably responsible for the increased growth hormone secretion early in the stress session, whereas depletion of hypothalamic DA and NE during more protracted stress results in the reduced growth hormone secretion evident later in the stress session (Terry & Martin, 1978).

It should be noted that with a chronic stress regimen, the hormonal alterations induced by acute stress are observed (Feldman & Brown, 1976; Keim & Sigg, 1976; Kvetnansky et al., 1977; Mikulaj et al., 1976, Tache et al., 1978). As mentioned earlier, during chronic stress synthesis of transmitters increase to meet the high utilization rates. Accordingly, hypothalamic depletions do not occur and the secretion of hormones such as β-endorphin, ACTH and adrenal corticosteroids is returned to normal (see Sklar & Anisman, 1981).

Social stressors also modify hormonal activity. However, the endocrine changes during social stress persist and do not appear to undergo adaptation. For example, the increased levels of corticosterone produced by isolation persist even after chronic isolation (Henry & Stevens, 1977). Similarly, the

increased release of corticosterone provoked by acute predator exposure is
evident even after long-term predator exposure (Hamilton, 1974).

Finally, acute exposure to uncontrollable physical insults will also enhance
peripheral NE and epinephrine (E) secretion from the adrenal medulla and from
the sympathetic nerve endings in blood vessels and in several organs (Draskoczy,
Pulley & Burack, 1966; Goldstein & Nakajima, 1966; Kvetnansky & Mikulaj, 1970).
Unlike the endocrines previously discussed, the pituitary is not involved in
this phenomenon, and the release is due to increased activity in sympathetic
preganglionic ACh neurons. Adaptation to chronic physical stress also occurs
in the sympathetic system; however, the adaptation results from increased synthesis of NE and E, rather than from decreased release as evidenced by the fact
that high plasma levels of these transmitters are still observed (e.g., Barrett
& Cairncross, 1976; see Kvetnansky et al., 1980). These peripheral changes in
catecholamine secretion may be important in determining the tumorigenic effects
of stress and we will return to this point in a later section.

Immune mechanisms

Exposure to traumatic events influences cellular and humoral immune functioning. These effects are the topic of several chapters in this volume and will be
only briefly mentioned here. Suffice it to say that among infrahumans acute
uncontrollable physical stress will result in immunosuppression in both the T-
and B-cell systems, whereas chronic stress will result in immunofacilitation
(Monjan & Collector, 1977; see also reviews in Riley, 1981; Rogers, Dubey &
Reich, 1979; Solomon & Amkraut, 1979). Moreover, acute uncontrollable physical
stress will produce profound lymphocyte population changes which are reminiscent
of massive antigen activation (Nieburgs et al., 1979).

Among humans, both surgical stress and bereavement depress lymphocyte function (Bartrop et al., 1977; Pees, 1977). Furthermore, stress due to suspected
cancer was associated with a preponderance of large lymphocytes and a reduction
in the number of smaller lymphocytes (regardless of whether cancer was present
or not), a finding similar to the stress effects observed in rodents (Nieburgs
et al., 1979).

While there is evidence that some of the immunosuppressive effects of stress
exposure are due to the central catecholamine alterations causing increased
plasma levels of adrenal corticosteroids (see reviews in Riley, 1979, 1981;
Rogers et al., 1979), the exact mechanisms mediating the other immunological
consequences of stress have yet to be elucidated. However, growth hormone has
been reported to facilitate T-cell activity (Pandian & Talwar, 1971) and trans-

formed lymphocytes contain specific β-endorphin receptor sites (Hazum, Chang & Cuatrecases, 1979), indicating that these centrally controlled hormones may also play a role in determining the stress-induced immunological alterations.

Unfortunately, there have been no reports which specifically examined the role of coping factors on stress-induced immune alterations. Nonetheless, among women given mammography for suspected breast cancer, the finding that those with the largest lymphocyte population changes displayed repressed hostility (Nieburgs et al., 1979), suggests that coping processes are involved in this phenomenon. Moreover, as in the case of central NE, DA, ACh and enkephalin activity, cues associated with an acute stressor in infrahumans can later successfully induce immunosuppression by themselves (Ader & Cohen, 1975; Rogers et al., 1979).

It is noteworthy that as in the case of the neurochemical and hormonal consequences of social stress, the immunosuppressive effects of social stressors are not altered by chronic conditions. Handling, social isolation, overcrowding and predator stress suppress the responsiveness of both the T- and B-cell systems even if chronically applied (Brayton & Brain, 1974; Nieburgs et al., 1979; Solomon & Amkraut, 1979). Moreover, handling appeared to increase the number of large lymphocytes and reduce the number of uncommitted smaller lymphocytes just as physical stress did (Nieburgs et al., 1979). The fact that adaptation to chronic social stress does not occur in both the neurochemical and immunological systems, while adaptation to physical stress does occur again suggests that the neurochemical changes are associated with the ultimate physiological consequences.

Summarizing briefly, behavioral coping, stress chronicity, stress type, and social conditions appear to be the major factors determining the neurochemical consequences of exposure to traumatic stressors. Of course, these factors also determine the hormonal and immunological alterations induced by stress, since these changes appear to be secondary to the neuronal effects. Thus acute uncontrollable physical stress results in depletion of hypothalamic catecholamines, and increased brain concentrations of ACh, increased synthesis and secretion of hormones and immunosuppression. Adaptation in these biological mechanisms is observed following long-term physical stress exposure such that normal levels of functioning or alterations opposite to those provoked by acute stress are observed. In addition, the social environment onto which the stressor is imposed can alter the consequences of physical stress resulting in accentuated or attenuated neurochemical changes depending on the stress parameters and species employed.

The ability to cope behaviorally with a stressor, rather than the imposition of the stressor per se, appears to be fundamental in determining these physiological alterations. If control over an aversive experience is possible, then the neuronal and hormonal variations are not observed. There is some indication that the immunological consequences of physical stressors are also influenced by coping factors, however, this has not as yet been adequately evaluated.

STRESS AND NEOPLASIA

The same variables which influence the neurochemical alterations induced by stress also influence stress-provoked tumorigenic alterations. Indeed, coping factors, stress chronicity, and the social environment of the organism all appear to be fundamental in determining the tumorigenic changes. Interestingly, such effects are seen across a wide variety of tumor types including carcinogen-induced, viral, and transplanted tumors. In view of this parallel, the possible role of the central nervous system in determining the ultimate physiological changes which culminate in the variations of tumor growth will be discussed.

Tumorigenic consequences of acute physical stress

Several investigators reported that acute physical insults enhanced the development of viral-induced and transplanted tumors, and increased the incidence of tumors among mice that received a $TD_{50}$ dosage of tumor cells (Jamasbi & Nettesheim, 1977; Peters, 1975; Peters & Kelly, 1977; Riley, 1981; Sklar & Anisman, 1980; Sklar, Bruto & Anisman, 1981). Several of these studies involved transplantation of non-immunogenic cells syngeneic with the host animal, suggesting that the effects of the stress were not due to alterations in the classical T- and B-lymphocyte immune system (Jamaski & Mettesheim, 1977; Peters & Kelly, 1977). Indeed, irradiation enhanced the $TD_{50}$ provided that cell transplantation occured within 48 hours following the irradiation. Yet, the immunosuppressive properties of this treatment persisted for as long as 2 weeks, suggesting that stress effects on tumorigenesis and the T- and B-immune systems are independent of one another. Further to the same point, immunologic reconstitution by transplantation of syngeneic spleen cells after stress exposure did not influence the stress provoked enhancement of the $TD_{50}$ (Jamasbi & Nettesheim, 1977). Finally, Peters and Kelly (1977) showed that the enhancement of the $TD_{50}$ by surgical stress (laparotomy) was not modified by bilateral adrenalectomy, a treatment which ordinarily would prevent the suppression of T- and B- systems provoked by stress-induced corticosterone release. Curiously, these investigators did observe that ACTH or dexamethasone treatment enhanced tumorigenicity in non-stressed animals. Thus it appears that while not a necessary factor, corticoid changes might contribute to the stress-induced enhancement of tumorigenicity; however, such an effect appears to occur through mechanisms other than corticoid related changes in T- and B-cell functioning. Of course, this does not imply that the effects of aversive stimuli on other immune system, such as macrophages and natural killer cells, are not essential in the stress-related enhancement of tumorigenesis.

In contrast to these formulations, Riley (1981) argued that acute physical stress will only enhance tumor growth if the tumor is ordinarily under partial or complete control of the T- and B-immune systems. According to this view, the effect of stress exposure is to release the tumor from the inhibiting influence of the immune systems. In fact, Riley (1981) reported that in two substrains of C3H mice rotational stress enhanced the growth of transplanted lymphosarcoma only if the tumor and host animal were nonhistocompatible. While the differential effects of stress in these two sub-strains might have been related to histocompatibility factors, it should also be considered that the particularly rapid rate of tumor growth in the histocompatible sub-strain (C3H/Bi) may have precluded detection of a further increase in tumorigenicity provoked by the aversive stimulation. This is particularly the case since the effects of stress on isogenic tumor systems, while reliable, are generally relatively small (see for example Peters & Kelly, 1977; Sklar & Anisman, 1979). A second consideration concerns possible differences between these sub-strains in response to aversive stimulation. That is, strain differences in emotionality, as well as in neurochemical and hormonal activity may have contributed to the differential effects on tumor development. To be sure, strain and sub-strain differences in these variables have often been reported (see reviews in Wahlsten, 1978; Wimer, Reid & Eleftheriou, 1973). In yet another study, Riley (1981) found that within a single strain(C57BL/6), stress in the form of exposure to LDH virus enhanced the growth of a non-pigmented melanoma while it had no effect on a more histocompatible pigmented melanoma. However, in the absence of the stressor, the rate of growth of the pigmented melanoma was considerably greater than that of the non-pigmented melanoma, making it difficult to determine if the absence of a stress effect was due to the isogenicity of the tumor or merely to the rapid growth rate preventing detection of the LDH effect. Such a question, of course, could be examined by employing various doses of the pigmented tumor so as to equate the growth rates between the pigmented and non-pigmented melanomas.

The aforementioned comments should not be misconstrued to imply any detraction of the work conducted by Riley and his associates. To the contrary, these data show clearly that stress as well as manipulations of adrenal corticosteroids will influence tumor growth, and it is certainly possible that such effects are related to immunocompetence. It should be considered, however, that tumor systems in humans are syngeneic and autochtonous and thus these effects may not be analogous to human neoplastic disease (for a further discussion of this issue see Hewitt, 1978).

It seems that acute stress may enhance tumorigenesis; however, one important feature in this respect is related to the organism's ability to cope with the stress through behavioral means. As in the case of the differential effects of escapable shock and inescapable shock on central NE levels, such treatments have been shown to differentially influence the growth of transplanted syngeneic tumors (P815 mastocytoma). Sklar and Anisman (1979) and Sklar et al. (1981) reported that escapable footshock applied 24 hours after cell transplantation did not appreciably influence tumor size relative to nonshocked mice. In contrast, mice that received an identical amount of uncontrollable shock (in a yoked paradigm) developed larger tumors than nonshocked animals.

In addition to the effects of stress on tumor growth, acute uncontrollable physical stress has been shown to increase the frequency of metastases. As indicated previously, such effects were seen using $TD_{50}$ model of metastases. In addition, various forms of acute stress increased the incidence of liver and pulmonary tumors following intravenous injections of malignant cells (Fisher & Fisher, 1979; Saba & Antikatzides, 1976; Van den Brenk et al., 1976). Moreover, Maruyama and Johnson (1969) found that irradiation stress increased the incidence of tumors among mice that received only a single syngeneic lymphosarcoma cell. Finally, it was shown that surgical stress enhanced the frequency of metastases in a tumor which spontaneously metastasized (Lundy et al., 1979).

## Tumorigenic consequences of chronic physical stress

The consequences of repeated aversive experiences can be distinguished from that of a single stress session. Repeated exposure to physical stressors inhibited the induction and growth of DMBA and 20-methylcholanthyrene-induced tumors (Newberry, 1978; Newberry & Sangbusch, 1979; Newberry et al., 1972, 1976; Nieburgs et al., 1979, Pradhan & Ray, 1974; Pradham, 1974; Molomut, Lazere & Smith, 1963) and retarded the growth of several different transplantable tumor systems as well (Pradhan & Ray, 1974; Ray & Pradham, 1974; Gershen, Benuck & Shurrager, 1974). For example, within a single experiment it was shown that aversive stimulation applied for 5 min a day at 4 day intervals over

90 days increased the number of tumors engendered by DMBA administration while reduced size and number of tumors were evident in rats that received the same stress treatment over 150 days (Nieburgs et al., 1979).

The timing of stress application appears to be a critical variable in the inhibition of carcinogenesis and tumor growth provoked by chronic exposure to physical stressors. Chronic cold stress inhibited the induction of radiation-induced tumors only if it was applied after exposure to the carcinogen (Baker & Jahn, 1976). Similarly, Newberry (1978) found that chronic restraint inhibited tumor incidence only if applied after DMBA administration. Moreover, Newberry (1978) demonstrated that stress applied prior to this period will not have carry-over effects that influence carcinogenesis. It seems that a critical period exists during which chronic physical stress will inhibit tumor incidence. The existence of this critical period following carcinogen exposure Newberry (1978) and Newberry and Sengebush (1979) to suggest that the inhibitory effects of chronic stress were due to reduction of cell proliferation rates rather than modification of the initial neoplastic change.

In considering the effects of chronic stressors on the inhibition of tumor growth it should be emphasized that more than a single mechanism might be operative in determining the observed effects. On the one hand, the depletion of central amines that occur after an acute stress session are not evident following chronic stress. Moreover, although basal levels of NE and DA are seen after chronic stress, the rate of turnover of these amines is greatly increased both centrally and peripherally, and receptor sensitivity is substantially altered as well. Any one of these alterations could theoretically influence tumorigenesis either through effects on immune systems or some other mechanism. On the other hand, aversive stimulation, particularly of a chronic nature, applied during a later phase of tumor development, may have been responsible for the tumor inhibition. That is, rather than the stress chronicity itself, the observed tumor inhibition may have resulted from stress application after some critical developmental change in the tumor (e.g., angiogenesis).

## Social stress

Social conditions have been shown to influence tumorigenesis and modify the effects of other stressors on tumor development. Several investigators, for example, reported that individual housing in mice increased the frequency of spontaneous tumors and enhanced the growth of transplanted tumors (Adervont, 1944; Dechambre & Gosse, 1973; Sklar & Anisman, 1980). It seemed, however, that to a great extent the effect of the individual housing was a consequence of a change in housing conditions. To be more explicit, animals that were group housed and then transferred to individual housing exhibited greater tumor development than did mice that had been continuously housed individually after weaning. When mice were transferred from individual to group housing, tumor growth was also enhanced; however, the enhanced tumor growth was not evident among mice that engaged in fighting (Sklar & Anisman, 1980). The latter effect may have been a reflection of the influence of coping factors, since fighting, as previously mentioned, will ameliorate other stress-related neurochemical events. Alternatively, it should be considered that both isolation and fighting represented stress events and a combination of these stressors resulted in an effect comparable to that engendered by chronic physical stress.

Among the social conditions that influence tumorigenesis, Riley (1981) indicated that ordinary laboratory conditions (e.g., noises, smells) will influence tumor growth, ostensibly because of the effects on corticoid levels and immune responsivity. In addition to the direct effects, such conditions will also modify the effects of other stressors on tumor growth. For example, Sklar and Anisman (1980) reported that the tumor enhancing effects of uncontrollable shock were not evident if mice were housed in isolation. Similarly, Nieburgs et al. (1979) reported that immunosuppression produced by experimental stressors were not detected within the first few days of arrival from the breeding laboratories. In effect, all of these studies point to the fact that the tumorigenic effects of stress must be considered within the context of the social conditions in which animals are housed, and even subtle environmental events may obscure or modify the effects of stress on tumorigenesis.

CENTRAL NEUROCHEMICAL INFLUENCES ON TUMORIGENESIS

The basic thesis of the present paper is that exposure to aversive insults may influence tumorigenesis through alterations in central neurochemical mechanisms. The central neurochemical changes, in turn, will influence hormonal and/or immunological processes as well as peripheral neurotransmitters. Ultimately, one or more of these mechanisms probably govern the alterations of tumor growth evident after exposure to a stressor. It follows from such a position that neurochemical manipulations which mimic the effects of stressors should have predictable effects on tumor growth. That is, those pharmacological treatments that decrease central (probably hypothalamic) catecholamine activity should enhance tumor growth, whereas those pharmacological treatments that increase catecholamine activity should have an opposite effect. Caution, however, must be taken in considering the consequences of pharmacological treatments since secondary effects, such as receptor supersensitivity or sub-sensitivity, as well as serial and parallel effects of the drug treatments could potentially confound or obscure the predicted outcomes.

As detailed in the chapter by Stein in this volume, anterior hypothalamic lesions which presumably reduce catecholamine levels, resulted in a depression of T- and B-cell functioning (see Janakovic & Isakovic, 1973; Konovalov, Korneva & Khai, 1971; Stein et al., 1976; Stein, Keller & Schleifer, 1981). In a similar fashion, systemic injection of the catecholamine storage granule depleter, reserpine, produced immunosuppression (Dukor et al., 1966), whereas stimulation of DA receptors and increased activity of DA sensitive cAMP was shown to enhance immune function (Cotzias & Tang, 1977; Tang & Cotzias, 1977).

With respect to the tumorigenic consequences of drugs influencing catechol-amines, it has been reported that amphetamine or L-DOPA, which increase neuronal activity, inhibited the growth of DMBA-induced tumors, as well as transplanted syngeneic tumors (Driscoll et al., 1978; Quadri, Kledzik & Meites, 1973; Wick, 1977, 1978a, b, 1979). Conversely, reduction of catecholamine levels or blockade of catecholamine receptors enhanced the growth of tumors induced by DMBA as well as spontaneous mammary tumors and transplanted syngeneic tumors (Lacasagne & Duplan, 1959; Lapin, 1978; Quadri, Clark & Meites, 1973; Sklar & Anisman, 1981b; Welsch & Meites, 1970). However, if toxic doses of receptor blockers were employed or if animals received repeated neuroleptic treatments, tumor inhibition rather than exacerbation was observed (Belkin & Hardy, 1957; Gottlieb et al., 1960; Van Woert & Palmer, 1969). As indicated earlier, firm conclusions cannot be drawn on the basis of the latter studies since altera-tions in receptor sensitivity following chronic drug administration or secondary factors associated with toxic drug doses may have contributed to the observed effects. Furthermore, and this applies to all of the aforementioned studies, the tumorigenic consequences of the drug treatments may have resulted from peripheral rather than central alterations. Indeed, systemic injections of epinephrine increased suppressor T-cell function (see the chapter by Borysenko), and Wick (1979) observed that several catecholamine agonists with exclusive peripheral properties inhibited tumor growth. Wick (1979) suggested that the inhibition of enzymes associated with DNA synthesis was principally responsible for the antitumor action. It should be noted, however, that this does not exclude some contribution of the central catecholamines, since alterations of these transmitters will have peripheral repercussions which may ultimately influence neoplasia.

MEDIATING MECHANISMS

Reiterating, it is our contention that the neurochemical alterations provoked by stressful events are fundamental to the variations of tumor growth. These neurochemical alterations presumably have their effects through their action on hormonal, immunological, or metabolic processes. The evidence in favor of a role for T- and B- lymphocyte alterations in the stress provoked tumor enhancement is at best equivocal. As will be recalled, Riley (1981) provided evidence suggesting that corticoid changes induced by stress inhibit these immune mechanisms thereby enhancing tumor growth. In addition to the reservations expressed earlier concerning such a proposition, it has been reported that both growth hormone and thyroxine enhance immune functioning (Denckla, 1974; Ritter, 1977). Indeed, thyroxine and growth hormone restore immunocompetence in immune deficient animals (Denckla, 1974). Since the secretion of these hormones is increased by stress, it might be expected that the immunosuppression provoked by the increased corticoid release would be offset by the growth hormone and thyroxine secretion, and thus tumor enhancement would not be evident. In fact, among humans undergoing stressful experiences there appears to be no relationship between immunosuppression and serum cortisol, growth hormone, or thyroxine (Bartrop et al., 1977; Dorian et al., 1981; Schleifer et al., 1980).

While the aforementioned data suggest that changes in the classical T- and B-cell immune systems are not responsible for the tumorigenic consequences of stressful experiences, a role for other immunological systems should not be dismissed. It has been proposed that natural killer cells and macrophages are fundamental to the host defense against neoplasia (Alexander, 1977; Herberman & Holden, 1978; Oehler & Herberhman, 1978; Oehler et al., 1978, see also the chapter by Herberman in this volume), and thus changes in these systems may be responsible for the stress-provoked alterations of tumorigenicity. Indeed, in mice, immobilization stress has been shown to inhibit macrophage mediated cytotoxicity (Pavlidis & Chirigos, 1980). Moreover, in humans stressful life event changes were associated with decreased natural killer cell activity, and this effect was only evident among individuals who did not cope adequately with the stress (see Locke in this volume). This finding is congruent with the infrahuman work which indicated that the inability to cope was the essential feature for stress induced NE depletion and enhanced tumor growth (see Sklar & Anisman, 1981).

In addition to immunological factors, metabolic changes associated with stressful events may also contribute to the enhanced tumorigenicity. For example, the increased secretion of peripheral catecholamines and adrenal corticosteroids will increase metabolic rate and induce lipolysis, proteolysis and glycogenolysis (Guyton, 1980). If nutrient supply is one of the limiting factors of tumor cell proliferation, then the mobilization of these nutrient stores could ostensibly be responsible for the enhanced tumor growth. The finding that corticosterone is increaed to a greater extent by uncontrollable than by controllable stress (Weiss, 1971), coupled with the fact that corticosterone plays a permissive role in the catecholamine induced nutrient mobilization, is consistent with the differential effects of controllable and uncontrollable stress on tumor growth. Finally, it should be added that the increased catecholamine secretion in response to aversive insults will increase the activity of cAMP, which in turn, influences immunocompetence (see Stein, this volume), in addition to affecting metabolic rate. Either or both of these cAMP actions could conceivably contribute to the tumorigenic consequences of stress.

GENERAL CONSIDERATIONS

As outlined in several of the chapters in this volume, a great deal of data have pointed to stress as being one factor that may exacerbate human neoplasia. Moreover, it appears that the individual's ability to cope with stress is an essential feature in determining whether or not such an effect will occur. It is generally agreed that analysis of the relation between stress and cancer must consider a wide range of tumor types. In addition, however, particular attention must be devoted to the characteristics of the stressor, as well as the time of its occurrence, background social conditions and the organism's previous stress history. We have emphasized repeatedly that acute and chronic stressors would not be expected to yield similar outcomes. Moreover, in considering the effects of any given stressor it would be propitious to consider also early life stresses. As indicated previously, the neurochemical response to a particular stressor will be greatly increased provided that the organism had previously been exposed to a similar stressor. Likewise, Brown (1979) reported that the affective and emotional consequences of a stressful experience while certainly dependent on coping factors, are most dramatic among individuals who had encountered early life trauma. Accordingly, it might be considered that early life stress may sensitize the individual to later life stresses, thus allowing ordinarily innocuous events to have profound consequences on carcinogenesis.

Finally, in closing, one additional comment warrants attention. Much of the present paper has been concerned with stress effects on the development of primary tumors. Some of the infrahuman research suggests that stressful events will also influence metastases. It will be recalled that the effects of stress on tumor development are most detectable when only small colonies of cells are present. Once the tumor is sufficiently large, the effects of aversive events appear to be minimal. As such, it may be the case that stressful events are particularly important in influencing the formation of secondary neoplasms. During the formation of metastases, when the colony of cells is relatively small, acute uncontrollable stress may allow these cells to escape from the control exerted by hormones, macrophages, natural killer cells and other metabolic factors, thereby increasing the probability of secondary tumor formation.

## REFERENCES

Ader R, Cohen N (1975) Behaviorally conditioned immunosuppression. Psychosom Med 37:333-340.

Akiskal HS, McKinney WT (1973) Depressive disorders: Toward a unified hypothesis. Science 183:20-29.

Alexander GJ, Kopeloff LM (1977) P-chlorophenylalanine-mediated decrease in susceptibility to audiogenic seizures in inbred mice. Neuropharm 16:405-410.

Alexander P (1977) Innate host resistance to malignant cells not involving specific immunity. In Day SB, Myers WPL, Stansley P, Garattini S, Lewis MG (eds.), Cancer Invasion and Metastasis: Biologic Mechanisms and Therapy. New York: Raven Press.

Amkraut A, Solomon GF (1972) Stress and murine sarcoma virus (Maloney)-induced tumors. Cancer Res 32:1428-1433.

Andervont EB (1944) Influence of environment on mammary cancer in mice. J Natl Cancer Inst 4:579-581.

Anisman H (1978) Neurochemical changes elicited by stress: Behavioral correlates. In Anisman H, Bignami G (eds.), Psychopharmacology of Aversively Motivated Behavior. New York: Plenum Press.

Anisman H, Sklar LS (1979) Catecholamine depletion upon re-exposure to stress: Mediation of the escape deficits produced by inescapable shock. J Comp Physiol Psychol 93:610-625.

Anisman H, Sklar LS (1981) Social housing conditions influence escape deficits produced by uncontrollable stress: Assessment of the contribution of norepinephrine. Behav Neur Biol 32: 406-427.

Anisman H, Kokkinidis L, Sklar LS (1981) Neurochemical consequences of stress: Contributions of adaptive processes. In Burchfield S (ed.), Physiological and Psychological Interactions in Response to Stress. New York: Hemisphere.

Anisman H, Pizzino A, Sklar LS (1980) Coping with stress, norepinephrine depletion and escape performance. Brain Res 191:583-588.

Baker DG, Jahn A (1976) The influence of a chronic environment stress on radiation carcinogenesis. Rad Res 68:449-458.

Bassett JR, Cairncross KD (1976) Endogenous levels of catecholamines in the rat myocardium following exposure to stress. Pharmacol Biochem Behav 4: 35-38.

Bartrop RW, Lazarus L, Luckhurst E, Kiloh LG, Penny R (1977) Depressed lymphocyte function after bereavement. Lancet 1:834-836.

Belkin M, Hardy WG (1957) Effect of reserpine and chlorpromazine on sarcoma 37. Science 125:233-234.

Blanc G, Herve D, Simon H, Lisoprawski A, Glowinski J, Tassin JP (1980) Response to stress of mesocortical-frontal dopaminergic neurones in rats after long-term isolation. Nature 284:265-267.

Brayton AR, Brain PF (1974) Studies on the effects of differential housing on some measures of disease resistance in male and female laboratory mice. J Endocrin 61:48-49.

Brown GW (1979) The social etiology of depression. London studies. In Depue RA (ed.), The Psychobiology of the Depressive Disorders. New York: Academic Press.

Chance WT, White AC, Krynock GM, Rosecrans JA (1978) Conditional fear-induced antinociception and decreased binding of (3H)N-leuenkephalin to rat brain. Brain Res 141:371-374.

Costa E, Tagliomonte A, Brunello N, Cheney DL (1980) Effect of stress on the metabolism of acetylcholine in the cholinergic pathways of extrapyramidal and limbic systems. In Usdin E, Kvetnansky R, Kopin IJ (eds.), Catecholamines and Stress: Recent Advances. New York: Elsevier.

Cassens G, Roffman M, Kuruc A, Orsulak PJ, Schildkraut JJ (1980) Alterations in brain norepinephrine metabolism induced by environmental stimuli previously paired with inescapable shock. Science 209:1138-1140.

Cherek DR, Lane JD, Freeman ME, Smith JE (1980) Receptor changes following shock avoidance. Soc Neurosci Abs 6:543.

Cotzias GC, Tang L (1977) An adenylate cyclase of brain reflects propensity for breast cancer in mice. Science 197:1094-1096.

Dechambre RP, Gosse C (1973) Individual versus group caging of mice with grafted tumors. Cancer Res 33:140-144.

Denckla WD (1974) Role of the pituitary and thyroid glands in the decline of minimal $O_2$ consumption with age. J Clin Invest 53:572-581.

Dorian BJ, Keystone E, Garfinkel PE, Brown GM (1981) Immune mechanisms in acute psychological stress. Psychosom Med 43:84.

Draskoczy PR, Pulley KK, Burack WR (1966) The effect of cold environment on the endogenously labeled catecholamine (CA) stores. Pharmacologist 8:178-184.

Driscoll JS et al. (1978) Psychotropic drugs as potential antitumor agents: A selective screening study. Cancer Treat Rep 62:45-73.

Dukor P, Salvin SB, Dietrich FM, Gelzer J, Hess R, Loustalot P (1966) Effect of reserpine on immune reactions and tumor growth. Europ J Cancer 2:253-261.

Feldman J, Brown GM (1976) Endocrine responses to electric shock and avoidance. Conditioning in the rhesus monkey: Cortisol and growth hormones. Psycho-neuroendocrinology 1:231-242.

Fisher B, Fisher ER (1959) Experimental studies of factors influencing hepatic metastases: II. Effect of partial hepatectomy. Cancer 12:929-932.

Fox BH (1978) Premorbid psychological factors as related to cancer incidence. J Behav Med 1:45-133.

Galosy RA, Gaebelein CJ (1977) Cardiovascular adaptation to environmental stress: Its role in the development of hypertension, responsible mechanisms and hypotheses. Biobehav Rev 1:165-175.

Goldstein M, Nakajima K (1966) The effect of disulfiram on the biosynthesis of catecholamines during exposure of rats to cold. Life Sci 5:175-179.

Ganong WF (1980) Participation of brain monoamines in the regulation of neuroendocrine activity under stress. In Usdin E, Kvetnansky R, Kopin IJ (eds.), Catecholamines and Stress: Recent Advances. New York: Elsevier/North Holland.

Gershben LL, Benuck I, Shurrager PS (1974) Influence of stress on lesion growth and on survival of animals bearing parenteral and intracerebral leukemia L1210 and Walker tumors. Oncology 30:429-435.

Gottlieb LS, Hazel M, Broitman S, Zamcheck N (1960) Effects of chlorpromazine on a transplantable mouse mastocytoma. Fed Proc 19:181 (Abstract).

Guillemin R (1978) Peptides in the brain: The new endocrinology of the neuron. Science 202:390-402.

Guyton AC (1971) Textbook of Medical Physiology. Toronto: W.B. Saunders Co.

Hamilton DR (1974) Immunosuppressive effects of predator induced stress in mice with acquired immunity to Hymenolepis Nana. J Psychosom Res 18:143-153.

Hazum E, Chang KJ, Cuatrecases P (1979) Specific non-opiate receptors for β-endorphin. Science 205:1033-1035.

Henry JP, Stevens PM (1977) Stress, Health and the Social Environment. Berlin: Springer.

Herberman RB (1978) Natural cell-mediated cytotoxicity in nude mice. In Klein G, Weinhouse S (eds.), The Nude Mouse in Experimental and Clinical Research. New York: Academic Press.

Herberman RB, Holden HT (1978) Natural cell-mediated immunity. In Klein G, Weinhouse S (eds.), Advances in Cancer Research (Vol. 27). New York: Academic Press.

Hewitt HB (1978) The choice of animal tumors for experimental studies of cancer therapy. In Klein G, Weinhouse S (eds.), Advances in Cancer Research (Vol. 27). New York: Academic Press.

Hibbs JB (1973) Macrophage nonimmunological recognition: Target cell factors related to contact inhibition. Science 180:868-870.

Hingtgen JN, Smith JE, Shea PA, Aprison MH, Gaff TM (1976) Cholinergic changes during conditioned suppression in rats. Science 193:332-334.

Jamasbi RJ, Nettesheim P (1977) Non-immunological enhancement of tumor transplantability in x-irradiated host animals. Brit J Cancer 36:723-729.

Janakovic BD, Isakovic K (1973) Neuro-endocrine correlates of immune response: I. Effects of brain lesions on antibody production. Arthus reactivity, and delayed hypersensitivity in the rat. Inter Arch Aller Appl Immun 45:360-372.

Karczmar AG, Scudder CL, Richardson DL (1973) Interdisciplinary approach to the study of behavior in related mice types. In Ehrenpreis S, Kopin IJ (eds.), Chemical Approaches to Brain Function. New York: Academic Press.

Keim KL, Sigg EB (1976) Physiological and biochemical concomitants of restraint in rats. Pharmacol Biochem Behav 4:289-297.

Kobayashi RM, Palkovits M, Kizer JS, Jacobowitz DM, Kopin IJ (1976) Selective alterations of catecholamines and tyrosine hydroxylase activity in the hypothalamus following acute and chronic stress. In Usdin E, Kvetnansky R, Kopin IJ (eds.), Catecholamines and Stress. Oxford: Pergamon.

Konovalov GV, Korneva EA, Khai LM (1971) Effect of destruction of the posterior hypothalamic area on experimental allergic polyneuritis. Brain Res 29:383-386.

Lacassagne A, Duplan JF (1959) Le mécanisme de la cancérisation de la mamelle chez les souris, considéré d'après les résultats d'expériences au moyen de la réserpine. Compte Rendus 249:810-812.

Kvetnansky R (1980) Recent progress in catecholamines under stress. In Usdin E, Kvetnansky R, Kopin IJ (eds.), Catecholamines and Stress: Recent Advances. New York: Elsevier/North Holland.

Kvetnansky R, Mikulaj L (1970) Adrenal and urinary catecholamines in rats during adaptation to repeated immobilization stress. Endocrinology 87:738-743.

Kvetnansky R, Mitro A, Palkovits M, Brownstein M, Torda T, Vigas M, Mikulaj L (1976) Catecholamines in individual hypothalamic nuclei in stressed rats. In Usdin E, Kvetnansky R, Kopin IJ (eds.), Catecholamines and Stress. Oxford: Pergamon Press.

Lundy J, Lovett EJ, Wolinsky SM, Conran P (1979) Immune impairment and metastatic tumor growth. Cancer 43:945-951.

Maruyama Y, Johnson EA (1969) Quantitative study of isologous tumor cell inactivation and effective cell fraction for the LSA mouse lymphoma. Cancer 23:309-312.

Mazurkiewicz-Kwilecki DM, Taub H (1978) Effect of stress on brain histamine. Pharmacol Biochem Behav 9(4):465-468.

Mikulaj L, Kvetnansky R, Murgas K, Parzikova J, Vencel P (1976) Catecholamines and corticosteroids in acute and repeated stress. In Usdin E, Kvetnansky R, Kopin IJ (eds.), Catecholamines and Stress. Oxford: Pergamon Press.

Modigh K (1976) Influence of social stress on brain catecholamine mechanisms. In Usdin E, Kvetnansky R, Kopin IJ (eds.), Catecholamines and Stress. Oxford: Pergamon Press.

Molomut N, Lazere F, Smith, LW (1963) Effect of audiogenic stress upon methyl-cholanthrene-induced carcinogenesis in mice. Cancer Res 23:1097-1011.

Monjan AA, Collector MI (1977) Stress-induced modulation of the immune response. Science 196:307-308.

Newberry BH (1978) Restraint-induced inhibition of 7, 12-dimethylbenz(a)anthracene-induced mammary tumors: Relation to stages of tumor development. J Natl Cancer Inst 61:725-729.

Newberry BH, Sengbush L (1979) Inhibitory effects of stress on experimental mammary tumors. Cancer Detect Prevent 2:225-233.

Newberry BH, Frankie G, Beatty PA, Maloney BD, Gilchrist JC (1972) Shock stress and DMBA-induced mammary tumors. Psychosom Med 34:295-303.

Newberry BH, Gildow J, Wogan J, Reese RL (1976) Inhibition of Huggins tumors by forced restraint. Psychosom Med 38:155-162.

Nieburgs HE et al. (1979) The role of stress in human and experimental oncogenesis. Cancer Detect Prevent 2:307-336.

Oehler RJ, Herberman RB (1978) Natural cell-mediated cytotoxicity in rats: III. Effects of immunopharmacologic treatments on natural reactivity and on reactivity augmented by polyinosinic-polycytidylic acid. Int J Cancer 21:221-229.

Oehler RJ, Lindsay LR, Nunn ME, Herberman RB (1978) Natural cell-mediated cytotoxicity in rats: I. Tissue and strain distribution, and demonstration of a membrane receptor for the Fc portion of IgG. Int J. Cancer 21:204-209.

Oehler JR, Lindsay, LR, Nunn ME, Holden HT, Herberman RB (1978) Natural cell-mediated cytotoxicity in rats: II. In vivo augmentation of NK-cell activity. Int J Cancer 21:210-220.

Palkovits M, Brownstein M, Kizer JS, Saavedra JM, Kopin IJ (1976) Effect of stress on serotonin concentration and tryptophan hydroxylase activity of brain nuclei. Neuroendocrinology 22:298-304.

Pandian MR, Talwar GP (1971) Effect of growth hormone on the metabolism of thymus and on the immune response against sheep erythrocytes. J Exper Med 134:1095-1113.

Pavlidis N, Chirigos M (1980) Stress induced impairment of macrophage tumoricidal function. Psychosom Med 42:47-54.

Pees HW (1977) Influence of surgery and dexamethasone on cell-mediated immune responses in patients with meningiomas. Br J Cancer 35:537-545.

Peters LJ (1975) Enhancement of syngeneic murine tumor transplantation by whole body irradiation--A non-immunological phenomenon. Br J Cancer 31:293-300.

Peters LJ, Kelly H (1977) The influence of stress and stress hormones on the transplantability of a non-immunogenic syngeneic murine tumor. Cancer 39:1482-1488.

Pradhan SN, Ray P (1974) Effects of stress on growth of transplanted 7,12-dimethylbenz(a)anthracene-induced tumors and their modification by psychotropic drugs. J Natl Cancer Inst 53:1241-1245.

Quadri SK, Clark JL, Meites J (1973) Effects of LSDm Oargyline and Haloperidol on mammary tumor growth in rats. Proc Soc Exper Biol Med 124:22-26.

Quadri SK, Kledzik GS, Meites J (1973) Effects of L-DOPA and methyldopa on growth of mammary cancers in rats. Proc Soc Exper Biol Med 142:759-761.

Ray P, Pradhan SN (1974) Growth of transplanted and induced tumors in rats under a schedule of punished behavior. J Natl Cancer Inst 52:575-577.

Riley V (1979) Cancer and stress: Overview and critique. Cancer Detect Prevent 2:163-195.

Riley V (1981) Psychoneuroendocrine influences on immunocompetence and neoplasia. Science 212:1100-1109.

Ritter MA (1981) Embryonic mouse thymocyte development. Enhancing effect of corticosterone in acute psychological stress. Psychosom Med 43:84.

Ritter S, Pelzer NL (1978) Magnitude of stress-induced brain norepinephrine depletion varies with age. Brain Res 152:170-175.

Ritter S, Pelzer NL (1980) Age related changes in norepinephrine neuron function during stress. In Usdin E, Kvetnansky R, Kopin IJ (eds.), Catecholamines and Stress: Recent Advances. New York: Elsevier/North Holland.

Rogers MP, Dubey D, Reich P (1979) The influence of the psyche and the brain on immunity and disease susceptibility: A critical review. Psychosom Med 41: 147-164.

Rossier J, French EP, Rivier C, Ling N, Guillemin R, Bloom FE (1977) Footshock induced stress increases beta-endorphin levels in blood but not brain. Nature 270:618-620.

Saba TM, Antikatzides TG (1976) Decreased resistance to intravenous tumor cell challenge during reticuloendothelial depression following surgery. Br J Cancer 34:381-389.

Saito H, Morita A, Miyazaki , Takagi (1976) Comparison of the effects of various stresses on biogenic amines in the central nervous system and animal symptoms. In Usdin E, Kvetnansky R, Kopin IJ (eds.), Catecholamines and Stress. Oxford: Pergamon Press.

Schleifer SJ, Keller SE, McKegney FP, Stein MI (1980) Bereavement and lymphocyte function. Paper presented at the Annual Meeting of the American Psychiatric Association, San Francisco, May.

Schmale AH Jr, Iker HP (1966) The psychological setting of uterine cervical cancer. Ann NY Acad Sci 125:807-813.

Seligman MEP (1975) Helplessness: In depression, development and death. San Francisco: Freeman.

Selye H (1956) The Stress of Life. New York: McGraw-Hill.

Sklar LS, Anisman H (1979) Stress and coping factors influence tumor growth. Science 205:513-515.

Sklar LS, Anisman H (1980) Social stress influences tumor growth. Psychosom Med 42:347-365.

Sklar LS, Anisman H (1981) Stress and cancer. Psychol Bull 89:369-406.

Sklar LS, Anisman H (1981) Contributions of stress and coping to cancer development and growth. In Bammer K, Newberry BH (eds.), Stress and Cancer. Toronto: C.J. Hogrefe.

Sklar LS, Bruto V, Anisman H (1981) Adaptation to the tumor-enhancing effects of stress. Psychosom Med 43: 331-342.

Solomon GF, Amkraut AA (1979) Neuroendocrine aspects of the immune response and their implications for stress effects on tumor immunity. Cancer Detect Prevent 2:197-223.

Stein M, Schiavi RC, Camerino M (1976) Influence of brain and behavior on the immune system. Science 191:435-440.

Stein M, Keller SE, Schleifer SJ (1981) The hypothalamus and the immune response. In Weiner H, Hofer MA, Stunkard AJ (eds.), Brain, Behavior and Bodily Disease A.R.N.M.D. 59:45-66. New York: Raven Press.

Stolk JM, Conner RL, Levine S, Barchas JD (1974) Brain norepinephrine metabolism and shock-induced fighting behavior in rats: Differential effects of shock and fighting on the neurochemical response to a common footshock stimulus. J Pharm Exp Ther 190:193-209.

144

Stone EA (1975) Stress and catecholamines. In Friedhoff AJ (ed.), Catecholamines and Behavior. 2. New York: Plenum Press.

Stone EA (1979) Subsensitivity to norepinephrine as a link between adaptation
to stress and antidepressant therapy: An hypothesis. Res Comm Psychol
Psychiat Behav 4:241-255.

Taché Y, Ruisseau PD, Ducharme JR, Collu R (1978) Pattern of adenohypophyseal
hormone changes in male rats following chronic stress. Neuroendocrinology
26:208-219.

Tang L, Cotzias GC (1977) Quantitative correlation of dopamine-dependent adenylate cyclase with responses to levodopa in various mice. Proc Natl Acad Sci
USA 74:1242-1244.

Telegdy G, Vermes I (1976) Changes induced by stress in the activiy of the
serotoninergic system in limbic brain structures. In Usdin E, Kvetnansky R,
Kopin IJ (eds.), Catecholamines and Stress. Oxford: Pergamon Press.

Terry LC, Martin JB (1978) Hypothalamic hormones: Subcellular distribution and
mechanisms of release. In George R, Okun R (eds.), Annual Review of Pharmacology and Toxicology (Vol. 18). Palo Alto, CA: Annual Reviews.

Thierry AM (1973) Effects of stress on the metabolism of serotonin and norepine-
phrine in the central nervous system of the rat. In Nemeth S (ed.), Hormones,
Metabolism and Stress: Recent Progress and Perspectives. Bratislava:
Publishing House of the Slovak Academy of Sciences.

Thierry AM, Fekete M, Glowinski J (1968) Effects of stress on the metabolism
of noradrenaline, dopamine and serotonin (5-HT) in the central nervous system
of the rat. II. Modifications of serotonin metabolism. Eur J Pharmacol 4:
384-389.

Thierry AM, Tassin JP, Blanc G, Glowinski J (1976) Selective activation of
the mesocortical DA system by stress. Nature 263:242-244.

Thoa NB, Tizabi Y, Jacobowitz DM (1977) The effect of isolation on catecholamine
concentration and turnover in discrete areas of the rat brain. Brain Res 131:
259-269.

Thomas CB (1976) Precursors of premature disease and death: The predictive
potential of habits and family attitudes. Ann Intern Med 85:653-658.

Thomas CB, Duszynski KR (1974) Closeness to parents and the family constella-
tion in a prospective study of five disease states: Suicide, mental illness,
malignant tumor, hypertension and coronary heart disease. Johns Hopkins
Med J 134:251-270.

Van Den Brenk HAS, Stone MG, Kelly H, Sharpington C (1976) Lowering of innate
resistance of the lungs to the growth of blood-borne cancer cells in states
of topical and systemic stress. Br J Cancer 33:60-78.

Van Woert MH, Palmer SH (1969) Inhibition of the growth of mouse melanoma by
chlorpromazine. Cancer Res 29:1952-1955.

Wahlsten D (1978) Behavioral genetics and animal learning. In Anisman H,
Bignami G (eds.), Psychopharmacology of Aversively Motivated Behvaior. New
York: Plenum Press.

Weber E, Voigt KH, Martin R (1978) Concomitant storage of ACTH and endorphin-
like immunoreactivity in secretory granules of anterior pituitary cortico-
trophs. Brain Res 157:385-390.

Weiss JM, Stone EA, Harrell N (1970) Coping behavior and brain norepinephrine
level in rats. J Comp Physiol Psychol 72: 153-160.

Weiss JM, Glazer HI, Pohorecky LA (1976) Coping behavior and neurochemical
changes: An alternative explanation for the original "learned helplessness"
experiments. In Serban G, Kling A (eds.), Animal Models in Human Psychobiology. New York: Plenum Press.

Weiss JM, Glazer HI, Pohorecky LA, Brick JT, Miller NE (1975) Effects of
chronic exposure to stressors on avoidance-escape behavior and on brain
norepinephrine. Psychosom Med 37:522-534.

Welch BL, Welch AS (1970) Control of brain catecholamines and serotonin during acute stress and after d-amphetamine by natural inhibition of monoamine oxidase: An hypothesis. In Costa E, Garattini S (eds.), Amphetamines and Related Compounds. New York: Raven Press.

Welsch CW, Meites J (1970) Effects of reserpine on development of 7,12-dimethyl-benzanthracene-induced mammary tumors in female rats. Experentia 26:1133-1134.

Wick MM (1977) L-dopa methyl ester as a new antitumor agent. Nature 269:512-513.

Wick MM (1978) L-dopa methyl ester: Prolongation of survival of neuroblastoma-bearing mice after treatment. Science 199:775-776(a).

Wick MM (1978) Dopamine: A novel antitumor agent active against B-16 melanoma in vivo. J Invest Dermatol 71:163-164(b).

Wick MM (1979) Levodopa and dopamine analogs: Melanin precursors as antitumor agents in experimental human and murine leukemia. Cancer Treat Rep 63:991-997.

Wimer RE, Norman R, Eleftheriou E (1973) Serotonin levels in hippocampus: Striking variations associated with mouse strain and treatment. Brain Res 63:397-401.

Zajaczkowska MN (1975) Acetylcholine content in the central and peripheral nervous system and its synthesis in the rat brain during stress and post stress exhaustion. Acta Physiol Pol 26:493-497.

# THE ROLE OF BRAIN AND THE NEUROENDOCRINE SYSTEM IN IMMUNE REGULATION-POTENTIAL LINKS TO NEOPLASTIC DISEASES

Marvin Stein, M.D., Steven E. Keller, Ph.D., Steven J. Schleifer, M.D.

Mount Sinai School of Medicine, Department of Psychiatry, 1 Gustave L. Levy Place, New York, New York 10029.

## INTRODUCTION

Numerous studies have suggested that psychological factors contribute to the course and development of cancer. Stressful life experiences, particularly experiences of separation and loss, are reported to frequently precede the clinical onset of various neoplasias (Le Shan, 1959), particularly cancer of the cervix (Paloucek and Graham, 1959), leukemia and lymphoma (Greene, 1966). While a relationship between life experience and onset of cancer of the breast (Schonfield, 1975; Muslin et al, 1966) or bladder (Pond, 1977) has not been demonstrated, associations have been found between life events and both benign breast disease (Schonfield, 1975) and benign prostatic hypertrophy (Pond, 1977).

Psychological states have also been related to cancer onset. Schmale and Iker (1966) found that women who had reacted to life stress with feelings of hopelessness were more likely to have positive cone biopsies for cervical cancer. Breakdown in coping has also been associated with findings of malignancy following breast biopsy (Katz et al., 1970). Prospective studies have found that subjects scoring high on scales associated with depressive mood were at higher risk for the subsequent development of cancer (Hagnell, 1966; Shekelle et al., 1981), although findings in studies attempting to relate clinical depression and cancer risk have been primarily negative (Kerr, 1969; Malzberg, 1950; Odegaard, 1952; Niemi and Jaaskelainen, 1978).

Other personality traits have been related to cancer susceptibility. Kissen and co-workers (1964, 1967; Kissen and LeShan, 1964) have repeatedly observed that patients with lung cancer have a more restricted ability for emotional discharge than patients without cancer. Thomas and Greenstreet (1973), in a thirty year prospective study of medical students, similarly found that individuals who later developed cancer tended not to readily express emotions. Greer and Morris (1975) found that extreme suppression of emotions, particularly anger, as well as extreme expression of emotions was characteristic of women presenting for breast biospy who subsequently were found to have malignancies. Bahnson and Bahnson (1969) have noted excessive utilization of the defenses of denial and repression in cancer patients. The personality trait of extraversion has also been found to be associated with cancer (Coppen and Metcalfe, 1963; Hagnell, 1966).

Clinical studies such as these suggest that psychosocial factors are associated with the onset of some malignancies. These observations are supported by a variety of experimental studies. Differential housing, restraint and sex-segregated groupings have been found to modify the incidence of sarcomas (Amkraut and Solomon, 1972), mammary carcinomas (Newberry et al, 1976; Henry, et al. 1975), and leukemia (Ebbeson and Rask-Nielsen, 1967) in mice. Chronic handling stress reduces the latency for development of maternally transmitted mammary tumors in mice (Riley, 1975) and infantile stimulation has been found to modify the course of Walker-256 sarcomas in rats (Ader and Friedman, 1965) as well as the survival of mice after transplantation of lymphoid leukemia (Levine and Cohen, 1959). Sklar and Anisman (1979) have shown that a psychological state can modify a stress induced increase in tumor growth in rats.

The evidence suggesting a causal link between psychosocial factors and the development of neoplasia has led to much speculation concerning the nature of the biological processes which may be involved. Immune function is one of many factors which could play a role in the mediation of psychosocial influences on cancer susceptibility and outcome (Fox, 1978). Altered immunity has long been implicated in the pathogenesis of cancer and both cell mediated and humoral immune responses may be involved in the etiology and course of neoplasia (Baldwin, 1973; Levy and Wheelock, 1974; Stutman, 1975). A decrease in cell mediated immune function may permit neoplastic cells to proliferate and thereby enhance tumor growth. On the other hand, alterations in B cell function may result in the production of blocking antibodies and, thus, protect tumors from host defenses.

A number of studies have demonstrated associations between psychological factors and both cell mediated and humoral immune function. In man, exposure to stressors such as one or two month space flights (Kimzey et al., 1976), 48 hour sleep deprivation (Palmblad et al., 1979), running a marathon (Eskola et al., 1978), or bereavement (Bartrop et al., 1977; Schleifer et al., 1980) has been associated with altered lymphocyte activity. Life stress has also been associated with altered immunoglobulin levels (Fessel, 1962). Personality factors may also be associated with immune function. For example, a subgroup of women with breast disease who tended to suppress anger had higher levels of IgA than those who did not (Pettingale et al., 1977).

In animals, changes in humoral immunity, measured by the reduced or increased production of specific antibody, has been described following various stressors in mice (Hill et al., 1967), rats (Solomon, 1969), rabbits (Medunitsyn, 1960), dogs and baboons (Petrovskii, 1961). Stress effects on cellular immune function were reported by Monjan and Collector (1977) who provided evidence that both B and T lymphocyte function may be altered in mice exposed to sound stress. We have demonstrated (Keller et al., 1981) that lymphocyte stimulation by the T cell mitogen, phytohemagglutinin, in the rat can be suppressed by electric shock.

In summary, there is considerable evidence suggesting that psychosocial factors may play a role in the development and course of neoplasia, effects which may be associated with altered immunity. This chapter will review studies concerned with the role of the brain in the regulation of immune function. Immune modulation by the central nervous system (CNS) may provide a link between psychological state, immune function, and the development of pathological states such as neoplasias.

## BRAIN EFFECTS ON HUMORAL IMMUNITY

Systematic investigation of the relationship between the brain and immune function was initiated in a series of studies concerned with the effects of brain lesions on lethal anaphylaxis. In 1958, Freedman and Fenichel (1958) reported that bilateral midbrain lesions in the guinea pig inhibited anaphylactic death. In the same year, Szentivanyi and Filipp (1958) demonstrated that lethal anaphylactic shock in the guinea pig and in the rabbit can be prevented by bilateral focal lesions in the tuberal region of the hypothalamus. The hypothalamus is an area of the brain of particular interest for the study of CNS and immune relationships due to its critical role in the regulation of a wide range of peripheral functions including endocrine, neurotransmitter and visceral processes, and behavior. Endocrine and neurotransmitter activity, in turn, may participate in the modulation of immune processes.

In our initial studies, Luparello et al. (1964) found that anterior but not posterior hypothalamic lesions inhibited development of lethal anaphylaxis in the rat. Further studies in our laboratory investigated the effect of hypothalamic lesions on guinea pig anaphylaxis (Macris et al., 1970). Bilateral electrolytic lesions were placed in the anterior, median, or

151

posterior basal hypothalamus of male Hartley strain guinea pigs (Figure 1).
Anterior hypothalamic lesions damaged the anterior hypothalamic region and the
suprachiasmatic nuclei, with the lesions impinging, in some animals, on the
preoptic area and on the rostral portion of the ventromedial nuclei. Median
hypothalamic lesions damaged the ventromedial nuclei and the arcuate nuclei.
Posterior hypothalamic lesions resulted in damage to the premammillary region
and to the medial mammillary nuclei. Controls included sham-operated and
unoperated animals. Each group was senzitized with picryl chloride, a hapten
or incomplete antigen, in Freund's adjuvant, 1 week after operation.
Circulating antibodies to the picryl hapten were determined and picryl-induced
anaphylaxis was studied.

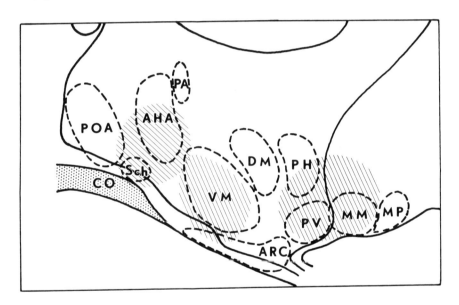

Fig. 1. Sagittal diagram of guinea pig hypothalamus. Lightly shaded areas
correspond to regions damaged by lesions. (reprinted with permission from
Macris NT, Schiavi RC, Camerino MS, and Stein M (1970) Effect of hypothalamic
lesions on immune processes in the guinea pig. Am. J. Physiol. 219:
1205-1209.)

Significant protection against lethal anaphylaxis was found in the animals with electrolytic lesions in the anterior hypothalamus. Lethal anaphylaxis occurred in 71 percent of control animals and in only 19 percent of the guinea pigs with anterior hypothalamic lesions. The median and posterior hypothalamic lesions had no significant effect on lethal anaphylaxis (Macris et al., 1970).

Anterior hypothalamic lesions in the guinea pig were also found to protect against anaphylactic death using ovalbumin as the antigen (Schiavi et al., 1975). Among sensitized sham-operated guinea pigs challenged with 0.25, 0.5, and 1.5 mg of ovalbumin, 17, 25, and 73 percent of the animals suffered anaphylactic death. In contrast, among the animals with anterior hypothalamic lesions, no deaths occurred with the two lower doses of antigen and only 36 percent of the animals injected with 1.5 mg of ovalbumin died.

While these studies indicate that antigen induced anaphylaxis may be modified by hypothalamic lesions, a major question has been concerned with the nature of this effect. Modification of anaphylaxis could be related to altered humoral immunity, to non-immune changes in tissue production of mediators of anaphylaxis, to altered target organ responsivity, or to a combination of effects.

Several investigators have attempted to demonstrate changes in the levels of circulating antibodies following brain lesions. Filipp and Szentivanyi (1958) reported reduced circulating and tissue-fixed antibodies in tuber-injured guinea pigs. Korneva and Khai (1964) found that lesions in the posterior hypothalamus, but not in other areas of the diencephalon, completely suppressed the production of complement-fixing antibodies to horse serum in rabbits. Stimulation of the posterior hypothalamus resulted in enhanced antibody titers (Korneva, 1976). Jankovic and Isakovic (1973) reported lower bovine serum albumin antibody levels in rats with bilateral lesions in either the hypothalamus or the reticular formation. Other investigators have also found changes in antibody levels with medial and posterior hypothalamic manipulations (Polyak et al., 1969; Tsypin and Maltsev, 1967). In addition, posterior hypothalamic lesions in young rats were reported to be associated with subsequent depressed humoral immunity in mature animals (Paunovic et al., 1976). Anterior hypothalamic lesions may also influence antibody production. We (Marcis et al., 1970) found that anterior hypothalamic lesions in the guinea pig were associated with significantly lower antibody titers to the hapten picryl chloride. Lesions in other areas of the hypothalamus did not alter antibody levels. Tyrey and Nalbandov (1972) reported that ovalbumin antibody production was depressed in rats with anterior hypothalamic lesions.

Other studies have found no changes in antibody levels in lesioned animals. Ado and Goldstein (1973) reported that anterior, medial, and posterior hypothalamic lesions in rabbits had no effect on the titer of complement binding and hemagglutinating antibodies to ovalbumin. Thrasher et al. (1971) reported similar negative findings with ovalbumin in the rat. In our laboratory, we observed no difference in ovalbumin titers between sham-operated guinea pigs and animals protected against anaphylactic death by anterior hypothalamic lesions (Schiavi et al., 1975).

The variability in the findings with respect to the effect of hypothalamic lesions on antibody levels may result from the heterogeneity of the study designs. Hypothalamic lesions may affect some components of humoral immunity and only under certain conditions of sensitization and challenge. Antibody studies have utilized different animal species, a wide range of sensitizing and test doses, variable time schedules, and different antigens. For example, differences were found by our group between studies using picryl chloride and those using ovalbumin. In these studies, antibody titers were assessed 7 days after exposure to booster doses of picryl chloride while 20 days elapsed between sensitization and assessment of ovalbumin antibody levels. Similarly, studies which have found depressed antibody levels following hypothalamic lesions, including studies with ovalbumin (Tyrey and Nalbandov, 1972), have found that the differences obtained were most marked during the first 10 days following sensitization, diminishing thereafter (Tyrey and Nalbandov, 1972; Jankovic and Isakovic, 1973; Isakovic and Jankovic, 1973). Time effects, however, do not fully explain the lack of change in ovalbumin titers since both Ado and Goldstein (1973) and Thrasher et al. (1971) found no differences in ovalbumin antibody levels in lesioned animals during the first 10 days after sensitization. Differences between the type of immune responses elicited could also explain differences in the two studies from our laboratory. Antibody production to the hapten picryl chloride is dependent upon recognition by T lymphocytes while ovalbumin does not require carrier recognition.

While the hypothalamus may influence certain aspects of antibody production, it has also been demonstrated that lesion-induced changes in circulating antibody levels are not required for the protective effect of hypothalamic lesions in anaphylaxis. In studies of passive anaphyalxis, animals are immunized by providing them with sufficient exogenous antibody to produce lethal anaphylaxis. Szentivanyi and Filipp (1958) reported that guinea pigs passively sensitized with homologous as well as with heterologous (rabbit) serum were protected from anaphylactic death by hypothalamic lesions. Our group (Macris et al., 1972) found significant protection against lethal anaphylaxis in guinea pigs passively immunized with heterologous (rabbit) antibody to ovalbumin after placement of anterior but not posterior hypothalamic lesions. These findings led to a series of studies investigating the effect of hypothalamic lesions on target tissue responsivity and mediator release in the course of anaphylaxis.

Studies from our laboratory have shown that anterior hypothalamic lesions do not alter tissue responsivity when ileum and skin are the target organs (Schiavi et al., 1975). Antigen-induced contraction of isolated ileum from animals actively sensitized with ovalbumin and of ileum from nonimmunized animals, passively sensitized in vitro, was investigated. Anterior hypothalamic lesions of size and location comparable to those providing protection against lethal anaphylaxis did not modify the anaphylactic response of ileum from actively sensitized guinea pigs or from isolated ileum passively sensitized in vitro. In passive cutaneous anaphylaxis studies, there were significant differences in the cutaneous anaphylactic responses to ovalbumin between lesioned animals and sham and non-operated controls 18 hours after intradermal passive sensitization. Thrasher et al. (1971) similarly reported that anterior, medial, and posterior hypothalamic lesions in the rat had no effect on passive cutaneous anaphylaxis to ovalbumin 4 hours after sensitization.

The findings in these studies do not support the hypothesis that the protective effect of anterior hypothalamic lesions in the guinea pig is due to impairment of antibody binding capacity or due to interference with the intracellular processes responsible for the release of histamine or other mediators of anaphylaxis. However, bronchial and bronchiolar smooth muscle, the primary shock organ in the guinea pig, have yet to be studied using this experimental paradigm.

Several studies have suggested that hypothalamic lesions may alter both the release of mediators of anaphylaxis and target organ responses to these agents. Mathe and his co-workers found that the release of prostaglandin $PGF_{2a}$ following anterior hypothalamic lesions was significantly reduced during ovalbumin induced anaphylaxis in the guinea pig as compared to control, sham, and posterior lesioned animals (Mathe et al., 1978). Several investigators have reported that the CNS modifies the susceptibility of animals to histamine, a primary mediator of anaphylaxis in the guinea pig (Przybylski, 1962; Whittier and Orr, 1962). Szentivanyi and Szekely (1958) found that lesions in the tuberal region of the guinea pig hypothalamus provided protection against lethal histamine shock. We have reported (Schiavi et al., 1966) that lesions in the anterior but not the posterior medial hypothalamus of guinea pigs afforded significant protection against histamine toxicity.

Lesion effects on the bronchospastic reaction may be related to vagal parasympathetic activity which may play an important role in the mediation of the physiological changes observed during anaphylaxis (Gold, 1973; Gold et al., 1972; Koller, 1968; Mills and Widdicombe, 1970; Parker, 1973). Damage to the region of the anterior hypothalamus, which is thought to mediate primarily parasympathetic responses, may decrease vagal bronchoconstrictor tone, resulting in the predominance of bronchial $\beta$-adrenergic activity. In keeping with this hypothesis, both vagal suppression and $\beta$-adrenergic enhancement reduce bronchospastic responses. Inhibition of vagal activity (Hexheimer, 1956; Widdicombe, 1963) or $\beta$-adrenergic stimulation (Aviado, 1970) decreases histamine-induced bronchoconstriction while blockade of $\beta$-receptors potentiates the histamine effect (McCulloch et al., 1967). Filipp (1972) has reported that propranolol and pertussis vaccine, both $\beta$-receptor blockers, diminish the protective effect of tuberal hypothalamic lesions in guinea pig anaphylaxis. Maslinski and Karczewski (1957) found similarly that reduced guinea pig anaphylaxis following stimulation of the temporal lobes was accompanied by a depression of vagal activity.

These studies suggest that tissue responses in the lung may be altered by hypothalamic lesions. The role of altered immunity in the hypothalamic modulation of anaphylaxis remained to be established. We have recently completed a study to determine if changes in immune function or tissue responses play a role in the protective effect of anterior hypothalamic lesions on guinea pig anaphylaxis. In this study, animals were sensitized to ovalbumin 21 days prior to placement of bilateral anterior hypothalamic lesions and subjected to anaphylactic challenge either 7 or 28 days following the stereotactic procedure. No differences were found between lesion, sham operated, or non-operated animals in the incidence of lethal anaphylaxis or in the severity of anaphylaxis in surviving animals. These findings suggest that the protective effect of anterior hypothalamic lesions found in our previous studies may be related to altered antigen sensitization following the placement of lesions and cannot be explained on the basis of target tissue responsivity. These findings appear to differ from those of Filipp and Mess (1969) who found that lesions in the tuberal region of the guinea pig hypothalamus placed 10 days after sensitization with horse serum afforded protection against anaphylactic challenge 21 days thereafter. It may be, however, that lesions placed 10 days after the initiation of sensitization may still affect the sensitization process.

Anaphylaxis has been utilized as a model to study the effect of the hypothalamus on the humoral immune response. The above review indicates that anterior hypothalamic lesions inhibit lethal anaphylactic shock in the guinea pig. The effects of hypothalamic lesions on anaphylaxis could be explained by changes in the immune system or by changes in tissue factors and target organ responsivity. Studies investigating the influence of hypothalamic lesions on antibody levels have been inconclusive but prior sensitization studies suggest that altered antigen sensitization may play a primary role in the effect of hypothalamic lesions on lethal anaphylaxis. In addition, however, hypothalamic lesions may diminish the responsivity of the lung, the target organ in guinea pig anaphylaxis, to the pharmacologic agents liberated by the antigen-antibody reaction. The modification of target organ responses may be related to changes in autonomic nervous system function.

Studies by Besedovsky and Sorkin (1977) have provided further evidence of a specific relationship between the hypothalamus and humoral immunity. These investigators found an increase in the firing rate of neurons in the ventromedial nuclei of the hypothalamus in rats after immunization with two different antigens. These results suggest the presence of a feedback loop between the immune response and the hypothalamus.

## BRAIN EFFECTS ON CELL-MEDIATED IMMUNITY

Cell mediated immune function is of particular importance in the control of neoplasia. The role of the brain in cell-mediated immunity has only recently become a focus of research. In 1970, we (Marcis et al., 1970) reported that anterior hypothalamic lesions in the guinea pig suppressed the delayed cutaneous hypersensitivity response to picryl chloride and to tuberculin. Median and posterior hypothalamic lesions did not alter the response. Jankovic and Isakovic (1973) reported that a lesion involving a large part of the hypothalamus in the rat resulted in a decreased delayed cutaneous response to bovine serum albumin. Hypothalamic stimulation was subsequently found to enhance the delayed cutaneous hypersensitivity response (Jankovic et al., 1979). These studies of hypothalamic effects on delayed cutaneous hypersensitivity suggest that the hypothalamus may modulate aspects of cell-mediated immunity.

We have recently investigated the effect of anterior hypothalamic lesions in the guinea pig on lymphocyte function utilizing in vitro correlates of cell-mediated immunity (Keller et al., 1980). Lymphocyte stimulation by the mitogen phytohemaglutinin (PHA) (a nonspecific T cell activator) and by the antigen tuberculin purified protein derivative (PPD) was studied following anterior hypothalamic lesions. The number of T and B lymphocytes was also determined. In addition, the effect of anterior hypothalamic lesions on delayed cutaneous hypersensitivity to tuberculin was investigated. As in previous studies, bilateral electrolytic lesions were placed in the anterior hypothalamus of male Hartley strain guinea pigs. Sham-operated and unoperated animals served as controls. One week postoperatively, the guinea pigs were sensitized to tuberculin by injection of complete Freund's adjuvant. Skin reactions were elicited 32 days following sensitization by intradermal injection of PPD and the delayed cutaneous response was measured at 24 hours. The guinea pigs with anterior hypothalamic lesions had significantly smaller cutaneous tuberculin reactions than the nonoperated or sham-operated controls while the response of the control groups did not differ significantly.

One week after skin tests were measured, aliquots of blood from each animal were used for the in vitro studies. No differences were found in the total number of white blood cells or in the total number of lymphocytes among the various groups. The percentage and absolute number of T and B cells were not significantly changed by the hypothalamic lesions.

160

Lymphocyte function was measured by means of in vitro lymphocyte stimulation assays using whole blood and using isolated lymphocytes. Dose response curves were determined for the antigen PPD and for the mitogen PHA. The response to lymphocyte stimulation was measured by the incorporation of $^{125}$IUdR. All lymphocyte stimulation results were expressed as counts per minute (cpm) in stimulated cultures minus the cpm in unstimulated cultures ($\Delta$ cpm).

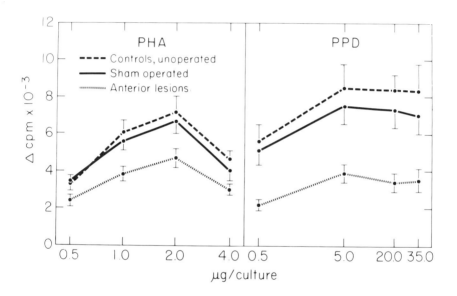

Fig. 2. In vitro whole blood lymphocyte stimulation with PHA and with PPD in unoperated control, sham operated, and anterior hypothalamic lesioned guinea pigs. Values are expressed as $\Delta$ cpm (mean ± standard error) (reprinted with permission from Keller SE, Stein M, Camerino MS, Schleifer SJ, and Sherman J (1980) Suppression of lymphocyte stimulation by anterior hypothalamic lesions in the guinea pig. Cellular Immunology, 52: 332-340.)

The lymphocyte stimulation data for PHA and PPD utilizing the whole blood technique are illustrated in Figure 2. Analysis of variance for repeated measures revealed that there were significant differences among the groups for both PHA and PPD. Multiple comparison tests showed that the responses of anterior hypothalamic lesioned guinea pigs to both PHA and to PPD were significantly lower than those of the nonoperated or of the sham-operated controls. The two control groups did not differ significantly for either PHA or PPD.

The dose response curves for PHA and PPD with the isolated lymphocyte cultures are shown in Figure 3. No significant differences were found among the groups for PHA or for PPD.

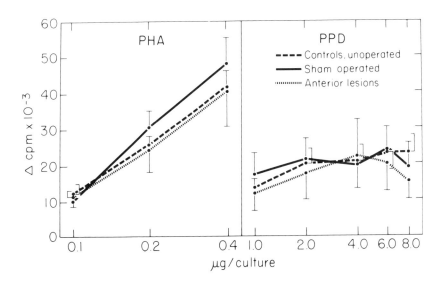

Fig. 3. In vitro isolated lymphocyte stimulation with PHA and with PPD in unoperated control, sham operated, and anterior hypothalamic lesioned guinea pigs. Values are expressed as $\Delta$ cpm (mean ± standard error) (reprinted with permission from Keller SE, Stein M, Camerino MS, Schleifer SJ, and Sherman J (1980) Suppression of lymphocyte stimulation by anterior hypothalamic lesions in the guinea pig. Cellular Immunology, 52: 332-340.)

162

The findings that anterior hypothalamic lesions suppress in vitro lymphocyte stimulation by the antigen PPD and by the mitogen PHA in whole blood cultures demonstrated that the hypothalamus can directly influence lymphocyte function. This effect did not appear to be related to a depletion of T lymphocytes. The lack of effect of anterior hypothalamic lesions on the isolated lymphocyte response to PPD further suggests that the lesions do not impair the primary acquisition of immunity to an antigen but rather modify the efferent limb of the cell-mediated immune system. The inhibition of both PHA- and PPD-induced lymphocyte stimulation in whole blood but not in isolated lymphocyte cultures in the anterior hypothalamic lesioned guinea pigs suggests that the modulating effect of anterior hypothalamic lesions may be related to humoral factors. A humoral inhibitory factor may be associated with neuroendocrine or autonomic processes since the hypothalamus is involved in the regulation of these functions (Martin et al., 1977; Porter, 1962; Reichlin et al., 1978). Depletion of a humoral growth factor could also explain the findings.

Lymphocyte responses to mitogens and antigens have been reported to be influenced by other cells such as marcophages, monocytes, erythrocytes, and platelets (Bach and Hirschhorn, 1965; Ferguson et al., 1976). Lymphocyte isolation procedures remove or alter the number of such cell types. The inhibition of lymphocyte stimulation in whole blood but not in isolated lymphocyte cultures of lesioned guinea pigs could be related to changes in these cell populations.

Cross et al (1980) recently studied cell mediated immune function in the rat. Animals with bilateral anterior hypothalamic lesions were compared with two groups of surgical controls 4 to 14 days after the surgical procedure. Both lymphocyte and spleen cell numbers were found to be lower in the animals with hypothalamic lesions 4 days following the procedure but did not differ 14 days after the procedure. Similarly, the response of spleen cell suspensions to Conconavalin A, a mitogen with both B and T cell activating properties, was suppressed 4 days after placement of the hypothalamic lesions but not at 7 or 14 days. These findings suggest that anterior hypothalamic lesions induce a short term suppression in the number of lymphoid cells which may then be reflected in a concomitant reduction in lymphocyte stimulation. This phenomenon appears to reflect a second, perhaps unrelated, lymphocyte effect of anterior hypothalamic lesions distinct from our findings of suppressed peripheral lymphocyte responses in guinea pigs 46 days following the placement of lesions. In our studies, suppression of total lymphocytes, T or B cells did not explain the suppressed responses (Keller et al., 1980).

A series of clinical studies utilizing patients with primary intracranial tumors have provided further evidence of brain effects on cell mediated immunity. Brooks et al. (1972) studied 23 patients with benign and malignant primary intracranial neoplasms who showed no evidence of significant weight loss, anemia, granulocytopenia, or lymphopenia. In contrast to 20 healthy hospital employees, patients with brain tumors showed diminished delayed cutaneous hypersensitivity to common skin test antigens. In addition, over two-thirds of the patients, in contrast to none of the controls, could not be sensitized to dinitrochlorobenzene (DNCB), a T cell antigen. Parallel findings were obtained with in vitro lymphocyte stimulation responses to antigens using a washed leukocyte assay. The investigators were able to identify a humoral factor, associated with the IgG fraction in the patients' sera, which inhibited lymphocyte stimulation both with PHA and in mixed lymphocyte cultures using lymphocytes from both patients and controls. In subsequent studies (Roszman and Brooks, 1981), the investigators demonstrated diminished PHA responsiveness using isolated peripheral lymphocytes from patients with malignant primary intracranial neoplasms and provided evidence for a qualitative lymphocyte abnormality in these patients.

While clinical studies of patients with neoplastic disorders are not readily comparable to experimental manipulation of otherwise healthy laboratory animals, both types of studies provide evidence for a link between the brain and cellular immune function which can be demonstrated both in vivo, with suppressed delayed cutaneous hypersensitivity, and in vitro, with evidence of altered lymphocyte function.

## MEDIATION OF BRAIN EFFECTS ON IMMUNE FUNCTION

Investigation of possible mechanisms of brain effects on immune function have focused on the hypothalamus with particular emphasis on the neuroendocrine axis. Hypophysectomy can depress both antibody production and delayed cutaneous hypersensitivity in rats (Nagy and Berczi, 1978). The studies of Filipp and Mess (1969) suggest that the protective effect of hypothalamic lesions on anaphylaxis may be related, at least in part, to changes in endocrine function. They found that thyroxine partially restored the sensitivity to anaphylaxis of actively immunized guinea pigs with tuberal hypothalamic lesions. They also reported that thyroxine together with metopirone, an inhibitor of adrenocortical hormone synthesis, completely abolished the protective action of the lesions, suggesting that the antianaphylactic effect of hypothalamic damage is due to the combined effect of decreased thyroid function and increase adrenocortical activity. Other studies have demonstrated the role of the thyroid in enhancing immune processes in the rat, mouse, and guinea pig (Denckla, 1978; Leger and Masson,

1947; Nilzen, 1955). Suppression of thyroid activity inhibits local and systemic anaphylaxis, abolishes circulating precipitins, and decreases the susceptibility of the animals to exogenous histamine.

Changes in corticosteroid levels may have a major role in the mediation of the effects of the hypothalamus on immunity. Tyrey and Nalbandov (1972) found that the antibody titer depression in the rat that follows anterior hypothalamic lesions can be significantly blocked by either hypophysectomy or adrenalectomy. Corticosteroid effects on the immune system are extensive and complex. Pharmacologic doses of corticosteroids have been shown to suppress primary and secondary antibody formation (Elliot and Sinclair, 1968; Petranyi et al., 1971), modify complement levels, protect against anaphylactic shock (Dews and Code, 1951), delay or prevent graft rejection, enhance tumor growth, control autoimmune disease, and increase the incidence and severity of bacterial infections. Both physiological and pharmacologic doses of corticoids diminish lymphocyte stimulation by PHA in vitro (Berenbaum et al., 1973; 1976; Fauci, 1975; Goodwin et al., 1979). Physiological doses of corticosteroids have been reported to enhance T-cell development (Ritter, 1977) and B-cell lymphocyte stimulation by pokeweed mitogen (Fauci et al., 1977). Physiological doses of corticoids also result in a redistribution of T cells from the circulating pool to the bone marrow (Claman, 1975; Fauci and Dale, 1975).

Aside from their direct effects on immune function, adrenocortical hormones may also alter immune phenomena such as anaphylaxis by means of their profound effects on the metabolism and actions of histamine. Corticosteroids inhibit histamine decarboxylase activity (Parrot and Laborde, 1955), tissue binding of newly formed histamine (Schayer et al., 1955), and the amount of histamine released by the tissues (Schmutzler and Freundt, 1975; Yamasaki and Yamamoto,

1963). Corticosteroid effects on histamine may further influence immune function since histamine itself has been shown to modulate lymphocyte activity (Goodwin et al., 1979; Roszkowski et al., 1977).

A number of other hormones which are regulated by the hypothalamus influence immune processes. Growth hormone (Brown and Reichlin, 1972; Rice et al., 1978; Alpert et al., 1976) appears to have an enhancing effect on the immune system. Gisler (1974) found that GH reversed the immunosuppressive effects of corticosteroids in the plaque-forming cell assay, a measure of humoral immunity. Growth hormone also enhances graft rejection (Comsa et al., 1975) and is required for the development of the immune system (Denckla, 1978). Sex hormones generally have an inhibitory effect on immune response. Estrogen, testosterone, and progesterone have all been found to inhibit lymphocyte stimulation (Mendelsohn et al., 1977; Wyle and Kent, 1977). Androgens and estrogens can suppress delayed cutaneous hypersensitivity (Kappas et al., 1963) and gonadectomy in male and female guinea pigs may enhance cell-mediated immune responses (Kittas and Henry, 1979). In contrast, estrogens may increase antibody responses to antigens (Eidinger and Garrett, 1972; Thanavala et al., 1973).

Endocrine modulation of immune function may result from the interaction of hormones. As previously noted, thyroid or growth hormone and corticosteroids may have antagonistic effects on immune function (Filipp and Mess, 1969; Gisler, 1974). Denckla (1978) reported that thyroxine, together with growth hormone, restored immunocompetence to immunologically deficient animals. A study by Pierpaoli and Maestroni (1978) showed that a specific combination of LH, FSH, and ACTH inhibits a blockade of antibody production produced by an alteration in neurotransmitter function.

Temporal factors may play an important role in hypothalamic effects on immune function. Circadian rhythms have been described for humoral and cell-mediated immune processes including immediate cutaneous hypersensitivity (Reinberg et al., 1965), resistance to infection (Feigin et al., 1969) and lymphocyte stimulation by PHA (Dionigi et al., 1973). A number of studies have demonstrated that anterior hypothalamic lesions alter or abolish the pattern of corticosteroid and thyroid hormone secretion (Abe et al., 1979; Moore and Eichler, 1972; Rice et al., 1978). The effects of anterior hypothalamic lesions on immune function may, therefore, be mediated, in part, by alterations in hormonal circadian rhythms.

In addition to the previously described effects on target tissues, the autonomic nervous system may also be involved in the mediation of hypothalamic influences on immune activity by direct effects on immunocompetent cells. Chemical sympathectomy has been associated with altered immune function (Kasahara et al., 1977; Williams et al., 1980). A number of studies have found that β-adrenergic stimulation is immunosuppressive, whereas β-blockade enhances immune function. Isoproterenol, a β-adrenergic agonist, decreases antigen-specific cutaneous hypersensitivity (Kram et al., 1975; Shereff et al., 1973), inhibits T-cell rosette formation (Galant and Remo, 1975), decreases immunoglobulin production (Sherman et al., 1973) and inhibits mitogen-induced lymphocyte stimulation at physiological doses (Goodwin et al., 1979; Smith et al., 1971). Propranolol, a β-antagonist, increases immediate cutaneous hypersensitivity (Shereff et al., 1973) and increases immunoglobulin production (Nakazawa et al., 1977), consistent with the general finding that β-adrenergic activity inhibits immune function. In contrast to these findings, Patterson et al. (1976) reported that isoproterenol increases in vitro IgE production.

168

Pierpaoli and Maestroni (1978) have suggested that neurotransmitters may interact in the modulation of immune function. The combination of an α-adrenergic antagonist, a serotonin precursor, and a dopamine blocker administered prior to exposure to an antigen was found to block antibody production completely and specifically. As previously noted, the combination of LH, FSH, and ACTH reversed the blockade.

The regulation of lymphocyte activity by hormones and catecholamines may be related to their ability to influence cellular cyclic nucleotide levels. Many studies have found that elevated cAMP levels can inhibit immune function while decreased levels enhance immune activity (Ferreira et al., 1976; Galant and Remo, 1975; Schmultzler and Derwall, 1973). Recently Watson (1975) and Ohara et al. (1978) have suggested that the ratio of cAMP to cGMP is important for the control of antibody synthesis, whereas the absolute concentration of cAMP is not critical. Kasahara et al. (1977) and Wang et al. (1978) found that, aside from its usual immunosuppressive effects, cAMP may be required to initiate lymphocyte responses. A biphasic cAMP pattern appears to be necessary, with an initial rise followed by a subsequent fall in cAMP levels.

CONCLUSION

The brain, and in particular the hypothalamus, modifies both humoral and cell-mediated immune processes. An extensive network of endocrine and autonomic processes may be involved in these effects. The multiple pathways linking limbic and higher cortical areas with the hypothalamus suggest that the hypothalamus may be of central importance in mediating psychosocial influences on endocrine, neurotransmitter and immune functions. Further research is required to determine if interactions among the hypothalamus, neuroendocrine and immune systems alter the development, onset, and course of neoplastic disorders.

REFERENCES

Abe K, Kroning J, Greer MA, Critchlow V, (1979). Effects of destruction of the suprachiasmatic nuclei on the circadian rhythms in plasma corticosterone, body temperature, feeding and plasma thyrotropin. Neuroendrocrinol 29:119-131.
Ader R, Friedman SB (1965). Differential early experiences and susceptibility to transplanted tumor in the rat. J Comp Physiol Psychol 59:361-364.
Ado A, Goldstein MM (1973). The primary immune response in rabbits after lesion of the different zones in the medical hypothalamus. Ann Alergy 31:585-589.
Amkraut A, Solomon GF (1972). Stress and murine sarcoma virus (Maloney) - induced tumors. Cancer Res 32:1428-1433.
Alpert LC, Brawer JR, Patel YC, Reichlin S (1976). Somatistatinergic neurons in anterior hypothalamus: Immunohistochmeical localization. Endocrinology 98:255-258.
Aviado DM (1970). Antiasthmatic action of sympathomimetics: A review of the literature on the bronchopulmonary effects. J Clin Pharmacol 10:217-221.
Bach FH, Hirschhorn K (1965). The in vitro immune response of peripheral blood lymphocytes. Semin Hematol 2:68.
Bahnson CB, Bahnson MB (1969). Role of ego defenses: Denial and repression in the etiology of malignant neoplasm. Ann NY Acad Sci 164:827-845.
Baldwin RW (1973). Immunological aspects of chemical carcinogensis. Adv Cancer Res 18:1-75.
Bartrop RW, Lazarus L, Luckhurst E, Kiloh LG (1977). Depressed lymphocyte function after bereavement. Lancet 1:834-836.
Berenbaum MD, Fluch PA, Hurst NP (1973). Depression of lymphocyte responses after surgical trauma. Brit J Exp Path 54:597-607.
Berenbaum MC, Cope WA, Bundick RA (1976). Synergistic effect of cortisol and prostanglandin E on the PHA response. Clin Exp Immunol 26:534-541.
Besedovsky H, Sorkin E (1977). Network of immuneneuroendrocrine interactions. Clin Exp Immunol 27:1-12.
Brooks WH, Netsky MG, Normansell DE, Horwitz DA (1972). Depressed cell mediated immunity in patients with primary intracranial tumors. J Exp Med 136:1631-1647.
Brown GM, Reichlin S (1972). Psychologic and neural regulation of growth hormone secretion. Psychosomat Med 34:45-61.
Claman HN (1975). How corticosteroids work. J Allerg Clin Immunol 55:145-151.
Comsa J, Leonhardt H, Schwartz JA (1975). Influence of the thymus-corticotrophin-growth hormone interaction on the rejection of skin allografts in the rat. Ann NY Acad Sci 249:387-401.
Coppen A, Metcalfe M (1963). Cancer and extraversion. Brit Med J 2:18-19.
Cross RJ, Markesbery WR, Brooks WH, Roszman TL (1980). Hypothalamic-immune interactions. The acute effect of anterior hypothalamic lesions on the immune response. Brain Res 196:79-87.
Denckla WD (1978). Interactions between age and neuroendocrine and immune systems. Fed Proc 37:1263-1266.
Dews PB, Code CF (1951). Effect of cortisone on anaphylactic shock in adrenalectomized rats. J Pharmacol Exp Therap 101:9.
Dionigi R, Zonta A, Albertario F, Galeazzi R, Bellinzonn G (1973). Cyclic variation in the response of lymphocytes to phytohemagglutinin in healthy individuals. Transplantation 16:550-557.
Ebbeson P, Rask-Nielsen R (1967). Influence of sex-segregated grouping and of innoculation with subcellular leukemic material on development of non-leukemic lesions in DBA/2, BALB/C and CBA mice. J Nat Cancer Inst 39:917-925.
Eidinger D, Garrett TJ (1972). Studies in the regulatory effects of the sex hormones on antibody formation and stem cell differentiation. J Exp Med 136:1098-1116.

Elliot EV, Sinclair NR (1968). Effect of cortisone acetate on 19S and 7S haemolysin antibody: A time course study. Immunol 15:643-652.

Eskola J, Ruuskanen O, Soppi E, Viljanen MK, Jarvinen M, Toivonen H, Kouvalainen K (1978). Effect of sport stress on lymphocyte transformation and antibody formation. Clin Esp Immunol 32:339-345.

Fauci AS, Dale DC (1975). The effect of hydrocortisone on the kinetics of normal human lymphocytes. Blood 46:235-243.

Fauci AS, Pratt KR, Whalen G (1977). Activation of human B lymphocytes IV. Regulatory effects of corticosteroids on the triggering signal in the plaque-forming cell response of human peripheral blood B lymphocytes to polyclonal activation. J Immunol 119:598-603.

Feigin RD, San Joaquin VH, Haymond MW, Wyatt RG (1969). Daily periodicity of the susceptibility of mice to pneumococcal infection. Nature 224:379-380.

Ferguson RM, Schmidtke JR, Simmons RL (1976). Inhibition of mitogen induced lymphocyte transformation by local anesthetics. J Immunol 116:627-634.

Ferreira GG, Massuda-Brascher HK, Javierre MQ, Sassine WA, Lima AO (1976) Rosette formation by human T and B lymphocytes in the presence of adrenergic and cholinergic drugs. Experientia 32:1594-1596.

Fessel WJ (1962). Mental stress, blood proteins, and the hypothalamus. Arch Gen Psychiat 7:427-435.

Filipp G (1973). Mechanism of suppressing anaphylaxis through electrolytic lesion of the tuberal region of the hypothalamus. Ann Allergy 31:272-278.

Filipp G, Mess B (1969). Role of the adrenocortical system in suppressing anaphylaxis after hypothalamic lesion. Ann Allergy 27:607-610.

Filipp g, Szentivanyi A (1958). Anaphylaxis and the nervous system. Part III Ann Allergy 16:306-311.

Fox BH, (1978). Premorbid psychological factors as related to cancer incidence. J Behav Med 1:45-133.

Freedman DX, Fenichel G (1958). Effect of midbrain lesion on experimental allergy. arch Neurol Psychiatry 79:164-169.

Galant SP, Remo RA (1975). B-adrenergic inhibition of human T lymphocyte rosettes. J Immunol 114:512-513.

Gisler (1974) Stress and the hormonal regulation of the immune response in mice. Psychother Psychosomat 23:197-208.

Gold WM, Kessler GS, Yu (1972) Role of vagus nerves in experimental asthma in allergic dogs. J appl Psysiol 33:719-725.

Gold WM (1973) Cholinergic pharmacology in asthma. In Austen KF, Lichtenstein LM, (eds.) Asthma Physiology, Immuno-Pharmacology and Treatment. Academic Press, p. 169, New York, New York.

Greene WA (1966) The psychosocial setting of the development of leukemia and lymphoma. Ann NY Acad Sci 129:794-806.

Greer S, Morris T (1975) Psychological attributes of women who develop breast cancer: A controlled study. J Psychosom Res 19:147-153.

Hagnell O (1966) The premorbid personality of persons who develop cancer in a total population investigated in 1947 and 1957. Ann NY Acad Sci 125:846-855.

Henry JP, Stephens PM, Watson FMC (1975) Force breeding, social disorder and mammary tumor formation in CBA/USC mouse colonies: A pilot study. Psychosom Med 37:277-283.

Hexheimer H (1956) Bronchoconstrictor agents and their antagonists in the intact guinea pig. Arch Intern Pharmacodyn 106:371-380.

Hill CW, Greer WE, Felsenfeld O (1967) Psychological stress, early response to foreign protein, and blood cortisol in vervets. Psychosom Med 29:279-283.

Isakovic K, Jankovic BD (1973) Neuro-endocrine correlates of immune response. Int Arch Allergy Appl Immunol 45:373-384.

Jankovic BD, Isakovic K (1973) Neuro-endocrine correlates of immune response. 1. Effects of brain lesions on antibody production, Arthus reactivity and delayed hypersensitivity in the rat. Int Arch Allergy Appl Immunol 45:360-372.

Jankovic BD, Jovanova K, Markovic BM (1979) Effect of hypothalamic stimulation on the immune reactions in the rat. Periodicum Biologorum 81:211-212.

Kappas A, Jones HEH, Roitt IM (1963) Effects of steriod sex hormones on immunological phenomena. Nature 198:902.

Kasahara K, Tanaka S, Hamashima Y (1977) Suppressed immune response to T-cell dependent antigen in chemically sympathectomised mice. Res Comm in Chem Path and Pharm 16:687-694.

Katz JL, Weiner H, Gallagher TF, Hellman L (1970) Stress, distress, and ego defenses. Arch Gen Psychiat 23:131-142.

Keller SE, Stein M, Camerino MS, Schleifer SJ, Sherman J (1980) Suppression of lymphocyte stimulation by anterior hypothalamic lesions in the guinea pig. Cellular Immunology 52:334-340.

Keller SE, Weiss JM, Schleifer SJ, Miller NE, Stein M (1981) Suppression of immunity by stress: Effect of a graded series of stressors on lymphocyte stimulation in the rat. Science 213:1397-1400.

Kerr TA, Schapira K, Roth M (1969) The relationship between premature death and affective disorders. Brit J Psychiatry 115:1277-1282.

Kimzey SL, Johnson PC, Ritzman SE, Mengel CE (1976) Hematology and immunology studies: The second manned skylab mission. Aviat Space Environ Med 47:383-390.

Kissen DM (1964) Relationship between lung cancer, cigarette smoking inhalation, and personality. Brit J Med Psychol 37:203.

Kissen DM, LeShan LL, eds. (1964) Psychosomatic aspects of neoplastic disease. Pitman, London.

Kittas C, Henry L (1979) Effect of sex hormones on the immune system of guinea-pigs and on the development of toxoplasmic lesions in non-lymphoid organs. Clin Exp Immunol 36:16-23.

Koller EA (1968) Atmung und kreislauf in anaphylaktisch-enasthma bronchiale des meerschweinchens. III. Die Lune veranderungen in asthmaanfall und die inspiratorische reaction. Helv Physiol Pharmac Acta 26:153-17.

Korneva EA (1976) Neurohumoral regulation of immunological hemeostasis. Fiziologa Cheloveka 2(3):469-481.

Korneva EA, Khai LM (1964) Effect of destruction of hypothalamic areas on immunogenesis. Fed Proc (Trans Supp) 23:88-92.

Kram J, Bourne H, Maibach H, Melmon K (1975) Cutaneous immediate hypersensitivity in man: Effects of systematically administered adrenergic drugs. J Allerg and Clin Immunol 36:387.

Leger J, Masson G (1947) Factors influencing an anaphylactoid reaction in the rat. Fed Proc 6:150-151.

LeShan L (1959) Psychological states as factors in the development of malignant disease: A critical review. J National Canc Inst 22:1-18.

Levine S, Cohen C (1959) Differential survival to leukemia as a function of infantile stimulation in DB A/Z mice. Proc Soc exp Biol Med 102:53-54.

Levy MH, Wheelock EF (1974) The role of macrophages in defense against neoplastic disease. Adv Cancer Res 20:131-163.

Luparello TJ, Stein M, Prk CD (1964) Effect of hypothalamic lesions on rat anaphylaxis. Am J Physiol 207:911-914.

Macris NT, Schiavi RC, Camerino MS, Stein M (1970) Effect of hypothalamic lesions on immune processes in the guinea pig. Am J Physiol 219:1205-1209.

Macris NY, Schiavi Rc, Camerino MS, Stein M (1972) Effect of hypothalamus on passive anaphylaxis in the guinea pig. Am J Physiol 222:1054-1057.

Malzberg B (1950) Mortality from cancer among patients with mental disease in New York civil state hospitals. Psychiat Q: Supplement 124.

Martin JB, Reichlin S, Brown GM (1977) Clinical Endocrinology FA Davis Company, Philadelphia.

Maslinski C, Karczewski W (1957) The protective influences of brain stimulation by electric currents on histamine shock in guinea pigs. Bull Acad Polon Sci 5:57-62.

Mathe AA, Yen SS, Sohn RJ, Kemper T (1978) Effect of hypothalamic lesions on anaphylatic release of PSs from guinea pig lung. Proc 7th Int Congress Pharmacol, Paris.

McCulloch MW, Proctor C, Rand MJ (1967) Evidence for an adrenergic homeostatic bronchodilator reflex mechanism. Eur J Pharmacol 2:214-223.

Medunitsyn MV (1960) Unspecific stimulation of the process of antibody formation. Zh Mikrobiol Epidemiol Immunobiol 31:132-135.

Mendelsohn J, Multer MM, Bernheim JL 91977) Inhibition of human lymphocyte stimulation by steroid hormones: Cytokinetic mechanisms. Clin Exp Immunol 27:127-134.

Mills JE, Widdicombe JG (1970) Role of the vagus nerves in anaphylaxis and histamine-induced bronchoconstriction in guinea pigs. Brit J Pharmacol 39:724-731.

Moore RY, Eichler VB (1972) Loss of a circadian adrenal corticosterone rhythm following suprachiasmatic lesions in the rats. Brain Res 42:201-206.

Muslin HL, Gyarfas K, Pieper WJ (1966) Separation experience and cancer of the breast. Ann NY Acad Sci 125:802-806.

Nagy E, Berczi I (1978) Immunodeficiency in hypophysectomized rats. Acta Endocrinologica 89:530-537.

Nakazawa H, Hobday J, Townley R, Chaperon E (1977) Effect of B-adrenergic blockage, Pertussis vaccine and Freund's adjuvant on reaginic antibody response in mice. Int Archs Allergy Appl Immun 53:197-205.

New berry BH, Gildow J, Wogan J, Reese RI (1976) Inhibition of Huggins tumors by forced restraint. Psychosom Med 38:155-162.

Niemi T, Jaaskelainen J (1978) Cancer morbidity in depressive persons. J Psychosom Res 22:117-120.

Nilzen A (1955) The influence of the thyroid gland on hypersensitivity reactions in animals. Acta Allergol 7:231-234.

Odegaard O (1952) The excess mortality of the insane. Acta Psychiat Scand 27:353-367.

Ohara J, Kishimoto T, Yamamura Y (1978) In vitro immune response of human peripheral lymphocytes. 3. Effect of anti- anti- antibody on PWM-induced increase of cyclic nucleotides in human B lymphocytes. J Immunol 121:2058-2096.

Palmblad J, Petrini B, Wasserman J, Akerstedt T (1979) Lymphocyte and granulocyte reactions during sleep deprivation, Psychosom Med 41:273-278.

Paloucek FB, Graham JB (1959) Precipitating factors in cancer of the cervix. Ann Cov Am Coll Surgeons.

Parker CW (1973) Adrenergic responsiveness in asthma. In KF Austen, LM Lichtenstein, (eds.), A thma Physiology, Immunopharmacology, and Treatment. pp. 185-210, Academic Press Inc, New York, New York.

Parrot JL, Laborde C (1955) Inhibition d'histidine-decarboxylase par la cortisone et par le salicylate de sodium. J Physiol 53:441-442.

Patterson R, Suszko IM, Metzger WJ, Roberts M (1976) In vitro production of IgE by human peripheral blood lymphocytes: Effect of choleratoxin and B-adrenergic stimulation. J Immunol 117:97-101.

Paunovic VR, Petrovic S, Jankovic BD (1976) Influence of early postnatal hypothalamic lesions on immune responses of adult rats. Periodicum Biologorum 78:50.

Petranyi Jr G, Bengzur M, Alfoldy P (1977) The effect of single large dose hydrocortisone treatment on IgM and IgG antibody production, morphological distribution of antibody producing cells and immunological memory. Immunology 21:151-158.

Petrovskii IN (1961) Problems of nervous control in immunity reactions II. The influence of experimental neuroses on immunity reactions. Zh Mikrobiol Epidemiol Immunobiol 32:63-69.

Pierpaoli W, Maestroni GJM (1978) Pharmacological control of the hormonally modulated immune response II. Blockade of antibody production by a combination of drugs acting on neuroendocrine functions. Its prevention by gonadotrophins and corticotrophin. Immunology 34:419-430.

Polyak AI, Rumbesht LM, Sinichkin AA (1969) Antibody synthesis following electroagulation on the posterior hypothalamic nucleus. Zh Microbiol Epidemiol Immunobiol 46(3):52-56.

Pond DA, Maratos J (1977) Psychosocial inter-relations of benign prostatic hypertrophy. J Psychom Res 21:201-206.

Porter JC (1962) Hypothalamic Peptide Hormones and Pituitary Regulation. Plenum Press, New York.

Przybylski A (1962) Effect of the removal of cortex cerebri and the quadrigeminal bodies region on histamine susceptibility of guinea pigs. Act Physiol Polon 13:535-541.

Reichlin S, Baldessarini RJ, Martin JB (1978) The Hypothalamus. Raven Press, New York.

Reinberg A, Sidi E, Ghata J (1965) Circadian reactivity rhythms of human skin to histamine or allergen and the adrenal cycle. Journal of Allergy 36:273-283.

Rice RW, Abe K, Critchlow V (1978) Abolition of plasma growth hormone response to stress and of the circadian rhythm in pituitary-adrenal function in female rats with preoptic-anterior hypothalamic lesions. Brain Research 148:129-141.

Riley V (1975) Mouse mammary tumors: Alteration of incidence as apparent function of stress. Science 189:465-467.

Ritter M (1977) Embryonic mouse thymocyte development enhancing effect of corticosterone at physiological levels. Immunol 33:241-246.

Roszkowski W, Plaut M, Lichtenstein LM (1977) Selective display of histamine receptors on lymphocytes. Science 195:683-685.

Roszman TL, Brooks WH (1980) Immunobiology of primary intracranial tumours III. Demonstration of a qualitative lymphocyte abnormality in patients with primary brain tumours. Clin Exp Immunol 39:395-402.

Schayer RW, Davis JK, Smiley RL (1955) Binding of histamine in vitro and its inhibition by cortisone. Am J Physiol 182:54-56.

Schiavi RC, Adams J, STein M (1966) Effect of hypothalamic lesions on histamine toxicity in the guinea pig. Am J Physiol 211:1269-1273.

Schiavi RC, Macris NT, Camerino MS, STein M (1975) Effect of hypothalamic lesions on immediate hypersensitivity. Am J Physiol 228:596-601.

Schleifer SJ, Keller SE, McKegney FP, STein M (1980) Bereavement and lymphocyte function (Abstract) American Psychiatric Association, San Francisco, Ca.

Schmale A, Iker H 91966) The psychological setting of uterine cervical cancer. Ann NY Acad Sci 125:807-815.

Schmutzler W, Derwall R (1973) Experiments on the role of Cyclic AMP in guinea pig anaphylaxis. Int Arch Allergy Appl Immunol 45:120-122.

Schmutzler W, Freundt GP (1975) The effect of glucocorticoids and catecholamines on Cyclic AMP and allergic histamine release in guinea pig lung. Int ARch Allergy Appl Immunol 49:209-212.

Schonfield J (1975) Psychological and life-experience differences between Israeli women with benign and cancerous breast lesions. J Psychosom Res 19:229-234.

Shekelle RB, Raynor WJ, Ostfeld AM, et al. (1981) Psychological depression and 17 year risk of death from cancer. Psychosom Med 43:117-125.

Shereff R, Harwell W, Leiberman P, Rosenberg EW, Robinson H (1973) Effects of beta adrenergic stimulation and blockade on immediate hypersensitivity skin test reactions. J Allergy Clin Immunol 52:254-259.

Sherman NA, Smith RS, Middleton Jr E (1973) Effect of adrenergic compounds aminophylline and hydrocortisone, on in vitro immunoglobulin synthesis by normal human peripheral lymphocytes J Allergy and Clin Immunol 52:13-22.

Sklar LS, Anisman H (1979) Stress and coping factors influence tumor growth. Science 205:513-515.

Smith JW, Steiner AL, Parker CW (1977) Human lymphocyte metabolism. Effects of cyclic and non-cyclic nucleotides on stimulation by phytohemagglutinin. J Clin Invest 50:442-448.

Solomon GF (1969) Stress and antibody response in rats. Int Arch Allergy 35:97-104.

Stutman O (1975) Immunodepression and malignancy. Advances in cancer Res 22:261-422.

Szentivanyi A, Filipp G (1958) Anaphylaxis and the nervous system. Part II Ann Allergy 16:143-151.

Szentivanyi A, Szekely J (1958) Anaphylaxis and the nervous system. Part IV Ann Allergy 16:389-392.

Thanavala YM, Rao SS, Thakur AN (1973) The effect of an aestrogenic steroid on the secondary immune response under different hormonal environments. Act Endocrinologica 72:582-586.

Thomas CB, Greenstreet RL (1973) Psychobiological characteristics in youth as predictors of five disease states. Johns Hopkins Med J 132:16-43.

Thrasher SG, Bernardis LL, Cohen S (1971) The immune response in hypothalamic-lesioned and hypophysectomized rats. Int Arch Allergy 41:813-820.

Tsypin AB, Maltsev VN (1967) The effect of hypothalamic stimulation on the serum content of normal antibodies. Patol Fixiol Eksp TEr 11:83-84.

Tyrey L, Nalbandov AV (1972) Influence of anterior hypothalamic lesions on circulating antibody titers in the rat. Am J Physiol 222:179-185.

Wang T, Sheppard JR, Foker JE (1978) Rise and fall of cyclic AMP required for onset of lymphocyte DNA synthesis. Science 201:155-159.

Watson J (1975) The influence of intracellular levels of cyclic nucleotides on cell proliferation and the induction of antibody synthesis. J Exp Med 141:97-111.

Whittier JR, Orr A (1962) Hyperkinesia and other physiologic effects of caudate deficit in the adult albino rat. Neurol 12:529-539.

Widdicombe JG (1963) Regulation of tracheobronchial smooth muscle. Physiol Rev 43:1-37.

Williams JW, Peterson RG, Shea PA, Schmedtje JF, Bauer DC, Felten Dl (1980) Sympathetic innervation of murine thymus and spleen: Evidence for a functional link between the nervous and immune systems. Brain Res Bulletin 6:83-94.

Wyle FA, Kent JR (1977) Immunosuppression by sex steroid hormones. Clin Exp Immunol 27:407-415.

Yamasaki H, Yamamoto T (1963) Inhibitory effect of adrenal glucocorticoids on histamine release. Jap J Pharmac 19:223-224.

Published 1982 by Elsevier Science Publishing Co, Inc.
Sandra M. Levy, ed.
Biological Mediators of Behavior and Disease:
Neoplasia

IMMUNOCOMPETENCE AND NEOPLASIA: ROLE OF ANXIETY STRESS

VERNON RILEY, M.A. FITZMAURICE, AND DARREL H. SPACKMAN
Pacific Northwest Research Foundation and The Fred Hutchinson Cancer Research Center, Seattle, Washington.

"Stress" is a somewhat loosely used term for describing emotional and biological responses to novel or threatening situations. There is, thus, an extensive variety of experimental or other circumstances in which "stress" serves as a convenient term to express complex and incompletely understood psychological and physiological phenomena (Mason, 1975; Selye, 1975; Riley, 1979a).

## PHYSIOLOGICAL PARAMETERS OF STRESS

In the studies reported here, we have used the term "stress" within a more restricted experimental framework, largely to describe the stimuli and their consequences which include specific biochemical, cellular, and tissue alterations that are associated with an emotional activation of the adrenal cortex by way of the pituitary and its ACTH secretion (Turner and Hagnara, 1971; Mason, 1974). Within the biological systems that we have employed, several key parameters reflect or describe the physiological manifestations of stress, and relate to pathological and other changes that may be observed in experimental animals.

Although emotional stress brings about many biochemical changes in the experimental rodent, in these studies we have focused our attention on the adrenal cortex and have measured with precision the most conspicuous, and what appears at this time to be the most relevant of the biochemical substances elaborated by this remarkable organ in response to anxiety, namely corticosterone(CSR). Immediately following an emotional stimulus, or the perception of a situation that generates anxiety, the adrenal cortex in response to signals from the hypothalamus, via the pituitary, produces increased quantities of corticosterone. The rapidity of its appearance in the plasma and the quantitative extent of this biochemical product can be readily measured by appropriate microassay techniques (Glick, et al., 1964; Riley and Spackman, 1976a; Spackman, et al., 1978).

## IMMUNOLOGICAL AND PATHOLOGICAL CONSEQUENCES OF STRESS

Secondary manifestations resulting from an elevation of the corticosterone concentration in the blood plasma that are readily observed are: (1) lymphocytopenia, (2) thymus involution, and (3) an analogous loss of tissue mass of the spleen and peripheral lymph nodes. Details of these cellular and tissue stress effects will be discussed in other sections of this article. It is relevant to note, however, that the physiological consequences of such stress-mediated events have significant adverse effects upon important elements of the immunological apparatus. By appropriate experimental designs using mice, it is possible to demonstrate the pathological effects of a stress-associated decrease in immune competence upon cancer processes, virus titers, and other diseases that are subject to immunological control.

Although we favor a conservative attitude in extrapolating biological findings from mice to other species, it is not reasonable to ignore classical biology which has demonstrated that there are many physiological similarities and analogous biochemical relationships among animals belonging to an evolutionary phylum in which they have a common descent. A logical expectation associated with this thesis is that fundamental biological principles that are further delineated through the study of animal studies may have application to man.

## EARLY STUDIES

Many careful investigators have examined the relationships between various forms of "stress" and neoplastic processes. The formidable difficulties inherent in the establishment of authentic quiescent baseline conditions for experimental animals, however, complicated the interpretation of some of these earlier studies. In addition, in many cases there was a lack of access to the biochemical and cellular measurements which provide an objective assessment of the basic physiological manifestations of stress.

The resulting failure to obtain consistent results between laboratories tended to undermine confidence in the reliability of research in this difficult but vital field. However, rapid developments in the past few years delineating and characterizing many new facets of immunology, endocrinolgy, and neurobiology now provide a more effective base for re-examining and determining both the potentialities and the limitations of the effects of "stress" upon various neoplastic and other disease processes.

Our original incentive for studying stress and its manifestations was the need to understand better the seemingly mysterious uncontrolled factors that contributed to the accuracy and reproducibility of experimental results. The unexpected enlightening consequences of these experiments made us increasingly aware that the primary factors involved in the pathological effects of stress produce an impairment of the immunological apparatus. Thus, our present perspective in the study of behavioral and stress phenomena calls for an emphasis on the interrelationships between stress and immune competence. This is the biological basis for the entry of a new discipline, psychoneuroimmunology (Ader, 1981), as an important ingredient of an emergent field, behavioral medicine (Holden, 1980).

## THE BIOCHEMICAL NATURE OF STRESS

Anxiety or other varieties of emotional or psychosocial stresses in experimental animals produces the series of neuroendocrine and biochemical events that are illustrated in Figure I. At least one of these biochemical responses has an easily demonstrable destructive effect upon specific cells and tissues that are required for optimum immunological defense. As a consequence, the stress-compromised animal is less capable of defending itself against cancer cells, infectious agents, and other disease processes that are responsive to cell-mediated immunity. Thus, uncontrolled stress factors are important elements to be reckoned with in designing and carrying out most biological experiments.

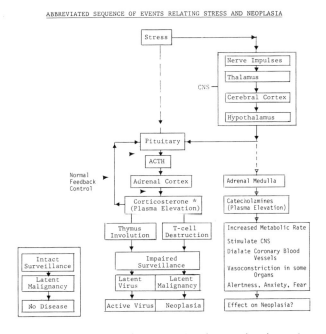

Figure I. Abridged diagram of the physiological pathways whereby anxiety stress signals are transmitted to the adrenal cortex, which responds to produce an increased level of adrenal cortical hormone in the blood.

There are, ot course many varieties of stress, some of which may activate separate physiological systems, either singly or as complexes. For purposes of simplification, the discussion and data presented in this article deal largely with the effects of uncomplicated anxiety and emotionally aroused stress associated with the activation of the adrenal cortex.

A characteristic biochemical expression of such stress is an abrupt and dramatic increase of "stress" hormones in the blood plasma. In rodents, this is corticosterone (CSR); in primates and man, it is largely cortisol. As illustrated in Figure I, such stress-induced hormone elevations produce secondary stress effects involving T cells and thymic components, and thus vital elements of the immunological apparatus. Relevant metabolic and biochemical alterations also occur, of course, through the influences of increased glucocorticoid action.

Within the framework of this limited definition of stress, it is assumed that the adrenal medulla is either not significantly activated by mild stress, or, in any case, does not greatly alter the specific stress effects associated with the adrenal cortical activation. However, participation of the adrenal medulla, with a release of potent CNS-active catecholamines, occurs in rodents under more intense stressful conditions, especially where fear or rage is the inciter (Cannon, 1929; Harlow and Selye, 1937; Henry, 1977; Henry and Stephens, 1977).

The rationale of stress-mediated disease follows logically from this series of well-known physiological events that bring about immunological impairment. Although the overall biochemical phenomena associated with stress are complex and have many subtle consequences, the primary events relevant to disease processes appear to be straightforward, at least those involving the adrenal cortex, as depicted in the abbreviated neuroendocrine pathways (Figure I) and by the following experimental data.

## LOW-STRESS ANIMAL HOUSING: AN ESSENTIAL RESEARCH FACILITY

Critical experimental studies cannot be carried out with confidence using conventional animal facilities, since such housing is not suitable for the maintenance of quiescent baseline values of the stress-associated hormonal and cellular elements that influence or control immunological and thus pathological processes. We have designed animal facilities which not only serve the experimental needs of stress research, but in addition, provide safer facilities for working with infectitious or allergenic agents, (Riley, 1972; Riley and Spackman, 1976b, 1977)

From the standpoint of the low stress environment that is essential for most in vivo biological research, these individually ventilated shelf units offer several beneficial features. For example, the enclosed shelves provide a substantial amount of soundproofing, which is of significance since it has been established that animals are stressed by a wide variety of noises which stimulate neuroendocrine reactions that have subsequent adverse effects upon immunocompetence (Jensen and Rasmussen, 1963; Henry, 1967; Sze, 1970; Sales, 1972; Monjan and Collector, 1977; Anisko, et al., 1978). Stressful cage motion and a variety of noises are prevalent in most conventional animal rooms, particularly where there are rolling metal racks, metal cages, transitor radios, shouting, frequent cage cleaning with rough handling, and other unappreciated stress-inducing practices.

The most essential features required for protective low-stress animal housing are: (a) No recirculation of noxious air that has been in previous contact with animals; (b) partial sound-proofing of animal storage shelves; (c) elimination of animal room vibrations and high pitched sounds of centrifuges, vacuum cleaners, ventilation fans, and other noisy laboratory or building equipment; d) elimination of drafts, air turbulence, and wind tunnel effects; (e) precise light control to stabilize circadian rhythms and to regulate light intensity exposure; (f) segregation of males and females with respect to transmissible odors, pheromones, and other stress-inducing signals (Gleason, et al., 1969; Riley, et al., 1981) (g) segregation of experimental animals that are experiencing stress from normal or control animals; (h) introduction of special minimal-stress animal handling techniques and cage cleaning procedures; and (i) avoidance of drafty, uncomfortable, and stressful wire-bottom cages.

Such quiescent housing conditions permit low baseline values of 0 to 35 ng/ml for plasma corticosterone. In contrast, corticosterone values observed in mice maintained in conventional communal animal rooms where the animals are rountinely exposed to chronic or intermittent stress have usually been in the range of 150 ng/ml. This constitutes an elevation of ten to twenty times the quiescent plasma corticosterone level.

## CONSIDERATIONS RELEVANT TO THE EXPERIMENTAL DESIGN OF ANIMAL STUDIES

Experimental contradictions. It is apparent from an examination of the inconsistent results obtained in earlier studies, that the experimental nuances and complexities of the effects of various forms of stress on cancer exceeded our ability to evaluate the relative potencies of the experimental variables involved and to provide all of the necessary experimental conditions and controls. It apears that these difficulties have arisen, at least partially, from a variety of unappreciated experimental factors.

The rapid physiological response to "handling"-induced stress. One troublesome aspect has been a failure to appreciate the extreme sensitivity and rapidity of the physiological response of animals exposed to experimental, manipulative, or enviromental-induced stress. Critical phases of the stress syndrome are initiated immediately following the slightest disturbance of mice. The physiological consequences of this stress may continue for hours or even days, depending upon the nature, severity, and duration of the stressful stimulus.

The rapid physiological response to handling-induced anxiety stress is indicated by the measurable elevation of plasma corticosterone levels observed only minutes after the animals have been agitated by simple capturing procedures. This is illustrated by the rapidly ascending corticosterone curve in Figure 2, which demonstrates that the response to handling is so rapid that its biochemical manifestation in the form of plasma corticosterone elevation is detectable after three and one-half minutes post-stimulus. This imposes a rigorous time limitation upon the investigator for obtaining the blood

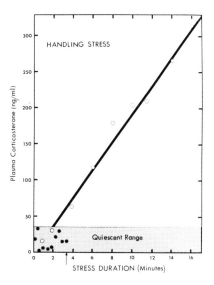

Figure 2.   Influence of animal capture and handling upon the concentration of stress-induced corticosterone in the plasm of "normal" mice as a function of time.

The unconnected points falling within the unstressed range of corticosterone concentration represent ten animals whose blood samples were obtained within a three and one-half minute period.

The ascending linear curve shows the systematic increase in plasma corticosterone with time following removal of the mice from their low-stress storage shelf and the capturing of individual animals.   The mice were selected randomly and bled at the periodic intervals indicated.   This curve demonstrates the rapidity of the physiological response to stress as measured by the corticosterone parameter.   Both groups of mice were bled by the orbital bleeding technique.

samples which establish the baseline levels for plasma corticosterone in control animals, as well as for measuring the physiological effects of experimentally induced stress. Rapid rises in plasma corticosterone can be generated by the routine practice of capturing animals for injections, cage transfer, bleeding, or other experimental procedures, or even by simply transporting the animals from their protective holding facilities to the laboratory bench. Unless these operations are completed within a 3.5 minute period, anxiety stress will be manifested by initiation of the typical stress syndrome resulting in elevated plasma corticosterone levels. After sufficient time elapses, leukopenia and eventually thymus involution will occur.

Under the circumstances illustrated by Figure 2, the corticosterone elevation is not induced by the bleeding procedure itself, but by the contageous anxiety induced in the entire cage population during the sequential capture of each mouse. Similar effects have been observed in each of four different mouse strains tested (BDF, BAF, C3H, and CBA, as well as in mice of different ages, ranging from seven weeks to 24 months of age. These data have led to the realization that accurate quiescent corticosterone levels can be obtained only when the blood samples are removed within three and a half minutes following the initial disturbance produced by transferring the animals from protective storage to the bleeding area.

These phenomena further demonstrate the dual need for quiescent protective animal facilities and the employment of appropriate animal handling techniques in biological studies, especially if optimal immunocompetence and normal physiology is of relevance to the experiment (Riley, et al, 1975; Riley, 1972, 1978, 1979b; Riley and Spackman, 1976a, 1976b, 1977a, 1977b, 1978a).

## MALE-FEMALE PROXIMITY AND STRESS

When male mice are housed in the same cage with females, their plasma corticosterone is elevated several fold (80-100ng/ml) and does not return to a quiescent baseline level within a thirty day observation period. The corticosterone levels of females caged with males remain elevated (80-120 ng/ml) for more than 80 days.

Figure 3 demonstrates that mice housed in separate cages, but maintained in proximity to cages of mice of the opposite sex, exhibited a four-to seven-fold increase in plasma corticosterone levels. This Figure also shows that male mice were less affected than analogous females when observed over a prolonged period of time. Thus, the mixing of the sexes within the same vicinity, even if housed in separate cages, may have physiological consequences that can distort biochemical and immunological parameters. It should be recognized, of course, that these striking effects may not be detectable under the chronically stressful conditions of a conventional animal room where the mice usually have plasma corticosterone elevations 5-to 10-fold above the quiescent level.

182

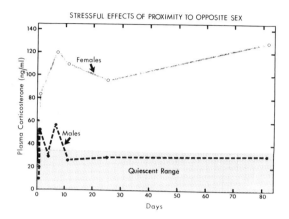

STRESSFUL EFFECTS OF PROXIMITY TO OPPOSITE SEX

Figure 3. Stressful effects of male-female proximity. Plasma corticosterone alterations occur in mice that are exposed to the presence of the opposite sex housed in the same vicinity, even though caged separately. All mice were housed five per cage in standard plastic units with corncob bedding, and were maintained in a low-stress animal facility.

These observations are relevant to immunological and neoplastic studies in which rigorous control of plasma adrenal corticoid levels are important. These data indicate the risk that females especially will respond differently to a tumor challenge when housed separately than when housed in the vicinity of cages of male mice.

POPULATION DENSITY AND STRESS

Several investigators have described the seemingly stressful effects of "cage crowding," and the apparent influences on the growth or incidence of various tumors, or upon other disease processes, presumably due to alterations in the immunological competence of the stressed mice (Vessey, 1964; Glenn and Becker, 1969; Dechambre and Gosse, 1973)

We have undertaken experiments to re-examine this question utilizing protective, low-stress facilities, and minimal-stress-inducing animal handling techniques. These facilities, plus this experimental approach, have provided an opportunity to control a number of the newly appreciated aspects of environmental stress in carrying out population density studies.

The experiments were designed to determine the different levels of emotional or anxiety stress that might occur among mice caged in groups of either 1,2,3,4,5,10,15, or 20, and held for relatively long periods in standard plastic cages. There were no mice of the opposite sex either in the cages or in the immediate vicinity, and thus there were no obvious sources of pheromones or other signals that can provide uncontrolled stress-inducing circumstances within the low-stress protective shelves. See Figure 3 for the stress effects associated with proximity to the opposite sex.

## ABSENCE OF EFFECTS OF POPULATION DENSITY UPON PLASMA CORTICOSTERONE LEVELS

It has been shown in these studies that various population densities of caged mice do not constitute in themselves a basis for "cage-crowding stress". This was demonstrated by a failure to detect differential levels of plasma corticosterone in female mice housed either 1,2,3,5,10,15, or 20 per standard plastic cage for various time intervals. It was expected, however, that quite different effects would be observed when employing more competitive and quarrelsome male mice under analogous experimental circumstances. It was thus surprising to observe that increasing cage population densities of males also failed to exhibit elevated plasma corticosterone levels. Figure 4 illustrates the similarity of plasma corticosterone levels in both male and female C3H/He mice when housed in various population densities.

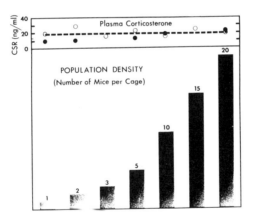

Figure 4. Absence of any differential concentration of stress-associated hormones in mice, either males or females, housed in various population densities.

## POPULATION DENSITY AND TUMOR GROWTH

Testing procedures for detecting possible effects of cage-crowding included challenging the mice with tumor transplants, and then monitoring the animals for percent tumor incidence, tumor latent periods, tumor growth rates and host survival times. One of the tumor types that had been reported by Dechambre and Gosse (1971) to be responsive to "cage crowding" was the transplantable B-16 mouse melanoma. An experiment similar to theirs, using the same tumor type, was carried out as follows: On experimental day 29 following initiation of a population density experiment involving multiple cages containing 1,2,3,5, 10, 15, or 20 BDF female mice, they were implanted with the B-16 pigmented melanoma. Three dimensional tumor measurements were made twice a week for determining relative tumor growth rates. Tumor latent periods were also determined, as well as the survival times of the hosts. In contrast to the report of Dechambre and Gosse, under the low-stress circumstances of our experiment there was no significant influence of population density on the tumor latent periods, growth rates, or the survival times of the hosts (Riley and Spackman, 1977b). Thus, in this experiment, the growth behavior of this particular tumor was essentially the same in mice housed individually as in those mice that were housed 20 to a cage, as well as in the other intermediate population densities. This is consistent with our independent observation which showed no effect of LDH-virus-induced stress upon the pigmentd B-16 melanoma.

## TUMOR REGRESSIONS AND POPULATION DENSITY

Since tumor regression in a properly balanced tumor-host model is a good index of immune competence, and thus of stress status, we utilized that parameter as one means for determining the optimal number of mice per standard plastic cage. The results of these experiments were unexpected. The tumor regression rate found with the 6C3HED lymphosarcoma implanted in C3H/He female mice in cages having only one animal per cage was 60 percent. This was in contrast to all other population densities tested consisting of 2,3,5,10,15, or 20 mice per cage, which had a range of 80 to 100 percent regressions, with an average of 93 percent (p $<$.001). Thus, based upon the imunological ability of femal mice to reject a tumor challenge, all tested densities of group housing were preferable to that of the single animal per cage.

Despite the significant difference in tumor regressions, housing male mice one or two per cage had no observable influence upon daytime plasma cortiocosterone levels. It was noted, however, that male mice housed two per cage exhibited a lower food consumption and somewhat lighter body weights than did those housed one or three per cage.

An experiment similar to the one above employed male mice. As shown in Table 2, male C3H/He mice that were housed one or two per cage had less ability to reject the 6C3HED lymphosarcoma than did those housed 3,5,10,15, or 20 per cage. Unlike female mice, male mice housed 2 per cage exhibited no advantage over isolated mice, with respect to tumor growth. It therefore appears that for optimum immunocompetence, male mice should not be housed either one or two per cage. However, any number over two per cage, up to 20 per cage, yielded similar results, with no optimum number per cage within this range detected.

Despite the significant difference in tumor regressions, housing male mice one or two per cage had no observable influence upon daytime plasma corticosterone levels. It was noted, however, that male mice housed two per cage exhibited a lower food consumption and somewhat lighter body weights than did those housed one or three per cage.

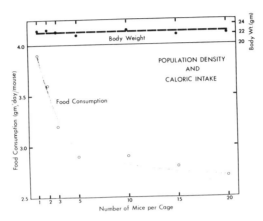

Figure 5.    Influence of mouse population density upon food consumption.    The interpretation is that in the higher density mouse populations there is less body heat loss with a consequential relative reduction in caloric requirements for the maintenance of normal body weight.

TABLE I

EFFECTS OF ISOLATION UPON PERCENT TUMOR REGRESSIONS IN FEMALE C3H/He MICE

| Number of Mice Per Cage | Tumor Regressions[a] (Percent) | Probability [b] |
|---|---|---|
| 1 | 60% | $P < .001$ |
| 2,3,5,10,15, or 20 | 93% | |

a)   The Gardner 6C3HED lymphosarcoma was implanted into C3H/He female mice 56 days after initiation of the various population densities.  Percent tumor regressions were determined on day 25 after tumor implantation.
b)   The probability value was determined by the chi-square method, comparing the data from one mouse per cage with the combined data from 2, 3, 5, 10,15, or 20 mice per cage.

186

## POPULATION DENSITY AND METABOLIC EFFECTS

Another experimental factor that needs to be considered in deciding upon the optimum number of animals per cage is shown in Figure 5. These data indicate that a sensitive homeostatic thermal mechanism appears to be operating, based upon a thermal regulatory feed-back that controls caloric intake as a function of body weight maintenance requirements. This mechanism is influenced by the caloric requirements of mice that retain or lose body heat depending upon the population density in their cage. Among the multiple influences affecting tumor growth and carcinogenic processes that have been reported include the consequences of various caloric intakes (Tannenbaum, 1940; Tannenbaum and Silverstone, 1953; Sprunt and Flanigan, 1956; and Riley, 1979a) and environmental temperatures (Fuller, et al., 1941; Wallace et al., 1944; Young, 1958). These observations are relevant to the selection of appropriate experimental population densities.

TABLE 2

EFFECTS OF POPULATION DENSITY UPON PERCENT TUMOR REGRESSIONS IN MALE C3H/He MICE

| Number of Mice Per Cage | Tumor Regressions[a] (Percent) | Probability[b] |
|---|---|---|
| 1 | 70% | |
| 2 | 65% | |
| 1 or 2 (combined data) | 67.5% | |
| 3,5,10,15, or 19 (combined data) | 84.6% | P .01 |

a) The Gardner 6C3HED lymphosarcoma was implanted into C3H/He male mice 56 days after initiation of the various population densities. Tumor regressions were determined on day 25 after tumor implantation.
b) The probability value was determined by the chi-square method, comparing the data from 1 to 2 mice per cage (combined data) with the combined data from 3,5,10,15,or 19 mice per cage.

## BENIGN STRESS-INDUCING MACHINE

The disconcerting, contradictory results of some previous studies demonstrated the need for a simple, reproducible, and non-traumatic means for the quantitative induction of simple anxiety stress in experimental animals.

Such stress should preferably be produced without significantly activating hormonal systems other than those of the adrenal cortex, or depriving the animals of free access to food and water by restraint or other means, or subjecting them to unnecessary harsh treatment. We have developed a simple stress-inducing device that provides a controllable readily reproducible form of quantifiable stress, and further, permits automatic programming of a wide variety of intermittent stress/rest intervals.

This stress-inducing instrument is a modified phonograph turntable having the four standardard speeds of 16, 33.3, 45, and 78 rpm. The instrument has been designed so that an entire cage of animals can be rotated without changing the familiar arrangement of their living quarters. Thus, with this benign stressing device it is not necessary to submit the animals to a disturbing novel environment, to restrain them, or to alter the availability of their food and water, inasmuch as the slow rotational speeds permit the animals to move about their cage and to continue eating and drinking. The maximum lateral gravitational force experienced by the mice is less than one G. This stress-inducing instrument is thus not a centrifugal device, but is essentially a mechanical means for inducing mild spatial disorientation, and possibly vertigo or dizziness, with an associated anxiety that activates the adrenal cortex resulting in a prompt and predictable elevation of plasma corticosterone.

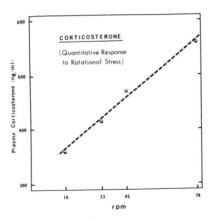

Figure 6. Linear relationship between speed of rotation (rpm) and the resulting corticosterone levels in the mouse plasma following 20 minutes of cage rotation. It should be noted that the maximum speed employed generates less than one G at the maximum radius of the cage. This is thus not a centrifugally-induced stress, but the instrument produces merely a spatial disorentation with an attending anxiety and a consequential systematic corticosterone increase.

CONTROLLED CORTICOSTERONE ELEVATIONS INDUCED BY SLOW ROTATION

The ability of this stress-inducing device to induce variable intensities of stress is illustrated in Figure 6, where plasma corticosterone values are plotted against the various rotational speeds. It may be seen that following the rotation of separate groups of mice at each of the four speeds, that a graded and systematic increase in plasma corticosterone was observed. For most stress-inducing purposes in the experiments reported here, the intermediate speed of 45 rpm has been employed. For prolonged stress exposures, the animals were usually rotated for 10 minutes followed by a 50-minute rest. This, or other on/off cycles, can be repeated for any desired periodicity, or for any time sequence by employing pre-programmed automation.

An ability to control the magnitude of the stress stimulus, and to actually quantitate stress-induction in terms of the biochemical and cellular response of the stressed subject has been an important development in placing our stress studies on a

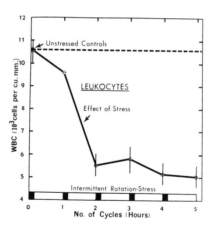

Figure 7. Leukocytopenia induced by mild, non-traumatic rotational stress at 45 rpm during five 60-minute cycles consisting of 10 minute of rotation followed by 50 minutes of rest.

A 50 percent leukocytopenia was produced by the end of the second cycle, and was maintained throughout the 5 hours of intermittent stress. Vertical lines through each point represent standard errors.

quantitive and easily reproducible basis. For example, the acquired data which will be described involving stress-associated lymphocytopenia, thymus involution, and other physiological and neoplastic responses have been accomplished with the aide of this simple but highly effective instrumentation.

## STRESS-INDUCED ANALYSIS OF CELLS AND TISSUES

Figure 7 shows the effect of programmed stress-inducing rotation on the leukocyte count employing a rotation schedule of 10 minutes out of the hour at 45 rpm. It is relevant to note that a stress-induced leukocytopenia immediately follows as a consequence of elevated plasma corticosterone concentration.

This alteration in an important cellular component is a key factor in bringing about an impairment of the rodent immunological apparatus. It is particularly relevant to note that the majority of the circulating mouse leukocytes are T cells, and this induced

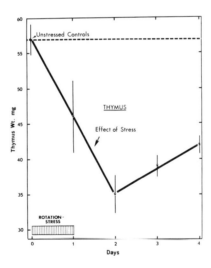

Figure 8. Thymus involution resulting from anxiety-stress induced by rotation. Evidence indicates that the thymocytes are lysed by the increased concentrations of plasma corticosterone which accompany stress. The anxiety-stress was induced by a mild spatial disorientation created by rotating the entire mouse cage slowly at 45 rpm for ten minutes out of each hour for a 24 hour period.

lymphocytopenia is thus indicative of a reduction of a critical component of the immunological defense system. This rapid loss of T cells acquires special significance in view of the substantial damage also done to the thymus, which prevents or delays processing of replacement T cells. Thus, in terms of the sequence of events, an increased concentration of corticosterone appears in the blood within a few minutes following anxiety stress stimuli· this, in turn, brings about circulating lymphocyte damage within one or two hours. Thymus involution follows; however, the disintegration of the solid organ requires more time, exhibiting a measurable weight loss within less than 24 hours. The time course of this hormonal action upon the thymus is shown in Figure 8.

## SELECTION OF EFFECTIVE TUMOR-HOST MODELS FOR STRESS STUDIES

For experiments that are intended to utilize measurements of the incidence and/or growth rate of a transplatable tumor in studying the effect of stress on immunocompetence and tumor behavior, selection of the proper tumor/host combination is critical. For example, tumors that are syngeneic with the host, such as the rapidly growing B-16 pigmented melanoma, are not visibly affected by stress or by other impairments of the immune system (Fig. 9A). However, the more slowly growing

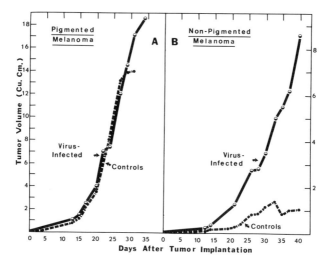

Figure 9. Comparison of the lack of influence upon tumor growth by an acute LDH-virus infection upon a rapidly growing pigmented B-16 melanoma, as shown in Panel A, in contrast to the virus-induced inhancement of the growth of a partially host-suppressed non-pigmented variant of B-16 origin, illustrated by Panel B.

non-pigmented B-16 variant is highly responsive to induced stress, indicating partial host control. This tumor/host combination is thus capable of responding to the biochemical and cellular events that are induced either by anxiety stress, by inoculation of a "stress-inducing" virus, or by injection of an exogenous corticoid.

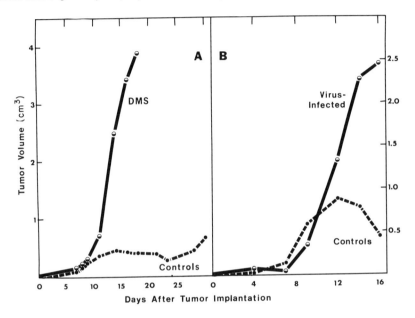

Figure 10. Tumor-enhancing effects of two varieties of "stress" on the 6C3HED lymphosarcoma. Panel A shows the consequences of synthetic corticoid administration by the implantation of a single dose of a long-acting preparation of dexamethasome (DMS). These data demonstrate the tumor enhancement that occurs following corticoid-induced impairment of the host's immunological apparatus. A similar tumor enhancement may be observed in Panel B, following inoculation of the "stress-inducing" LDH virus. The DMS and the LDH-virus injections were both administered on the same day as the implantation of the 6C3HED lymphosarcoma into the C3H/He mice.

Figure 10 shows another non-syngeneic tumor, the 6C2HED lymphosarcoma, growing in C3H/He mice, responding similarly to both dexamethasone (DMS) and LDH-virus infection. This tumor-host model is also responsive to rotational-induced mild anxiety stress, as will be shown later. However, as shown in Fig. 11, when the same tumor is implanted into C3H/Bi mice, a more histocompatible substrain, it grows rapidly even in unstressed animals, and its behavior is not significantly altered by stress, corticosterone, or DMS-induced immunoimpairment. Thus rapidly growing syngeneic tumors, such as the B-16 pigmented melanoma, or the Gardner lymphosarcoma growing in C3H/Bi mice, will not respond significantly to stress influences and represent examples of tumor/animal models that are not suitable for studying stress effects. Such differences in host-tumor compatibility and sensitivities may explain some of the experimental discrepancies and negative findings reported in the literature.

Table 3

EFFECT OF MOUSE SUB-STRAIN ON THE GROWTH BEHAVIOR OF THE 6C3HED GARDNER LYMPHOSARCOMA

| Parameter Measured | C3H/He Mice | C3H/Bi Mice |
|---|---|---|
| Tumor Regressions[a] | 100% | 0% |
| Tumor-Associated Deaths[b] | 0% | 100% |
| Maximum Tumor Volume ($cm^3$)[c] | $0.8 \pm 0.3$ | $2.3 \pm 0.8$ |
| Mean Tumor Latent Period[d] | $6.0 \pm 0.1$ | $6.1 \pm 0.3$ |

a) The median regression time of the tumors in theC3H/He mice was 21 days after implantation, and all tumors in this sub-strain had regressed by 35 days after implantation.
b) The median survival time of the C3H/Bi mice was 33 days following tumor implantation, and all 3CH/Bi mice were dead by 37 days after implantation.
c) In the C3H/He mice, maximum tumor volumes were attained between 16 and 19 days following implantation, after which the tumors in this sub-strain regressed.
In the c3H/Bi mice, maximum tumor volumes were observed just prior to the deaths of the mice, which occurred between 23 and 35 days afer implantation.
d) All mice were females, 9 weeks of age, housed 10 per cage in standard plastic cages with corn-cob bedding. The cages were maintained within low-stress, protective facilities.

An example of such phenomena is shown in Table 3, which compares various parameters of tumor behavior following implantation of the 6C3HED lymphosarcoma into C3H/He and C3H/Bi mice. As demonstrated by the dramatic differences in tumor regressions (0% versus 100%), this tumor is obviously more histocompatible with the C3'/Bi substrain than with the C3H/He mouse. The C3H/He mice are especially useful for detecting and measuring subtle, stress-induced impairments of immunocompetence, which is reflected by an enhanced growth of the 6C3HED tumor in this substrain. The C3H/Bi substrain is less useful in this respect, since there is less natural host capability for containment of the growth of this tumor, which progresses with equal rapidity in both stressed and non-stressed animals. The C3H/Bi mice are useful, however, for demonstrating an enhancement of immunological elements, which is expressed by a reduction in tumor growth or an increase in the percent of tumor regressions. These substrain features are illustrated in Figure 11.

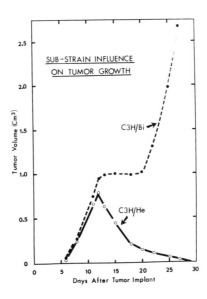

Figure 11. Differential tumor growth and regression behavior of a mouse lymphosarcoma transplanted into two different C3H substrains. The differences in histocompatibility provide useful tumor-host models for the detection of alterations of immunocompetence induced by stress or other factors.

ENHANCEMENT OF TUMOR GROWTH FOLLOWING ROTATION-INDUCED STRESS

Figure 12 shows the influence of intermittent rotation-induced stress on the subsequent growth rate of the 6C3HED lymphosarcoma in C3H/He mice. In this experiment half of the tumor-bearing mice were exposed to a mild disorienting rotation at 45 rpm for ten minutes out of each hour during days 4, 5, and 6 following subcutaneous implantation of the transplantable lymphosarcoma. Our interpretation of these observations assumes that those animals receiving such rotational stress had some elements of their immunological competence compromised which permitted this stress-sensitive tumor to grow at a more rapid rate than occurred in the control animals. The latter mice are known to possess an immunological capability for restraining the optimal growth of this tumor. Such a stress-induced decrease in immunological competence is consistent with the known consequence of T cell damage that is associated with plasma corticosterone elevation.

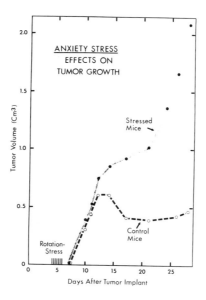

Figure 12. Stress-associated influences on tumor growth in mice exposed to an intermittent course of mild anxiety stress. The stress was induced by slow rotation at 45 rpm for 10 minutes out of each hour during days 4, 5, and 6 following tumor implantation. The tumor was the 6C3HED lymphosarcoma in C3H/He female mice. Food and water were available ad libitum during the course of the experiment.

BIOLOGICAL INTERACTIONS; STRESS AND VIRUS INFECTION

Specific influences imposed by the ubiquitous LDH-virus that may alter or compromise experiments involving neoplasia or immunological responses include the following: 1) elevations of plasma corticosterone during the acute phase of infection; 2) subsequent thymus involution; 3) lysis of circulating lymphocytes, largely T cells; 4) dual effects upon the spleen, with a destruction of small lymphocytes concomitant with a continuous immunoblast proliferation in the thymus-independent regions, resulting in a moderate splenic hyperplasia; 5) enhancement of spleen antibody-forming B cells during acute infection, followed by B cell inhibition during the subsequent life-long chronic phase of the infection; 6) an increase in the incidence of tumors induced by certain

Table 4

VARIOUS PHYSIOLOGICAL AND BIOCHEMICAL DIFFERENCES CAPABLE OF AFFECTING IMMUNOLOGICAL COMPETENCE, BETWEEN NORMAL MICE AND THOSE INFECTED WITH THE LDH-VIRUS

| Parameters Measured | Normal Mice (No LDH-Virus) | Virus-Infected Mice |
|---|---|---|
| Plasma Corticosterone | Normal | 2 to 20 fold[a] increase |
| Thymus Weight | Normal | 50% weight loss[b] |
| Peripheral Lymphocytes | Normal | 70% depletion[c] increase |
| Spleen Weight | Normal | 30% weight increase |
| Peripheral Nodes (Weight) | Normal | 50% weight increase |
| Carbon Clearance (K-rate) | 0.016 | 0.006 |
| Macrophage Integrity | Normal | Impaired |
| Spleen Anitbody-Forming Cells Plaques per Spleen) | | |
| Relative Numbers, | | |
| Acute Infection | 1 | 10 |
| Chronic Infection | 15 | 1 |
| Plasma LDH Level[d] | 200-400 | 2,00-4,000 |
| In Tumor-Bearing Mice | 200-2,000 | 10,000-100,000 |
| Clearance of Exogenous Enzymes ($T\frac{1}{2}$) | | |
| Lactate Dehydrogenase (LDH) | 12 hours | 24 hours |
| Asparaginase | 2-4 hours | 20-25 hours |

(a) First 48 hours following infection. (b) Four days following infection. (c) Four days following infection. (d) Wroblewski units.

196

oncogenic viruses; 7) reduction in regression rates of certain virus-induced tumors; 8) enhancement of growth rates of certain non-syngeneic transplantable tumors; 9) a three-fold to twenty-fold enhancement in the production of spleen tumor foci following intravenous inoculation of Friend virus; and 10) an impairment of the clearance of certain enzymes from the plasma, together with a concomitant increased influx of enzymes into the plasma, which persists for the lifespan of the infected mouse ( Riley, 1966, 1974; Howard, et al., 1969; Turner, et. al., 1978; Santisteban and Riley, 1973; Spackman and Riley, 1974..

In the presence of a growing tumor, these physiological alterations result in a

Table 5

VARIOUS DIFFERENCES IN TUMOR RESPONSES IN THE PRESENCE OR ABSENCE OF THE LDH-VIRUS

| Parameters Measured | Non-Infected Mice (No LDH-Virus) | LDH-Virus Infected Mice |
|---|---|---|
| Tumor Incidence | | |
| Harvey Sarcoma Virus | 25% | 100% |
| Moloney Sarcoma Virus | 34% | 83% |
| Tumor Regression Rates | | |
| Harvey Sarcoma | 100% | 0% |
| Moloney Sarcoma | 66% | 17% |
| 6C3HED Lymphosarcoma in C3H/He Mice | 100% | 0% |
| Tumor Growth Rate | | |
| Amelanotic Variant of -16 Melanoma | slow | rapid |
| Friend Virus Spleen Foci (No. per Spleen) | 8 | 24 |
| Host Survival following Treatment with 250 IU/kg of EC-2 Asparaginase (6C3HED Lymphosarcoma in C3H/Bi Mice) | 0 | 100% |

synergistic increase in the levels of certain endogenous enzymes, notably lactate dehydrogenase (LDH), that may amount to more than one hundred-fold over normal values (Riley, 1974; Riley and Spackmen, 1976b; Riley, et. al., 1978). These and other effects of LDH-virus infection are itemized in Tables 4 and 5. It would be presumptuous to assume that this is the only infectious entity capable of such physiological influences (Gotlieb-Stenatsky, et. al., 1966; Youn and Barski, 1966; Wheelock, 1967; Turner, et al., 1968).

## EFFECTS OF VARIOUS STRESS STIMULI ON THE BEHAVIOR OF MOLONEY SARCOMA VIRUS-INDUCED TUMORS

The Moloney sarcoma virus (MSV) tumor system provides a useful model for studying the rare phenomenon of spontaneous regression of autochthonous tumors (Fefer, et. al., 1968; Turner, et. al., 1971; Amkraut and Soloman, 1972; Soloman and AmKraut, 1979; Soloman, et. al., 198'). These experiments demonstrate the influence of induced anxiety-stress, and its endogenously produced biochemical products, upon this viral neoplastic system.

Enhancement of MSV-induced tumor incidence and tumor growth rate was observed, together with a delay in the usual tumor regressions, when programmed anxiety-stress was administered immediately following virus inoculation. Similar tumor enhancement was obtained by the biochemical simulation of the usual physiological consequences of stress, specifically by administering natural or synthetic corticoids. Single, slow-release repository doses of corticosterone or dexamethasone produced effects on the Moloney virus/tumor system similar to those produced by anxiety stress.

In order to examine the concomitant effect of a second virus as an additional biological stress-inducing factor, the LDH-virus (Riley, 1966, 1974; Howard et. al., 1969; Turner, et. al., 1971; Stantisteban and Riley, 1973; Spackman and Riley, 1974; Riley and Spackman, 1976b; Riley, et. al., 1978) was also examined in this system. When the benign, non-oncogenic LDH-virus was injected at an appropriate time in reference to the inoculation of the Moloney virus, tumor growth enhancement was obtained. Thus, three extraneous factors, all having the common capability of producing or simulating elevated adrenal corticoids, enhanced this neoplastic system.

Fig. 13 compares the effects of these three varieties of stress upon the growth behavior of tumors induced by the Moloney sarcoma virus. Tumor growth enhancement was expressed by significantly larger maximum tumor volumes attained in all three experimental groups as compared with the unstressed or untreated MSV-inoculated controls ($P \angle .001$ for all three experimental modalities).

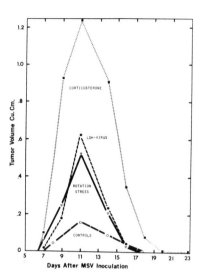

Figure 13. Enhanced growth of autohthonous tumors induced by the Mohoney sarcoma virus (MSV) following (1) rotation-induced stress, (2) infection with the LDH-virus, and (3) implantation of a single slow-release pellet of exogenous corticosterone.

The rotated group of mice was subjected to intermittent rotation (45 rpm, 10 minutes rotation, 50 minutes rest per hour) for a total period of 72 hours, starting on the day of MSV inoculation.

The LDH-virus infected group was inoculated with the LDH-virus on the same day that the MSV inoculation was performed.

The mice given exogenous corticosterone were implanted subcutaneously in the left hip with a slow-release corticosterone-spermaceti pellet, on the day of MSV inoculation.

The BALB/c female recipient mice were inoculated intramuscularly in the right hip with 0.05 ml of Moloney sarcoma virus inoculm.

All mice were housed in plastic cges, 10 per cage, within low-stress protective facilities.

The enhancing effects of these various forms of stress are all highly dependent upon the timing of the stressor relative to MSV inoculation. For example, rotation stress when applied from the fourth through the sixth day following MSV inoculation, resulted in a significant enhancement of tumor growth, but of lesser magnitude than that observed following rotation for the same length of time but initiated on the day of MSV inoculation. In contrast, rotation stress applied three days prior to MSV inoculation resulted in an inhibition, rather than enhancement, of the MSV-induced tumors. Similar timing effects may be responsible for the reported stress-induced inhibition of various tumors (Amkraut and Soloman, 1972; Crispens, 1976; Newberry, 1976; Nieburgs, et.al., 1976; Newberry and Sengbusch, 1979).

Our interpretation of these phenomena is consistent with other related data, namely, that all of the above stress stimuli cause an indirect impairment of immunocompetence. As a possible explanation for stress-associated tumor inhibition, such impairment may be followed by a homeostatic recovery of the immunological elements, followed by an overshoot resulting in a temporary immunological enhancement which could inhibit tumor growth if the timing is right (Monjan and Collector, 1977).

## EFFECTS OF CHEMICALLY STIMULATED STRESS UPON LDH-VIRUS TITERS

Figure 14 shows the physiological consequences of a single injection of the synthetic corticoid dexamethasone (DMS) upon thymus weights, as well as an inverse

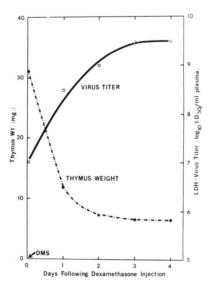

Figure 14. Effects of a single dose of the synthetic corticoid, dexamethasone, upon thymus weight and LDH-virus titers.
BDF female mice chronically infected with the LDH were injected with a slowly releasing pellet of dexamethasone seven days following infection with the virus. The low, chronic virus titers are increased to a level normally seen only during the acute phase of the infection when corticosterone levels are high.

DMS-induced enhancement of the equilibrated LDH-virus titer levels in mice chronically infected with this persistent virus.

The originally elevated endogenous corticosterone levels induced in the plasma during the acute phase of the LDH-virus infection return to normal in one or two days, which is followed by a drop in virus titer from approximately $10^{10}$ to $10^6$ $ID_{50}/ml$. The DMS-induced, or associated, secondary increase of the LDH-virus titer to the high level usually seen only during the acute infectious phase, suggests that stress-induced plasma corticosterone elevations may potentiate other viruses, possibly with pathological consequences; the question thus occurs as to whether stress may be directly or indirectly responsible for the appearance of certain virus-induced tumors, by activating latent carcinogenic viruses, or by increasing the titers of viruses that are present in a non-pathological low titer chronic state (Rasmussen, et al., 1963; Hirsch, 1974). The Bittner mammary tumor virus (MTV) in C3H mice is an example. The enhancement of oncogenic viruses and their neoplastic processes by the LDH-virus has been previously reported (Santisteban and Riley, 1973; Riley and Spackman, 1976). Of relevance to these phenomena are reports indicating that stress may suppress interferon production in virus-infected mice (Chang and Ramussen, 1965; Jensen, 1968a). A separate report describes the effects of stress on increasing susceptibility to viral infections (Jensen, 1968b).

## DIFFERENTIAL ENHANCEMENT OF MELANOMA GROWTH BY VIRUS-INDUCED OR BIOCHEMICALLY STIMULATED STRESS

Melanomas have a reputation for unpredictable clinical behavior. Cumulative data suggest that certain melanomas may generate an immunological response in the host that occasionally results in either a temporary or permanent regression (Cochran, et al., 1972). Similar regressions of benign pigmented lesions also occur (Nicholls, 1973). Thus it appears that such tumors are either capable of eliciting a specially vigorous host immunological response, or may at times exist in a more fragile histocompatible equilibrium with the host, and are therefore more susceptible to changes in immunological states of the host.

Figure 9 illustrates the differential influence of a stress-inducing LDH-virus infection upon the behavior of a slowly growing, non-pigmented variant of the B-16 malanoma, compared with its more rapidly growing, pigmented counterpart. Apparently, genetic transformation from the pigmented to a non-pigmented state results, in this case at least, in a tumor with different histocompatibility characteristics than the original pigmented tumor. The growth rates of the two tumors in C57 Black mice, the strain of origin, are significicaly different, as illustrated by Figure 9. Also, the tendency of the amelanotic variant to undergo spontaneous regression following limited tumor growth distinguishes it from the more syngeneic pigmented neoplasm. The immunologically suppressible non-pigmented melanoma thus is a suitable experimental model for detecting the influence of subtle immunological modifiers, which may include stress, synthetic corticoids, and certain viruses. An effect of the latter is demonstrated by the increased growth rate of this tumor in mice acutely infected with the LDH-virus, which has modulating effects upon host immunocompetence. In contrast, as shown in Figure 9, Panel A, the rapidly growing pigmented melanoma exhibited the same rate of growth in both virus-infected and control mice.

VIRAL INDUCTION OF STRESS

Figure 10 (Panel B) indicates that the LDH-virus has an enhancing effect upon the growth of the 6C3HED lymphosarcoma, whose degree of syngeneity with the C3H/He mice employed is imperfect. See Table 5. Again, in this instance acute infection with the LDH-virus enhanced tumor growth rate, and increased the percentage of progressively growing tumors following transplantation. At least 30 days following tumor implantation, 5 of 10 tumors in the non-infected mice had completely regressed, while in the virus-infected group, only one out of ten had regressed.

Figure 10 (Panel A) shows the enhancement of tumor growth produced by the direct administration of dexamethasone (DMS). This synthetic corticoid functions in a manner similar to the naturally elevated endogenous corticosterone that results from either anxiety stress or acute infection with the LDH-virus. Thus a significant enhancement of tumor growth resulted from infection with a benign virus, or the administration of synthetic hormone closely related to a natural hormone associated with stress. These results are consistent with the working hypothesis that all of these varied entities have similar damaging effects upon the immunological competence of these tumor-bearing hosts.

Since the LDH-virus will enhance the growth of certain stress-responsive tumors regardless of whether the virus is intentionally inoculated or transmitted as an inadvertent contaminant, it should be emphasized that efforts to study the effects of stress upon such an unsuspectedly contaminated tumor would probably be confusing and difficult to evaluate (Riley, 1966, 1974; Riley, et al., 1978).

IMMUNOSUPPRESSION FOLLOWED BY IMMUNOENHANCEMENT DURING CHRONIC STRESS

A stress experiment carried out by Monjan and Collector (1977) demonstrated that stress-induced immunosuppression occurred between one and 20 days following initiation of intermittent auditory stress. Of special note was the observation that this was followed by immunoehancement between 22 and 35 days, during chronic noctural exposure of mice to the intermttent auditory stress. When the responsiveness to mitogens of B and T cells obtained from the stressed mice were assayed in vitro, both types of cells displayed similar patterns of immunosuppression followed by immunoehancement. Plasma corticosterone levels were elevated during the immunosuppression phase, but had returned to nearly normal during the subsequent enhancement phase. The observed suppression of the T and B cells was undoubtly a consequence of elevated plasma corticosterone concentrations (Spackman, et al., 1974; Monjan and Collector, 1977). However, the mechansims underlying the subsequent immunoenhancement are less clear. Many humoral factors, including somatotrophin and thyroxin, have elevated plasma concentrations during long-term exposure to environmental stress (Pierpaoli and al., 1969; Riley, 1974; Mason, 1974; Monjan and Collector, 1977; Riley, 1974) It was postulated by Monjan and Collector that the delayed immunoenhancement during exposure to chronic stress might be due to the elevation of one or more such circulating factors which stimulate lymphocyte reactivity through activation of the cyclic nucleotide, guanosine 3', 5'-monophosphate.

The phenomenon of alternating immunosuppression and immunoenhancement during exposure to chronic environmental stress may account for some of the conflicting reports regarding enhancement versus inhibition of chemical carcinogenesis, tumor incidence, tumor growth, and regressions in experimental animals exposed to other varieties of chronic stress (Andervont, 1944; Ader and Friedman, 1964; Wheelock, 1967; Fefer, et. al., 1968; Ankraut and Solomon, 1972; Newberry, et. al., 1972; Seifter, et. al., 1973; Solomon and Amkraut Solomon, 1972; Fefer, et al., 1968; Solomon and Amkraut, 1979; Ader and Friedman, 1964; Andervont, 1944; Newberry, et al., 1972; Seifter, et al., 1973)

The data in Figure 15 illustrate another example of stress-associated impairment of immunological competence, depending upon the timing of the application of stress, or its stimulation by the injection of a synthetic corticoid such as dexmethasone. In this experiment, both tumor suppression and tumor enhancement were observed, depending upon the time of injection of DMS relative to tumor implantation. For example, if dexamethasone was administered seven days prior to tumor implantation, the immunocompetence of the host was enhanced approximately 21 days later, as judged by the observation that the growth rate of the developing tumors were suppressed in comparison with the growth of the untreated control tumors. However, when the DMS was administered seven days following implantation of the tumor, there was an overt immunological impairment since the tumor escaped host control, grew rapidly, killing the "stressed" hosts. This is further demonstration of the subtle factors that can change the end-result of an experiment; in this case a simple change in the timing of the various events.

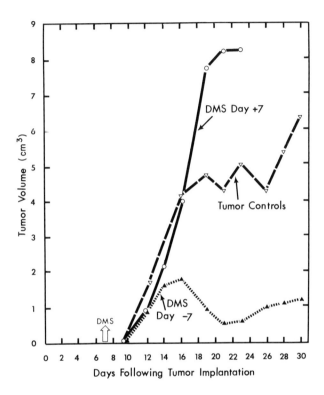

Figure 15. Comparative tumor response following administration of dexamethasone (DMS) at different times in respect to tumor implantation.

When DMS was injected one week prior to tumor implantation, an enhancement of the immunological competence of the host was observed as indicated by the increased suppression of tumor growth by the host compared with the untreated tumor-bearing controls. In contrast, when DMS was injected seven days following tumor implantation, host immunosuppression occurred as indicated by the enhanced growth rate of the tumors.

The 6C3HED lymphosarcoma was implanted as a cell suspension in the hip. Each point is the mean tumor volume of ten C3H/He female mice.

204

## EFFECTS OF THE TIMING OF SIMULATED STRESS ON TUMOR BEHAVIOR

It is possible to modulate the neoplastic process by administering a potent synthetic adrenocorticoid, fluocinolone acetonide (FCA). This hormone, like dexamathasone and corticosterone, induces an involution of the thymus, spleen, and lymph nodes, and a lymphocytopenia involving T and B cells. FCA also blocks the endogenous production of corticosterone by negative feedback to the pituitary. Of neoplastic relevance, a striking enhancement in the growth rate of the 6C3HED lymphosarcoma is produced when FCA is administered during the early stages of tumor growth. Also, the usual spontaneous tumor regressions observed in C3H/He mice implanted with this tumor are prevented or diminished. In contrast, administration of FCA seven days prior to tumor implantation produces an inhibition of subsequent tumor growth, which implies immunoenhancement. This may be an expression of a homeostatic, immunological rebound following suppression

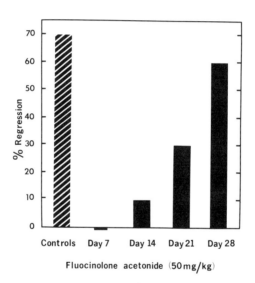

Fluocinolone acetonide (50 mg/kg)

Figure 16. The influence of a synthetic adrenocorticoid in preventing or inhibiting the normal regression of established 6C3HED lymphosarcomas transplanted in C3H/He female mice. The synthetic glucocorticoid was fluocinolone acetonide (FCA) implanted intraperitoneally as a slow release suspension of slight solubility, at the times indicated following tumor implantation. Ten mice were employed in each group.

of various elements of the immunological apparatus, which temporarily enhances the immunological competence of the host. These contrasting effects are both dose-and-time-dependent. Corticosteroids such as FCA, employed in conjunction with an experimental neoplastic system that is in tenous immunological equipoise with the host, provide a reliable model for examing the relationships between T ells, B cells, the pituitary-adrenal-thymus axis , and the cancer process.

Figure 16 provides information concerning the effects of the timing of biochemically simulated stress with respect to its influence upon neoplastic behavior. In this experiment, the neuroendrocrine stress pathways were intentionally bypassed and some of the biochemical and cellular characteristics of physiological stress were simulated by a single injection of FCA, which was administered to several similar tumor-implanted mouse groups at regular intervals following transplantation of the 6C3HED lymphosarcoma into C3H/He mice. When a single dose of the corticoid was administered seven days following tumor implantation, no tumor regressions occurred, which was indicative of an induced impairment of host immunocompetence. This was in contrast to 70% regressions observed in the untreated control mice, illustrating partial immunological control of the tumor by the host. However, this corticoid tumor-enhancing effect was systematically diminished when FCA was administered at later times during the course of tumor growth, as illustrated by Figure 17. These data may be interpreted as a demonstration of the impairment inflicted upon the host immunological apparatus by elevated adrenal corticoids, whether endogenously induced by stress, or directly administered subcutaneously. The quantitative expression of this immunological impairment by a systematic decrease in percent of tumor regressions is dependent upon the stage of the tumor development at the time of corticoid administration. The more advanced the tumor, the less corticoid enhancing effect.

This is further demonstrated by Figure 17, which shows the differences in tumor growth rates resulting from single FCA injections at various times following implantation. Maximum tumor growth enhancement occurred following a single FCA dose at 7 days following tumor implantation. Similar effects were observed when the compound was injected at 14 or 21 days post implantation, while no enhancing effect on the suppressed tumor growth was observed if treatment was delayed until 28 days after tumor implantation. These experiments illustrate that the timing of stressful stimuli may be critical with respect to their optimal or even tangible effects upon stress-responsive tumors.

## STRESS-LIKE EFFECTS IN MICE FOLLOWING EXPOSURE TO MICROWAVE RADIATION

Studies were undertaken in our laboratory, in collaboration with Guy and Chou

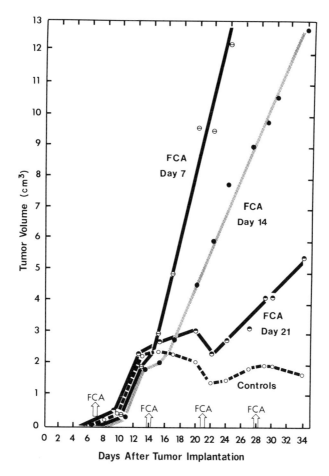

Figure 17. Systematically different tumor growth rates resulting from the injection of a single slow-release depot implant of synthetic corticosteroid at various times with respect to tumor implantation. Those mice receiving FCA on the 28th day post-implantation exhibited a tumor growth behavior that was indistinguishable from that of the untreated tumor-bearing controls.

(Riley, Guy, Spackman and Chou, 1978) to obtain information on possible interactions between non-ionizing radio frequency (RF) radiation and various biological materials. More specifically, we were interested in the possiblility of detecting authentic changes in cells, tissues, organs, and implanted tumors, following the exposure of mice to microwave fields (Riley and Spackman, 1978b).

In order to introduce and to maintain maximum environmental and handling control of the more critical experimental conditions in these studies, the sensitive 6C3HED lymphosarcoma tumor-host model was employed (Riley, Guy, Spackman and Chou, 1978). The logic that was followed in selecting this particular model stemmed from a widespread concern that some of the earlier reports ascribing certain physiological and pathological changes observed in humans and experimental animals exposed to RF radiation, may not have been adequately controlled with respect to anxiety and thus physiologically perturbing stress factors. These questions have arisen partly because some of the reported RF-associated changes were similar to known stress effects (Riley and Spackman, 1978)

Also of relevance, a number of reports concerning the physiological effects of microwaves and other RF frequencies, have implicated the immunological apparatus of experimental animals in vitro, or certain elements of the immune system in vitro (Czerski, 1975). As a consequence of the accumulating evidence that immunological competence might be modified during or following exposure to RF fields or to microwave radiation, experiments were designed to detect subtle RF influences on immunocompetence, employing the special mouse tumor model employed successfully in other stress studies.

The data reported here concern tumor regressions. Figure 18 illustrates the differential tumor regression behavior of the various experimental groups of C3H/He mice. This parameter seems to be the most sensitive in respect to the behavior of the tumors in the RF-radiation-exposed groups as compared to the sham-exposed controls. Tumor regressions occurred in a significally higher percentage of those animals that were previously exposed to either continuous wave (CW) or pulsed RF radiation than in the untreated controls or sham-exposed but non-irradiated animals.

Although there was a higher percentage of tumor regressions in mice exposed to the pulsed mode as compared to the CW mode, the differences beteen these two groups were not statistically significant.

A tentative explanation of the increased regressions assumes that there was an immunological impairment during RF exposure, and that this was followed by immunological recovery and overshoot that produced an enhancement of immunological competence, bringing about an increase in tumor regressions.

## PHYSIOLOGICAL STRESS AND BREAST TUMOR INCIDENCE IN MICE

Presumed identical groups of C3H/HeJ female mice carrying the mammary tumor virus have been monitored for mammary tumor incidence while housed under two different conditions in respect to chronic stress. Conventional open-rack facilities were

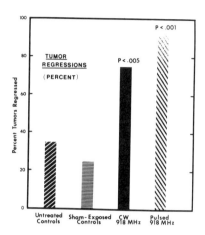

Figure 18. Tumor regressions associated with chronic exposure of C3H/He mice to microwaves (918 MHz RF radiation). The irradiated mice were exposed to 10 mW/cm² for 2 hours per day, 5 days per week, for an 8-week period. The 6C3HED tumors were implanted 8 days following discontinuance of the RF exposures. The regression percentages were observed on day 21 following tumor implantation. Probability values were determined by the chi-square procedure.

employed as a source of environmental stress for two groups of mice (A and B); whereas the protected group benefitted from specially designed low-stress facilities in order to minimize noises, odors, temperature fluctuations, and other stress-inducing factors. Although all of the mice were potential candidates for Bittner virus-induced breast cancer, the mice protected against excessive stress exhibited less than 10% tumor incidence at 13 months of age, as compared with 92% and 68% in those mice maintained under the conventional conditions.

In figure 19 stress-exposed experimental groups A and B are depicted by the two upper curves that show the differences found in mammary tumor latent periods and tumor incidence with time in both parous (A) and non-parous (B) C3H/HeJ mice housed on open movable racks in a communal animal room that was subject to the daily activities of cage cleaning, bleeding procedures, rack movement, and other stress-inducing

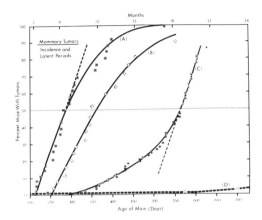

Figure 19.  Mammary tumor incidence and latent periods observed in C3H/He female mice housed under two enviromental conditions.  Group A consisted of parous mice housed under conditions of chronic stress, while Group B were nonparous females housed under the same stressful conditions.  Group C were nonparous females housed under environmental conditions of low stress. At 400 days of age both Groups A and B had high tumor incidences of 92 and 68 percent.  This was in contrast to less than 10 percent incidence for similar mice maintained in low stress protective facilities.  See text for a discussion of the increasing tumor incidence observed in Group C with increasing age.

experimental manipulations of animals in the same room.  Both groups were thus exposed to the usual noise, drafts, recirculating odors, and pheromones.

The experimental results obtained under these conventional environmental conditions are in contrast to the low incidence and extended mammary tumor latent periods observed in mouse group C, represented by the lower curve.  These animals were analogous to the nonparous mice of group B, but important modifications were made in their housing, and thus in their exposure to chronic stress.  Unlike groups A and B, group C mice were housed in plastic cages with bedding and were maintained within the specifically designed low-stress individually ventilated shelves previously described.

These low-stress residential changes are known to have a beneficial influence on the immunological surveillance capabilities of the mice in group C through a rentention of their thymus intearity and T cell population maintenance. Other known factors contributing to transformed cancer cell recognition and immunological competence may also have benefitted from the low-stress environment.

Thus, as a practical demonstration of the potential pathological effects of chronic environmental stress, the data of Figure 19 illustrate the significant differences obtained in mammary tumor incidence and latent periods in genetically susceptible mice carrying the Bittner mammary tumor virus when maintained under different environmental conditions. For example, the median tumor latent period for the parous mice in group A housed in conventional facilities was 276 days as compared to 358 days for the companion group B consisting of non-parous mice. In contrast, the non-parous group C mice housed in low-stress facilities had a median latent period of 566 days, a significant extension over both groups A and B (P$<$.001).

## MOUSE MAMMARY TUMOR INCIDENCE AND AGING

The experiment depicted by Figure 19 offers some useful implications concerning possible relationships between stress, immunocompetence, aging, and the cancer process. For example, a reasonable interpretation of the striking differences observed between 200 and 400 days in the slopes of the tumor incidence curves of the chronically stressed compared with the protected, low-stress animals, is that these diverse slopes are an expression of differences in immunological competence or transformed cell surveillance. This is consistent with the thesis that stress impairs the immunological process. Applying this principle to the case of the mice with the early high tumor incidence represented by curves A and B, it is reasonable to assume that these mice were at increased risk, and that the transformed malignant cells therefore had a greater opportunity to become progressively growing irreversible mammary tumors. These findings are in contrast to the reduced tumor incidence found in the low-stress animals (curve C) whose immune competence was preserved and was thus presumably adequate to prevent most of the transformed cells from reaching overt tumor status.

This interpretation is further supported by the steadily increasing mammary tumor incidence observed in the low-stress mice as they moved into old age, since it is known that immune competence systematically decreases as a function of age. The consequences of this immunological decline are demonstrated by the gradually increasing slope of their mammary tumor incidence curve. For example, between 550 and 600 days of age, the slope of curve C, during the period when immunological competence was obviously impaired by aging, was comparable to that of the stressed mice represented by curve A at 200 to 300 days of age.

These data indicate that protection against stress offers therapeutic or prophylactic benefits only when a potentially effective immunological system is available. Thus in older animals with a naturally reduced immune capability, protection against stress no longer results in a dramatically low tumor incidence.

AGE, IMMUNOCOMPETENCE AND TUMOR BEHAVIOR

Another example of an inverse correlation between increasing age and decreasing immunological competence is demonstrated in Figure 20, which shows that the growth rate of transplanted tumors is significantly enhanced in older mice. This illustration

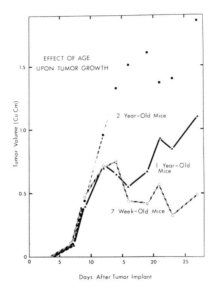

Days After Tumor Implant

Figure 20. Employment of tumor-host relationships for comparing immune competence in mice of various ages. These data confirm that young mice are more capable of restraining susceptible tumor growth than are older mice. This age-associated depreciation of immune competence is analogous to similar effects of emotional stress.

shows the relative tumor growth following identical subcutaneous injections of the 6C3HED lymphosarcoma into C3H/He mice of different ages. It is obvious that the youngest mice are the most capable of restraning the process of this tumor. Most of the tumors (80%) eventually regressed in these seven week-old mice, in contrast to the high lethality that occurred in the oldest animals (P < .005). In logical correlation with this age-associated differential tumor behavior, analogous groups of mice exhibited a corresponding decrease in their thymus weights with increasing age. For example, the average thymus weight of the 2 year-old mice was only 36 percent of that of the 7 week-

212

old mice (P < .001).

These data confirm that the normal aging process brings about an immunological impairment that is similar to the damaging effects of stress. Thus, in terms of inducing alterations in tumor behavior, aging and stress bring about similar pathological effects.

## IMMUNOLOGICAL SURVEILLANCE AGAINST NEOPLASIA

Although there is continuing controversy over the role of immunological surveillance in controlling cancer, accumulated data indicate that such protective monitoring is an immunological reality (see, for example, Herberman's chapter, this volume). It has been suggested that immune surveillance may be most effective against tumor-associated antigen systems that have been regularly encountered by the species during evolutionary processes. Of possible relevance, tumors induced by chemical carcinogens that are the result of the recent events of industrialization, are less affected by immunological mechanisms than other experimental tumors. Accumulated data also suggest that such chemically-induced tumors are less responsive to experimental stress than the more immunoresponsive tumors resulting from oncogenic viruses, such as murine mammary carcinoma or Moloney virus-induced sarcoma. These viruses may have been animal inhabitants during the latter stages of evolution.

## REQUIREMENTS FOR EFFECTIVE IMMUNOSURVEILLANCE

For immunosurveillance to function successfully at least two conditions must be met. Appropriate elements of the immunological system must be capable of recognizing foreign or neoplastic entities, and then be immunologically competent to effectively negate or to destroy the invaders. The present evidence appears to limit the role of stress to the immunocompetent phase of surveillance. Thus, immunological recognition of non-self is of little value if the host is not able to mount an effective attack with its T cells and related machinery. The function of a low-stress environment in assisting immunosurveillance is through maintenance of the integrity of the cellular constituents that permit cell-mediated immunity to function effectively once that non-self is recognized. This is persuasively demonstrated by the interrelationships between immunological status, the Bittner mammary tumor virus, malignant transformation, and the role of stress, or its absence, in permitting the formation of overt mammary tumors. See Figure 19.

## INCREASES IN CANCER INCIDENCE AS A CONSEQUENCE OF T CELL DEFICIENCY

Thymectomy or treatment with anti-lymphocytic serum results in an increased tumor incidence in animals innoculated with viruses such as polyoma or SV40. In contrast, if the ablated T cell system is replaced by thymus grafting, or by inoculation of syngeneic lymphocyte suspensions containing mature T cells, most of the tumors are suppressed, and the observed incidence is much lower. These results support the hypothesis that the increased tumor incidence of the immunologically impaired animals was related specifically to a T cell deficiency. Further supporting evidence, derived from the adverse effects of genetically determined immunodeficiency, is the increased tumor incidence in patients with the Wiskott-Aldrich syndrome, or with ataxia-telangiectasia. Both of these genetic diseases affect the T cell system adversely. Also, patients receiving long-term immunosuppression in order to maintain kidney transplants have an increased tumor incidence compared with the normal population. The accumulated data thus indicate that any compromise of T cell status predicts an increased risk of incipient neoplastic processes escaping immunological containment. This applies to immunosuppression induced by stress as well as by other means.

## DISCUSSION

The pathological effects of stress are dependent upon a variety of physiological and immunological conditions, and thus in many circumstances, no adverse consequences of stress are observed. In other cases, however, the physiological and hormonal changes induced by emotional or anxiety stress are capable of adversely shifting an immunological equipoise to induce lethal results. Various tumor-host and other models have been employed to illustrate the specificity of these circumstances.

Although an extensive variety of stimuli and their resulting physiological alteration are involved in the expression of the typical stress complex, there are certain common denominators that can account for many of the phenomena. The most conspicuous biochemical factor that is associated with stress in mice, whether it is induced by psychosocial confrontations, environmental factors, mechanically induced anxiety (rotation), or viral infections, is the increased concentration of corticosterone in the plasma. Closely related corticoid hormones are similarly involved in other species. The primary and early harm that corticoids cause when present in high plasma concentrations is damage to lymphocytes and thymus elements that are essential for optimum cell-mediated immune defenses, and possibly for effective immune surveillance involving NK lymphocytes when transformed cancer cells may be present (see Herberman's chapter, this volume).

A part of the confusion that is associated with studies of stress-related pathology stems from the two alternative concepts of direct stress-induction of pathologies, as opposed to stress-induced modulation of immune defense capabilities. There is consistent evidence that emotional stress can bring about an overt pathological state if an incipient or latent neoplasm or infection is either pre-existent or enters the picture during a period of acute or chronic stress. It further appears that neoplastic or viral pathologies that are clearly enhanced in the presence of stress are under partial or complete control of cell-mediated immunological defenses. Thus the enhancing effects of stress on these diseases occur as a consequence of the adverse effects of stress on specific immunological elements of the host. Such pathological effects of stress are thus indirect.

Further implications of this working hypothesis are: (1) Stress-associated infectious or neoplastic pathologies will not be observed, despite the presence of stress, if no underlying disease is present. (2) Even if latent pathologies exist, the enhancing effects of stress will not be observed unless the disease is under partial or complete control of the unimpaired immunological system. (3) Such adverse effects of stress will be observed only when the immunological defenses of the host and the resident pathological entity are in a state of equipoise that will permit the modulating forces of stress to be manifested by overt disease when the immunological competence of the host is impaired or otherwise altered.

## References

Ader, R. (1981). Psychoneuroimmunology. Academic Press, New York.

Ader, R., and Friedman, S.B. (1964). Social factors affecting emotionality and resistance to disease in animals: IV. Differential housing, emotionality and Walker 256 carcinosarcoma in the rat. Psychological Reviews 15, 535-541.

Amkraut, A., and Solomon, G.F. (1972). Stress and murine sarcoma virus (Moloney)-induced tumors. Cancer Res. 32, 1428.

Andervont, H.B. (1964). The influence of environment on mammary cancer in mice. J. Nat. Cancer Inst. 4, 579-581.

Anisko, J.J., Suer, S.F., McClintock, M.K., and Adler, N.T. (1978). Relation between 22-kHz ultrasonic signals and sociosexual behavior in rats. J. Comp. Physiol Psychol. 92, 821-829.

Cannon, W.B. (1929). "Bodily Changes in Pain, Hunger, Fear and Rage." Appleton, Second Edition, New York.

Chang, S.S., and Rasmussen, A.F., Jr. (1965). Stress-induced suppression of interferon production in virus-infected mice. Nature 205, 623.

Cochran, A.J., John, U.W., and Gothoskar, B.P. (1972). Cell mediated immunity in malignant melanoma. Lancet i, 1340-1341.

Crispens C.C., Jr. (1976). Apparent inhibitory influence of stress on SJL/JDg neoplasia. Psychology and Psychiatry 4, 169.

Dechambre, R.P., and Gosse, C. (1973). Individual versus group caging of mice with grafted tumors. Cancer Res. 33, 140-144.

Dechambre, R.P., and Gosse, C. (1971). Influence of an isolation stress on the development of transplanted ascites tumors in mice. Role of the adrenals. C. R. Acad. Sci. 272, 2720-2722.

Fefer, A., McCoy, J.L., Perk, K., and Glynn, J.P. (1968). Immunologic, virologic, and pathologic studies of regression of autochtonous Moloney sarcoma virus-induced tumors in mice. Cancer Res. 28, 1157.

Fuller, R.H., Brown, E., and Mills, C.A., (1941). Environmental temperatures and spontaneous tumors in mice. Cancer Res. 1, 130-133.

Gleason, K.K., et al. (1969). The behavioral significance of pheromones in vertebrates. Psychol. Bul. 71, 58-73.

Glenn, W.G., and Becker, R.E., (1969). Individual versus group housing in mice: Immunological response to time and phase injection. Physiol. Zool. 42, 411-416.

Glick, D., Von Redlick, D., and Levine, S. (1969). Fluorometric determination of coriteosterone and cortisol in 0.02-0.05 milliliters of plasma or submilligram samples of adrenal tissue. Endocrinology 74, 635-655.

Gotlieb-Stematsky, T., Karbi, S., and Allison, A.C., (1966). Increased tumor formation by polyoma virus in the presence of non-oncogenic viruses. Nature 212, 421-422.

Harlow, C.M., and Selye, H. (1937). The blood picture in the alarm reaction. Proc. Soc. Exp. Biol. Med. 36, 141-144.

Henry, K.R. (1967). Audiogenic seizure susceptibility induced in C57 BL/6J mice by prior auditory exposure. Science 158, 938-940.

Henry, J.P. (1967). Personal Communication.

Hirsch, M.S. (1974). Immunological Activation of oncogenic viruses: Interrelationship of immunostimulation and immunosuppression. Johns Hopkins Med. J. Supplement 3, 177-185.

Holden, C. (1980). Behavioral Medicine: An Emergent Field. Science 209: 479-481.

Howard, R.J., Notkins, A.L., and Mergenhagen, S.E. (1969). Inhibition of cellular immune reactions in mice infected with lactate dehydrogenase virus. Nature 221, 873-874.

Jensen, M.M. (1968a). Transitory impairment of interferon production in stressed mice. Proc. Soc. Exp. Biol. Med. 128, 174.

Jensen, M.M. (1968b). The influence of stress on murine leukemia virus infection. Proc. Soc. Exp. Biol. Med. 127, 610.

Jensen, M.M., and Rasmussen, A.F., Jr. (1963). Stress and susceptibility to viral infection. II. Sound stress and susceptibility to vesicular stomatitis virus. J. Immun. 90, 21.

Mason, J.W. (1975). Emotion as reflected in patterns of endrocrine regulation. In Emotions - Their Parameters and Measurements (L. Levi, ed.), pp. 143-181. Raven Press, New York.

Mason, J. W. (1974). Specificity in the organization of neuroendrocrine response profiles. In Frontiers in Neurology and Neuroscience Research (P. Seeman and G.M. Brown, ed.), pp. 68-80.

Mason, J.W. (1975). A historic view of the stress field, Parts I and II. J. Human Stress, March (pp. 6-11), and June (pp. 22-36).

Monjan, A.A., and Collector, M. I. (1977). Stress-induced modulation of the immune response. Science 196, 307-308.

Newberry, B.H. (1976). Inhibitory effects of stress on experimental mammary tumors. Abstracts, Third Int. Symposium on Detection and Prevention of Cancer, New York.

Newberry, B.H., and Sengbusch, L. (1979). Inhibitory effects of stress on experimental mammary tumors. Cancer Detection and Prevention 2 (2), 225-233.

Newberry, B.H., Frankie, G., Beatty, P.A., et al. (1972). Shock stress and DMBA-induced mammary tumors in mice. Psychosom. Med. 34, 295-303.

Nicholls, E.M. (1973). Development and elimination of pigmented moles, and the anatomical distribution of primary malignant melanoma. Cancer 32, 191-195.

Nieburgs, H.E., Weiss, J., Navarrete, M., Grillione, G., and Siedlecki, B. (1976). Inhibitory and enhancing effects of various stresses on experimental mammary tumorigenesis. Abstracts, Third Int. Symposium on Detection and Prevention of Cancer (No. 772), New York.

Pierpaoli, W., Baroni, C., Fabris, N., and Sorkin, E. (1969). Hormone and immunologic capacity. II. Reconstitution of antibody production in hormonally deficient mice by somatotrophic hormone, thyrotropic hormone, and thyroxin, Immunology 16, 217-230.

Rasmussen, A.F., Jr., Hildemann, W.H., and Sellers, M. (1963). Malignancy of polyoma virus infection in mice in relation to stress. J. Nat. Cancer Inst. 30, 101.

216

Riley, V. (1979a). Cancer and stress: overview and critique. Cancer Detection and Prevention, Vol 2, No. 2, 163-195.

Riley, V. (1979b). Introduction: Stress-cancer contradictions: a continuing puzzlement. Cancer Detection and Prevention, Vol 2, No. 2, 159-162.

Riley, V. (1978). Stress and cancer: fresh perspectives. Proc Third Int. Symp. on Det. and Prev. of Cancer, pp. 1769-1776.

Riley, V. (1974). Erroneous interpretation of valid experimental observations through interference by the LDH-virus. J. Natl. Cancer Inst. 52, 1673-1677.

Riley, V. (1972). Protective ventilated shelves for experimental animal storage. Proc. 23rd Annual Session, Amer. Assoc. Lab. Animal Sci., No. 22A. St. Louis.

Riley, V. (1966). Spontaneous mammary tumors: Decrease in incidence of mice infected with an enzyme-elevating virus. Science 153, 1657-1658.

Riley, V. , Fitzmaurice, M.A., and Spackman, D.H. (1981). Animal models in biobehavioral research. Proc. Acad. Behavioral Research. Academic Press, New York.

Riley, V., Guy, A.W., Spackman, D.H., and Chou, C.K. (1978). Neoplastic cells as sensitive targets for examining the biological and pathological effects of RF and microwave irradiation. Inter. Union Radio Science Abstr. OS:2, 93.

Riley, V., and Spackman, D.H. (1978a). Enhancing effects of anxiety-stress on the neoplastic process in mice. XII th International Cancer Congress Buenos Aires.

Riley, V., and Spackman, D.H. (1978b). Simulation of RF and microwave biological effects by handling and housing-induced stress of experimental animals. Inter. Union Radion Science Abstr. OS: 2, 63.

Riley, V., and Spackman, D.H. (1977a). Housing stress. Lab Animal 6, 16-21.

Riley, V., and Spackman, D.H. (1977b). Cage crowding stress: absence of effect on melanoma within protective facilities. Proc. Amer. Assoc. Cancer Res. 18, 173.

Riley, V., and Spackman, D.H. (1976a). Melanoma enhancement by viral-induced stress. In "The Pigment Cell; Melanomas: Basic Properties and Clinical Behavior" (V. Riley, ed.), pp. 163-173. Vol. 2, S. Karger, Basel.

Riley, V., and Spackman, D.H. (1976b). Modifying effects of a benign virus on the malignant process and the role of physiological stress on tumor incidence. Fogarty International Cancer Proceedings, No. 28, pp. 319-336, U.S. Government Printing Office, Washington, D.C.

Riley, V., Spackman, D.H., Santisteban, G.A., Dalldorf, G., Hellstrom, I., Hellstrom, K.E., Lance, E.M., Rowson, K.E.K., Mahy, B.W.J., Alexander, P., Stock, C.C., Sjorgren, H.O., Hollander, V.P., and Horzinck, M.C. (1978). The LDH-virus: An interfering biological contaminant. Science 200, 124-125.

Riley, V., Spackman, D.H., and Santisteban, G.A., (1975). The role of physiological stress on breast tumor incidence in mice. Proc. Amer. Assoc. Cancer. Res. 16, 152.

Santisteban, G.A., and Riley, V. (1973). Thymo-lymphatic organ response to the LDH-virus. Proc. Amer. Assoc. Cancer Res. 14, 112.

Seifter, E., Rettura, G., Zisblatt, M. et al. (1973). Enhancement of tumor development in physically-stressed mice innoculated with an oncogenic virus. Experimentia 29, 1379-1382.

Selye, H. (1975) Confusion and controversy in the stress field. Journal of Human Stress (June), pp. 37-44.

Solomon, G.F., and Amkraut, A.A. (1979). Neuroendrocrine aspects of the immune response and their implications for stress effects on tumor immunity. Cancer Detection and Prevention 2 (2), 197-224.

Solomon, G.F., Amkraut, A.A., and Rubin, R.T. (1981). Stress and psycho-immunological response. Proc. Acad. Behavioral Medicine Research Academic Press, New York.

Spackman, D.H., and Riley, V. (1974). Increased corticosterone, a factor in LDH-virus induced alterations of immunological responses in mice. Proc. Amer. Assoc. Cancer Res. 15, 143.

Spackman, D.H., Riley, V., and Bloom, J. (1978). True plasma corticosterone levels of mice in cancer/stress studies. Proc. Amer. Assoc. Cancer Res. 19, 57

Spackman, D.H., Riley, V., Santisteban, G.A., Kirk, W., and Bredburg, L. (1974). The role of stress in producing elevated corticosterone levels and thymus involution in mice. Abstracts, XI th International Cancer Congress 3, 382-383.

Sprunt, D.H., and Flanigan, C.C. (1956). The effect of malnutrition on the susceptibility of the host to viral infection. J. Exp. Med. 104, 687-706.

Sze, P., (1970). Neurochemical factors in auditory stimulation and development of susceptibility to audiogenic seizures. In Physiological Effects of Audible Sound. (B. Welch and A. Welch, ed.) Plenum Press, New. York.

Tannenbaum, A. (1940). The initiation and growth of tumors, I. The effects of underfeeding. Amer. J. Cancer 38, 335-350.

Tannenbaum, A., and Silverstone, H. (1953). Nutrition in relation to cancer. Advan. Cancer Res. 1, 451-501.

Turner, W., Chirigos, M.A., and Scott, D. (1968). Enhancement of Friend and Rauscher leukemia virus replication in mice by Guaroa virus. Cancer Res. 28, 1064-1073.

Turner, W., Ebert, P. S., Bassin, R., Spahn, G., and Chirigos, M.A. (1971). Potentiation of murine sarcoma virus (Harvey) (Moloney) oncogenicity in lactic dehydogenase-elevating virus-infected mice. Proc. Soc. Biol. Med. 136, 1314-1318.

Turner, C.D., and Hagnara, J.T. (1971) General Endocrinology, Fifth Edition, pp. 382-383. Sanders, Philadelphia.

Youn, J.K., and Barski, G. (1966). Interference between lymphocyctic choriomeningitis and Rauscher leukemia in mice J. Nat. Cancer Inst. 37, 381-388.

Young, S. (1958). Effect of temperature on the production of induced rat mammary tumors. Nature 219, 1254-1255.

Vessey, S.H., (1964). Effects of grouping on levels of circulating antibodies in mice. Proc Soc. Exptl. Biol. Med. 115, 252.

Wallace, E.W., Wallace, H.M., and Mills, C.A. (1944). Influence of environmental temperature upon the incidence and course of spontaneous tumors in C3H mice. Cancer Res. 4, 279-281.

Wheelock, E.F. (1967). Inhibitory effects of Sendai virus on Friend virus leukemia in mice. J. Nat. Cancer Inst. 38, 771-778.

Published 1982 by Elsevier Science Publishing Co, Inc.
Sandra M. Levy, ed.
Biological Mediators of Behavior and Disease:
Neoplasia

# BEHAVIORAL REGULATION OF IMMUNITY: IMPLICATIONS FOR HUMAN CANCER

JOHN WUNDERLICH
Immunology Branch, National Cancer Institute, National Institutes of Health,
Bethesda, Maryland  20205, USA

## Introduction

The basic issue considered in this volume concerns possible regulatory ties between behavior and cancer, especially human cancer.  My own interests lie in immunology and cancer; and from that viewpoint the general topic is intriguing, because one can seriously consider a triangular regulatory network consisting of the neoplasm, the immune system and the central nervous system (CNS).  Each of these three elements is clearly influenced by other factors, but the issue of particular interest is the extent to which they influence each other. Although only a limited portion of the network is considered here, namely possible influences of behavior on tumors via the immune system, it should be in the unspoken context of the broader network.

The nature of behavorial regulation of cancer via the immune system is a topic which has been addressed in depth in this volume from a variety of perspectives.  The purpose of this chapter is to consider issues which complicate exploration of the topic, particularly as it applies to human cancer. For me the fundamental difficulties involve how we define the extent of the immune system, limitations of tumor models as they apply to human cancer, contrasting effects of immune activity on tumor cells, the multiple options for CNS regulation of the immune system, and the challenges associated with clinical studies.  Each of these issues will be explored in turn.

## A Pragmatic Definition of the Immune System

Study of the immune system as a mediator of behavioral effects on tumor cells would be a rhetorical exercise, if there were no reason to believe that there is immune activity against spontaneously occuring tumors in man.  The issue of whether such immune activity exists is still a controversial one.  Part of the disagreement involves different viewpoints of what host mechanisms constitute the "immune system."

In defining the immune system it is useful to distinguish between sensitization and effector stages, because the former offers more

220

opportunity for host regulation. Sensitization refers to events which are involved in generation of immune activity. The sensitization stage either follows natural activation of the immune system, by means such as host exposure to environmental pathogens -- or follows treatment, such as immunization with vaccines. In either case a variety of different cell types are involved in generating immune activity (see below). The effector stage occurs after sensitization and concerns the reaction of the sensitized arm of the immune system with its target -- such as tumor cells. Actual delivery of the sensitized arm to the appropriate location, say lymphocytes from a lymph node to the tumor site, must fit into the scheme of events somewhere; and for our purposes it is arbitrarily included in the effector stage. The effector stage can be reached by a natural immune response or passively by treatment with previously formed immune activity (e.g. adoptive or passive immunotherapy). In the latter case, host regulation is limited to the effector stage, such as altering the traffic pattern of effector agents, changing the susceptability of tumor cells to injury or altering activity of the immune effector agent. Thus, with passive immunization a full host immune response is not necessary, because generation of immune activity occurs outside the host and is then provided as a form of treatment.

Traditionally, "immune system" has had connotations of antibody involvement-- that a specific immune reaction occurs in response to a specific antigen, which is recognized by antibody. This characteristic applies not only to humoral antibody responses, but also to antigen-specific T cell responses. Such T cells bear cell-surface determinants, which bind antigens connected to cell surfaces, and share combining sites with humoral antibody (Krawinkel et al., 1979). The fact that T cells recognize antigens on antigen-bearing cell surfaces is important, because certain cell-surface determinants on the antigen-bearing cells, coded by the major histocompatibility gene complex, restrict T-cell recognition of antigen (Berzofsky, 1981). The antigen-specific responses, both humoral antibody and T cell, are regulated by a complex network of interacting factors involving humoral antibody, antigen presenting cells (macrophages), suppressor lymphocytes and helper lymphocytes (Jerne, 1974; Broder and Waldmann, 1978; Tada and Okumura, 1979; Cantor, 1980; Berzofsky, 1981). This regulatory network can respond to signals not only from lymphoid cells, but also from cells outside the immune system (see below). The network can augment an immune response, provide a breaking action, or block its generation. The network probably has an important role in preventing responses against self (autoimmunity), which must be considered when manipulating it.

221

Three distinct types of cytotoxic immune responses against tumors involve tumor cell-surface antigens, defining "antigen" in the traditional sense of determinants which induce antibody responses: 1) complement-dependent cytotoxic humor antibody, 2) cytotoxic T cells, and 3) cell-dependent humoral antibody which can cooperate with a wide variety of nonimmunized cells (ADCC effector cells) to injure tumor cells. Regarding the last category, certain types of lymphocytes, macrophages, platelets and polymorphonuclear cells have all been implicated as potential host participants in this mechanism (Lovchik and Hong; 1977).

In contrast to the traditional immune system, there is a second category of host anti-tumor mechanisms, notable in that they are not yet known to involve antibody-like molecules for recognition of tumor cells. Thus, activated macrophages (Schultz and Chirigos, 1980) and natural killer (NK) cells (Herberman, 1980) preferentially injure tumor cells upon contact, but the recognition systems may entail components quite distinct from antibodies and antigens. This possibility is not distressing, since there are many examples of cell-cell recognition by mechanisms other than antigen and antibody (e.g. Beyer et al., 1979; Podleski and Greenberg, 1980; Gartner et al., 1981).

Regulation of cytotoxic macrophages and NK cells differs from that of antigen-specific immune responses. Activated macrophages, cytotoxic for tumor cells, are derived from resting, non-toxic macrophages by a variety of mechanisms (Schultz and Chirigos, 1980). Factors released by certain subclasses of sensitized lymphocytes stimulated by specific antigen will activate macrophages. Macrophages can also be activated nonspecifically and directly by antigen-antibody complexes, the lipid A component of bacterial endotoxin, double stranded RNA, some polysaccharides which occur naturally on the outer membranes of certain microorganisms, and activated complement. Macrophages can also be activated nonspecifically and indirectly by factors, such as interferon and certain lymphokines, which are released by other cell types. Inhibitors of cytotoxic macrophages have been identified, including glucocorticoids, substances which increase intracellular cyclic AMP, and factor(s) released by tumor cells which impede the accumulation of macrophages at the tumor site.

NK activity is augmented by viruses, tumor cells, bacterial adjuvants (e.g. Bacillus Calmette Guerin - BCG) and bacterial endotoxin, all of which may act by affecting levels of interferon (Herberman, 1980). Activity is diminished by hydrocortisone and by agents which elevate cyclic AMP, such as prostaglandin E and histamine.

In addition to the antitumor activity provided by activated macrophages and

NK cells, complement probably can be activated directly by cell surface viruses in the absence of antibody, and mediate tumor cell lysis (Bartholomew and Esser, 1980).

The major point here is that a variety of host antitumor mechanisms exist, which can loosely be included in the immune system. The factors which activate and regulate host antitumor activity are numerous, independent in many cases, and also involve activities of cells not included in the immune system. Thus, the opportunities for outside (e.g. behavior) modulation of an antitumor-immune network are extensive. However, the final result of modulation of the system from one source depends on the input of checks and balances from other sources of immune system regulation.

A distinction must be made between the immune system and other factors which influence it. Here, we are considering the following components to be part of the immune system: cells in the differentiation linage of lymphocytes or macrophages, products of such cells, and cells which cooperate with humoral antibody in host activity against tumor cells. As noted above, immune responses are regulated by cells which are part of the immune system. However, factors outside of the immune system also influence immune responses. Perhaps the best known example is the adrenal gland, whose hormonal products are able to modulate immune responses. Of interest here is the effect of behavior on adrenal function. The behavior-adrenal-immune system link is considered briefly in this chapter and in depth in other chapters. Direct links of the CNS and immune system will also be considered in this chapter. Not explored here is the possibility that other factors which regulate host antitumor immunity but are outside the immune system could also be modulated by behavior. For example, poor nutrition has been linked with immune responses (Fernandes et al., 1979), and behavior influences nutritional status. Also not explored here is the possibility of other forms of host antitumor defense mechanisms (e.g. regulation of tumor blood supply), which are affected by behavior or factors influencing behavior (see papers by Miller, Lippman, this volume).

## Tumor Models

Most of the data base supporting the concept of antitumor immune activity is derived from tumor models which predominantly involve 1) tumor cell lines or 2) animals in which tumors were induced by viruses or high doses of carcinogens. These points are frequently cited in critical analyses of studies dealing with possible relationships between the immune system and cancer in man (Baldwin and

Embleton, 1977; Klein and Klein, 1977; Hewitt, 1978). The main problem with tumor lines is that they can "drift" from the form of their predecessors and thus not reliably represent primary tumor cells growing in situ. A dramatic example of rapid drift between cultured tumor cells and their progenitors is expression on the cell surface of virus-related glycoproteins or intact viruses, which can occur within several serial passages of cells dispersed from the primary tumor (Brown et al., 1978; Cleveland et al., 1979). Also, selective survival and growth of a small subpopulation of the original tumor cells, perhaps encouraged by a semiphysiologic medium, is a clear possibility. Moreover, animal tumors commonly induced in the laboratory with carcinogens appear to be more "antigenic" than tumors which spontaneously arise (Prehn, 1975). Finally, there is no compelling evidence that human tumors are directly induced by infectious viruses in a fashion akin to the virus-induced animal tumors. Even if there is a common basic mechanism underlying neoplastic transformation in naturally occurring human cancer and the current tumor models, there will still be criticism of the immunologic relevance of tumor models because expression of new cell surface determinants (e.g. antigens) related to viruses or high-dose carcinogens may not occur with natural transformation of human cells.

The issue is reminiscent of a similar one which occurred in laboratories in the early 1900's. At that time investigators discovered that tumors transplanted between mice were rejected. The observers were optimistic that such host defense mechanisms could be used for treatment of human tumors. However, the mice used at that time were not inbred, and tumor rejection was mediated by histocompatibility antigens. Although recognition of the basis for these tumor rejections stimulated the field of transplantation biology, the reservations were clear about using histocompatibility differences to study host-tumor interactions as they occur in man. Tumors in natural hosts rarely express foreign histocompatibility antigens (Law et al., 1980). Thus, host mechanisms which reject grafted tissues because they express foreign histocompatibility antigens (e.g., mismatched kidney transplants), may not be involved in host responses against spontaneous tumors in man.

The historical issue of host-tumor histocompatiblity differences is relevant, because the immune system can also generate strong responses against viruses expressed by autologous or syngeneic cells (Zinkernagel and Doherty, 1979) and against chemically modified cells (Shearer and Schmitt-Verhulst, 1977) or against cells which have adsorbed foreign proteins (Forni and Green, 1976; Sulit et al., 1976; Golstein et al., 1978). Thus, the problem of "drift" of tumor cells from the progenitor cells occurring in the primary tumor involves not just genetic changes and selective survival but also viral contamination and adsorption of foreign tissue culture components, particularly from foreign serum used in tissue culture medium. These complications have contributed to the lack of unanimity on the question of whether man is capable of generating immune responses against spontaneously occurring tumors.

Despite these concerns, recent studies with monoclonal antibodies generated against human tumors have demonstrated antigens on tumor cells in tissue sections, antigens not apparent on normal cells from the patient (Schlom et al., 1980). The tumor cells were from primary tumor tissues which had not been passaged. These studies do not address the issue of whether there is host immune activity against tumor cells in man mediated by tumor antigens, but at least they establish a basis for possible tumor selective immune activity.

## Contrasting Effects of the Immune System on Tumor Cells

In general, the immune system should be more effective against human cancer after rather than before malignant transformation. This is because the immune system would have to recognize the transforming agents as foreign and inactivate it in order to prevent malignant transformation of cells. There is little evidence for such a possibility. With some possible exceptions, such as Epstein-Barr virus (Burkitt's lymphoma)(Klein, 1979), herpes simplex virus type 2 (cervical carcinoma)(Szmuness, 1978), and hepatitis B virus (hepatocellular carcinoma (Thomas and Rawls, 1978; Wilkie et al., 1980), infectious organisms do not appear to have a role in transformation of cells. If a direct and independent role, or even a collaborative role, could be established for infectious viruses in human cell transformation, tumor immunology research would rapidly expand in the direction of preventive immunization. However, up until now the major focus of tumor immunology has been on therapeutic interactions between the immune system and tumor cells rather than a preventive interaction of the immune system with transforming agents.

In animal models the immune system has been most effective against small tumor burdens, so the major interest of tumor immunologists has been in the role of the immune system in host surveillance for tumor cells shortly after transformation or in small clusters, and for metastasizing cells in contrast to large tumor masses.

What are the possible direct effects of the immune system on tumor cells? In short, probably both enhancing and inhibitory effects. Evidence exists that immune responses can make tumors grow faster and that immune responses can reject tumors. The possibility of these opposing outcomes has been supported by Prehn (1972), who used a mouse tumor model to show that relatively weak immune activity stimulates tumor growth whereas strong activity retards growth. Similar observations have been made by Kall and Hellstrom (1975), who used an in vitro model which allows detection of immune stimulation of tumor cell growth within several days rather than several weeks, thus reducing the possibility of intermediate events (e.g., effects of lymphokines on lymphocyte circulation patterns) linking the immune system to tumor cells.

Stimulation of the immune system may also promote tumor growth by indirect effects. For example, humoral immune responses alone are generally ineffective against solid tumors in animal models. However, they can inhibit antitumor cellular immune responses at any one of several stages of development. (Hellstrom and Hellstrom, 1974). Nontoxic humoral antibody may bind to tumor cells and protect them from cytotoxic immune cells; or immune serum factors may interfer with the activity or generation of cytotoxic cells.

To further complicate the issue of effects the immune system may have on a tumor, many independent immunological components have been identified which can interact with tumor cells (Haskill et al., 1978), such as macrophages, T lymphocytes, natural killer cells, humoral antibody, nonimmune cells which in cooperation with humoral antibody are cytotoxic, and various combinations thereof (see above). Different combinations of these effector mechanisms might be active against different individual tumors. Moreover, as noted above, these components and the cell differentiation pathways for generating them are under regulatory control, which can either augment or depress the responses. Since the components are generated along independent lines of cell differentiation, one would expect somewhat different mechanisms for their regulation. Thus, down regulation of one type of activity would not necessarily be accompanied by down regulation of other components. Some components of the immune system, such as natural antibody (Houghton et al., 1970), natural killer cells (Herberman, 1980) and activated macrophages (Schultz and Chirigos, 1980) occur in hosts which have not been intentionally immunized. These effector elements of the immune system, which are involved in cytotoxic reactions against many types of tumor cells in vitro, have been implicated in host surveillance against tumors.

Recent development of monoclonal antibodies against specific differentiation antigens on cell surfaces has greatly helped identification and isolation of the subclasses of immune effector cells and their regulating cell types (McKenzie and Potter, 1979; Reinherz and Schlossman, 1980). However, it is not yet clear how this complex network of immune activity against tumor cells is tipped in favor of tumor promotion or rejection. Also, it is not clear where the balance point lies between a particular tumor and the host influences which will promote or retard tumor growth. Perhaps this problem is a difficult one not just because of the heterogeneity between tumors but also because of heterogeneity of tumor cells within a single tumor and the heterogeneity of tumor growth sites.

## Multiple Facets of Central Nervous System Regulation of the Immune System

What is the basis for regulating immune activity and its development, particularly in the context of the CNS? Considerable evidence has been gathered for neuro-endocrine modulation of immune responses [e.g. see review by Strom and Carpenter (1980) and other chapters in this volume). T lymphocytes, which include cytotoxic effector cells, helper cells and suppressor cells, appear to express both adrenergic and cholinergic (muscarinic) receptors and thus are linked to the nervous system. The extent to which each of the functional subclasses of lymphocytes expresses these receptors at various stages of differentiation is not yet clear.

In general, activation of adrenergic receptors increases intracellular cyclic AMP and decreases cell proliferation and function whereas activation of cholinergic receptors increases cyclic GMP and increases cell proliferation and function. One or both of these effects apply to cytotoxic T cells, NK cells, ADCC effector cells and cytotoxic macrophages. Suppressor cells are an exception. They appear to be triggered by histamine (a cyclic AMP elevating agent) to release an immune suppressor factor (Rocklin et al., 1980). Thus, histamine activates suppressor cell function, but it also suppresses cytotoxic immune cell function, both of which reduce immune activity. Also an exception -- the activation roles of cyclic AMP and GMP may be reversed when one deals with early as opposed to the late stages of cell differentiation which are characteristic of cytotoxic effector cells (Scheid et al., 1978). Lymphocyte expression of receptors for neurotransmitters may fluctuate depending on whether cells are in a state of inactivity, early activation or late activation. Thus, CNS regulation includes not only multiple arms of the immune system but also different stages of immune cell differentiation.

Schwartz and colleagues (1980) have recently reported that histamine suppresses generation of cytotoxic T cells, thus establishing that both effector and sensitization stages of immune activity are sensitive to agents which modulate cyclic nucleotides. Corticosteroids, which are another source of CNS regulation of the immune system, are released by hypothalamic-pituitary-adrenal stimulation and redistribute human T cells in particular and inhibit at least some of lymphoid cell activities (Fauci et al., 1976; Haynes and Fauci, 1978). Thus, among the variables to consider in evaluating CNS effects on immune responses, are the subclass of target lymphoid cells, the type of neurotransmitter receptor expressed, and the state of activation or differentiation of the cells.

Apparently, immunosuppression via adrenergic receptors can occur directly from the sympathetic nervous system in addition to circulating adrenal catecholamines. Sympathetic innervation of both the thymus and the spleen has been reported (Williams et al., 1981). Chemical sympathectomy was associated with enhanced humoral immune responses. Of note, nerve fibers were seen in close proximity to mast cells, which release histamine following stimulation of their adrenergic receptors.

Thus, CNS regulation of the immune system is complex, in terms of both multiple regulators and multiple types of cells in the immune system which are subject to regulation. There can be intermediate steps in the regulatory chain, such as CNS modulation of mast cells or the adrenal gland which in turn regulate immune cells. The closer the tie, the more direct the regulation. The critical issue is what net effect particular forms of behavior or factors influencing behavior will have on cancer progression. Where the immune system is involved, the result will depend on whether humoral or cellular immunity is predominantly modulated, whether the modulation is stimulation or inhibition, whether the existing balance between the immune system and cancer growth sites is one of immunostimulation or one of immunosuppression, and whether there is such heterogeneity between tumor cells and types of immune activities at the growth sites that there can be no single outcome of modulation of the immune system (i.e., some growth sites will regress, others will progress and the remaining ones will not change).

## Challenges of Clinical Studies

Correlations between behavior, factors influencing behavior, and cancer have been analyzed by others in this volume. Including the immune system in

the analysis adds major complex challenges. The hypothesis to be tested is
that the immune system serves as an intermediate link between behavior and the
spread of cancer. The experimental approach to the problem is to correlate
behavior, antitumor activity and tumor progression or regression, preferably
in a prospective study. A major obstacle is that antitumor activity in man
detected by current tests is not clearly correlated with the fate of the tumor
for a variety of reasons: 1) both false negative and false positive tests for
immune activity, 2) unknown baseline levels of antitumor activity, and 3) non-
specific wasting effects of cancer or its treatment on immune activity.

False positive tests for immune activity may occur because of a) blocking
factors present in the host but inoperative in the test, b) development of
antitumor activity in vitro during the course of the test (some tests last 2-3
days) in spite of the absence of such activity in the patient, c) predominant
immunostimulation of tumor growth in the host, which is not detected by the
test, (some tests detect only cytotoxicity), d) antitumor activity in peripheral
blood cells (the usual source of cells for tests) but not in cells at tumor
sites, e) a temporary spike in antitumor activity which occurs at the time of
the test but is not of sufficient duration to be effective in the patient
against the tumor, f) positive activity in a tested segment of the immune
response (e.g. lymphocyte proliferation) which is not accompanied by cytotoxic
or cytostatic antitumor immune activity in the patient, or g) using for tests
sensitive tumor target cell lines which do not reflect immune susceptibility
of natural tumor cells in the patient.

False negative tests for immune activity may occur because a) the assay
time is inadequate to reveal tumor cell damage, b) cells in the peripheral
blood lack antitumor activity, whereas those at tumor sites have such activity,
c) immune cells in the patient only inhibit growth of tumor cells whereas the
assay is capable of detecting only tumor cell lysis, d) a brief dip in antitumor
activity which occurs at the time of the test but does not reflect the usual
level of activity, or e) the test is designed for the wrong arm of immune
activity (e.g. antitumor activity is present in macrophages but the test
samples only lymphocytes).

Unknown baseline levels of immune activity involve those which occur
naturally and are found in normal individuals: NK cells, cytotoxic macrophages,
and natural antitumor humoral antibody. Because these activities are found in
normal individuals and activities vary considerably between individuals, time
course studies which cover the period before and after tumor development are
desirable for correlating changes in activity with tumor development. Levels

of activity which existed in patients prior to appearance of the malignancy
are usually unknown.

Immuno-suppressive effects of cancer and many types of treatment have been
extensively described. In the same sense that patients may be anxious and
depressed as a consequence of cancer progression, immune activity may be low
in cancer patients as an effect of cancer or its treatment rather than a cause
of its progression.

Patient stratification for a clinical study is particularly difficult because
of factors outlined in the preceding paragraphs and the multitude of independent
factors which can affect immune activity or cancer progression. Moreover, the
immune system could be only one of several links between behavior and cancer.
In such a case, laboratory tests for antitumor immune activity could indeed
reflect events in the patient, but antitumor effects of the immune system might
be dominated in the patient by independent behavior-related mechanisms having an
opposite effect on cancer progression. Thus, a CNS-immune system-cancer link
could exist and yet be missed.

Stratification of patients could be simplified by directly controlling the
host antitumor response. Although neither passive or active immunotherapy in
its current form is generally considered useful for treatment of human cancer
(e.g. Rosenberg and Terry, 1977), a technique for treating human skin cancer
by sensitization against topically applied antigens has been used successfully
by Klein (1976). Correlating behavior with the efficiency of this form of
treatment, would not establish a behavior-immune system-cancer relationship,
because behavior could reflect the patient's reaction to the tumor. However,
the concept of intervention can be extended to psychological treatment.
Patients matched for the type of skin tumor and prognosis, as well as behavioral or personality type and form of local immunotherapy, could be randomly
assigned to a control group or to one receiving cognitive-behavioral intervention. This approach could provide a setting for correlating behavior, the
immune system and cancer in which the behavorial changes were not a result of
the cancer.

Positive correlations between behavior (e.g. depression and anxiety) and
cancer progression and between behavior (stress) and immune activity (peripheral
blood NK activity) have been reported (see other chapters, this volume); but
human behavior, immune activity and cancer progression have not been monitored
together in the same study, as far as I'm aware.

Conclusions

In summary, correlations between behavior and cancer have been noted. Animal model studies show that an immune response which develops against a tumor can either enhance or retard tumor growth. The response itself can be intensified or diminished by neuroregulation. Whether the immune system provides a link between behavior and cancer in man remains to be determined.

Facing such ambivalent outcomes of an antitumor immune response, namely either cancer progression or regression, what further information would be helpful in evaluating a CNS-immune system-cancer network? For starters, a more extensive description of neurotransmitters, their in situ half-lives and their regulation would be helpful. Do cancer cells express receptors for these transmitters, and if so what are the effects of receptor activation on tumor cells? Can various forms of CNS stimulation or discrete CNS lesions (Cross et al., 1980) be translated into reproducible changes in neurotransmitters which are relevant to lymphoid or cancer cells? Which functional subclasses of lymphoid cells express the receptors and what is the outcome of receptor activation? More information is needed regarding the effects of lymphoid cell differentiation on their expression of receptors for neurotransmitters. A critical issue is whether a particular form of CNS activity, such as adrenal stimulation, will have a uniform effect on various arms of antitumor immune activity at the tumor sites as reflected by generation, delivery and action of the immune effector arms. If the result of such CNS activity can be either cancer progression or regression, depending on the balance of effects on helper and suppressor regulatory cells and on effector cells and their precursors, then identification of a CNS-immune system-cancer link in man will clearly be difficult.

In contrast to testing biochemical and cellular parameters, tumor growth or incidence in the host could be monitored. For example, we could consider the effect of CNS stimulation on tumor growth in an animal model using as variables chemical sympathectomy or other forms of CNS depletion, and immunosuppression. However, the relevance of the tumor model to human neoplasia would be controversial, as noted above.

Would clinical studies be appropriate, such as an epidemiological analysis relating cancer incidence and immune activity to behavior--or even better, an analysis of the effects of behavioral or immunological intervention on the behavior-immune system-cancer network? Possibly, but a negative correlation could easily result from our inability to stratify patients into comparable groups.

## Acknowledgements

I am grateful to Dr. Philip Morrissey and Dr. Sandra Levy for comments on the manuscript and to Ms. Judith Steckel for her help in preparing the manuscript.

## References

Baldwin RW, Embleton MJ (1977) Assessment of cell mediated immunity to human tumor-associated antigens. Int Rev of Expt Path 17:49-95.

Bartholomew RM, Esser AF (1980) Mechanism of antibody-independent activation of the first component of complement (CL) on retrovirus membranes. Biochemistry 19:2847-2953.

Berzofsky JA (1981) Immune response genes in the regulation of mammalian immunity. In Goldberger RF (ed), Biological Regulation and Development 2:467-594 New York: Plenum.

Beyer EC, Tokuyasu KT, Barondes SH (1979) Localization of an endogenous lectin in chicken liver, intestine and pancreas. J Cell Biol 82:565-571.

Bourne HR, Lichtenstein LM, Melmon KL, Henney CS, Weinstein Y, Shearer GM (1974) Modulation of inflammation and immunity by cyclic AMP. Science 184:19-28.

Broder S, Waldmann TA (1978) The suppressor-cell network in cancer. N Eng J Med 299:1281-1284 and 1335-1341.

Brown JP, Klitzman JM, Hellstrom I, Nowinski RC, Hellstrom KE (1978) Antibody response of mice to chemically induced tumors. Proc Nat Acad Sci USA 75:955-958.

Cantor H (1980) Regulation of the immune system by lymphocyte sets; analysis in animal models. Clin Immunobiol 4:89-98.

Cleveland PH, Belnap LP, Knotts FB, Nayak SK, Baird SM, Pilch YH (1979) Tumor-associated antigens of chemically-induced murine tumors; the emergence of MuLV and fetal antigens after serial passage in culture. Int J Cancer 23:380-391.

Cross RJ, Markesbery WR, Brooks WH, Roszman RL (1980) Hypothalamic-immune interactions. I. The acute effect of anterior hypothalamic lesions on the immune response. Brain Res 196:79-87.

Fauci AS, Dale DC, Balow JE (1976) Glucocorticosteroid therapy: mechanisms of action and clinical considerations. Ann Int Med 84:304-315.

Fernandes G, West A, Good RA (1979) Nutrition, immunity, and cancer--a review. Part III: effect of diet on the diseases of aging. Clin Bull 9:91-106.

Forni I, Green I (1976) Heterologous sera: a target for in vitro cell-mediated cytotoxicity. J Immunol 116:1561-1565.

Gartner TK, Gerrand JM, White JG, Williams DC (1981) Fibrinogen is the receptor for the endogenous lectin of human platelets. Nature 19:688-690.

Golstein P, Luciani MF, Wagner H, Rollinghoff M (1978) Mouse T cell-mediated cytolysis specifically triggered by cytophilic xenogeneic serum determinants: a caveat for the interpretation of experiments done under "syngeneic" conditions. J Immunol 121:2533-2538.

Haskill JS, Hayry P, Radov LA (1978) Systemic and local immunity and allograft and cancer rejection. In Warner NL, Cooper MD (eds), Contemporary Topics in Immunobiology 8:107-170. New York:Plenum.

Haynes BF, Fauci AS (1978) The differential effect of in vivo hydrocortisone on the kinetics of subpopulations of human peripheral blood thymus-derived lymphocytes. J Clin Invest 61:703-707.

Hellstrom KE, Hellstrom I (1974) Lymphocyte-mediated cytotoxicity and blocking serum activity to tumor antigens. Adv in Immunol 18:209-277.

Henney CS, Bourne HR, Lichtenstein LM (1972) The role of cyclic 3'-5' adenosine monophosphate in the specific cytolytic activity of lymphocytes. J Immunol 108:1526-1534.

Herberman RB, Holden HT (1978) Natural cell mediated immunity. Adv in Cancer Res 27:305-377.

Herberman RB (ed)(1980) Natural cell-mediated immunity. New York:Academic Press.

Hewitt HB (1978) The choice of animal tumours for experimental studies of cancer therapy. Adv in Cancer Res 27:149-200.

Houghton AN, Taormina MC, Ikeda H, Watanabe T, Oettgen HF, Old LJ (1980) Serological survey of normal humans for natural antibody to cell surface antigens of melanoma. Proc Natl Acad Sci USA 77:4260-4264.

Kall MA, Hellstrom I (1975) Specific stimulatory and cytotoxic effects of lymphocytes sensitized in vitro to either alloantigens or tumor antigens. J Immunol 114:1083-1088.

Klein E, Holtermann O, Milgrom H, Case RW, Pharm B, Klein D, Rosner D, Djerassi I (1976) Immunotherapy for accessible tumors utilizing delayed hypersensitivity reactions and separated components of the immune system. In Terry, WB (ed), Medical Clinics of North America. Philadelphia: WB Saunders.

Klein G, Klein E (1977) Rejectability of virus-induced tumors and nonrejectability of spontaneous tumors: a lesson in contrasts. Transplant Proc 9: 1095-1104.

Klein G (1979) The role of viral transformation and cytogenic changes in viral oncogenesis. Ciba Found Symp 66:335-358.

Krawinkel U, Cramer M, Kindred B, Rajewsky K (1979) Isolated hapten-binding receptors of sensitized lymphocytes. V. Cellular origin of receptor molecules. Eur J Immunol 9:815-820.

Law LW, Rogers MJ, Appella E (1980) Tumor antigens on neoplasms induced by chemical carcinogens and by DNA- and RNA-containing viruses: properties of the solubilized antigens. Adv in Cancer Res 32:201-235.

Lovchik JC, Hong R (1977) Antibody-dependent cell mediated cytolysis (ADCC): analysis and projections. Prog Allergy 22:1-44.

McKenzie IFC, Potter T (1979) Murine lymphocyte surface antigens. Adv in Immunol 27:181-338.

Podleski TR, Greenberg I (1980) Distribution and activity of endogenous lectin during myogenesis as measured with antilectin antibody. Proc Natl Acad Sci 77:1054-1058.

Prehn R (1972) The immune reaction as a stimulator of tumor growth. Science 176:170-171.

Prehn R (1975) Relationship of tumor immunogenicity to concentration of the oncogen. J Natl Cancer Inst 55:189-190.

Reinherz EL, Schlossman SF (1980) The differentiation and function of human T lymphocytes. Cell 19:821-827.

Rocklin RE, Bendtzen K, Greineder D (1980) Mediators of immunity: lymphokines and monokines. Adv in Immunol 29:55-136.

Rocklin RE, Breard J, Gupta S, Good RA, Melmon KL (1980) Characterization of the human blood lymphocytes that produce a histamine-induced suppressor factor (HSF). Cell Immunol 51:226-237.

Roder JC, Klein M (1979) Target-effector interaction in the natural killer system IV. Modulation by cyclic nucleotides. J Immunol 123:2785-2790.

Rosenberg SA, Terry WD (1977) Passive immunotherapy of cancer in animals and man. Adv in Cancer Res 25:323-388.

Scheid MP, Goldstein G, Boyse EA (1978) The generation and regulation of lymphocyte populations. Evidence from differentiative induction systems in vitro. J Exp Med 147:1727-1743.

Schlom J, Wunderlich D, Teramoto YA (1980) Generation of human monoclonal antibodies reactive with human mammary carcinoma cells. Proc Natl Acad Sci USA 77:6841-6845.

Schultz RM, Chirigos MA (1980) Macrophage activation for nonspecific tumor cytotoxicity: a review. In Schuitzer R (ed), Advances in Pharmacology and Chemotherapy. 17:157-187. New York:Academic Press.

Schwartz A, Askenase PW, Gershon RK (1980) Histamine inhibition of the in vitro
induction of cytotoxic T-cell responses. Immunopharmacology 2:179-190.

Shearer GM, Schmitt-Verhulst AM (1977) Major histocompatibility complex
restricted cell-mediated immunity. Adv in Immunol 25:55-91.

Strom TB, Carpenter CB (1980) Cyclic nucleotides in immunosuppression--
neuroendocrine pharmacologic manipulation and in vivo immune regulation
of immunity acting via second messenger systems. Trans Proc 12:304-310.

Sulit HL, Golub SH, Irie RF, Gupta RK, Grooms GA, Morton DL (1976) Human
tumor cells grown in fetal calf serum and human serum:influences on the tests
for lymphocyte cytotoxicity, serum blocking and serum arming effects. Int J
Cancer 17:461-468.

Szmuness W (1978) Hepatocellular carcinoma and the hepatitis B virus: evidence
for a causal association. Prog Med Virol 24:40-69.

Tada T, Okumura K (1979) The role of antigen-specific T cell factors in the
immune response. Adv in Immunol 28:1-87.

Thomas DB, Rawls WE (1978) Relationship of herpes simplex virus type 2 antibodies and squamous dysplasia to cervical carcinoma in situ. Cancer 42:2716-
2725.

Wilkie NM, Eglin RP, Sanders PG, Clements JB (1980) The association of herpes
simplex virus with squamous carcinoma of the cervix, and studies of the virus
thymidine kinase gene. Proc R Soc Lond (Biol) 210:411-421.

Williams JM, Peterson RG, Shea PA, Schmedtje JF, Bauer DC, Felten DL (1981)
Sympathetic innervation of murine thymus and spleen: evidence for a functional link between the nervous and immune systems. Brain Res Bull 6:83-94.

Zinkernagel RM, Doherty PC (1979) MHC-restricted cytotoxic T cells: studies
on the biologic role of polymorphic major transplantation antigens determining
T-cell restriction-specificity, function, and responsiveness. Adv in Immunol
27:51-177.

Published 1982 by Elsevier Science Publishing Co, Inc.
Sandra M. Levy, ed.
Biological Mediators of Behavior and Disease:
Neoplasia

POSSIBLE EFFECTS OF CENTRAL NERVOUS SYSTEM ON NATURAL KILLER (NK) CELL ACTIVITY

RONALD B. HERBERMAN
Chief, Laboratory of Immunodiagnosis, National Cancer Institute, Bethesda, MD
20205, USA.

INTRODUCTION

Some of the influences of behavior on neoplasia may be mediated by interactions between the central nervous system and the immune system. In this
regard, it is important to recognize the complexity of the immune system. Until
recently, all attention was directed toward T and B cells. There is now a need
to consider a heterogeneous assay of potential effector mechanisms, each of
which, alone or in concert with other parts of the immune system, could play an
important role in host defenses against tumors.

One recently described type of effector cell is the natural killer (NK) cell.
Before considering the evidence for possible interactions between the central
nervous system and NK cells, it seems worthwhile to summarize briefly the
characteristics of these cells and the indications for their possible importance in protection against progressive growth of tumors.

CHARACTERISTICS OF NK CELLS

NK cells share a number of features with T cells, being nonadherent and
nonphagocytic and having some T cell-associated markers. However, NK cells are
not thymic-dependent, with high levels of activity being detectable in athymic
nude or neonatally thymectomized mice and rats (Herberman and Holden, 1978;
Herberman, 1980). NK cells also share some properties with macrophages and
polymorphonuclear leukocytes (PMNs) and they therefore represent a cell popu
lation that is quite difficult to categorize. NK cells have been found in most
normal individuals of a wide range of mammalian and avian species (Herberman and
Holden, 1978; Herberman, 1980). They express surface receptors for the Fc
portion of IgG and they thereby appear to also function as K cells, mediating
antibody-dependent cell-mediated cytotoxicity (ADCC) against tumor target cells
(Ojo and Wigzell, 1978; Landazuri et al., 1979). Although NK cells clearly are
not typical T cells, they have been found to share a variety of T cell-associated markers. About half of human NK cells express receptors for sheep

erythrocytes (West et al., 1977) and the majority react (Ortaldo et al., 1982) with some monoclonal antibodies (9.2 and 3A1) to T cell-associated antigens. Similarly, at least half of mouse NK cells were shown to express Thy 1 (Mattes et al., 1979) and about 20% reacted with a monoclonal antibody to LyT1 (Koo and Hatzfeld, 1980). Also the monoclonal antibody, OX8, directed against a subpopulation of rat T cells with suppressor activity has been shown to react with a large proportion of rat NK cells (Reynolds et al., 1981a). NK cells have also been shown both to grow in response to T cell growth factor (TCGF) (Dennert, 1980, Ortaldo and Timonen, 1982) and may also produce TCGF (Domzig et al., 1981). Furthermore, a highly enriched population of human NK cells has been shown to proliferate in response to T cell mitogens, phytohemagglutinin and concanavalin A (Timonen et al., 1981a). In contrast to such evidence for a relationship of NK cells to T cells, NK cells have also been shown to share some cell surface markers with macrophages and polymorphonuclear leukocytes (PMNs). In the human, each of these cell types reacts with OKM1 monoclonal antibodies and andibodies to asialo GM1 and Mac 1 (Zarling and Kung, 1980; Kay and Horwitz, 1980; Breard et al., 1981; Ault and Springer, 1981) and in the mouse, one group has detected a macrophage-associated antigen Mph 1, on a considerable portion of NK cells (Lohmann-Matthes and Domzig, 1980).

Particularly because of the conflicting evidence as to the relationship of NK cells to well-known categories of lymphoid cells, much effort has been directed toward the identification of markers restricted to, or at least highly selective for, NK cells. The best such marker to date has been a morphologic one: recent evidence has indicated that virtually all human and rat NK activity is mediated by large granular lymphocytes (LGL) (Timonen et al., 1981b, Reynolds et al., 1981b), which comprise only about 5% of the peripheral blood or splenic leukocytes in man and other species. LGL can be readily identified on cytocentrifuge preparations of lymphoid cells and they can be highly enriched by centrifugation on density gradients of Percoll (Timonen and Saksela, 1980; Timonen et al., 1981b; Reynolds et al., 1981b). It now appears that LGL account for a high proportion of human $T_G$ cells (Ferrarini et al., 1980) whose relationship to typical T cells also has recently been questioned (Reinherz et al., 1980b). A monoclonal antibody, OKT10, has been found to react with most human LGL but not with other peripheral blood leukocytes (Ortaldo et al., 1982). However, this antigen is not entirely specific for LGL, since it is also expressed on most thymocytes and a subpopulation of bone marrow cells (Reinherz et al., 1980a). Several surface antigens have also been found to be expressed, with some selectivity, on most or all mouse NK cells (Glimcher et al., 1977; Cantor et al.,

1979; Kasai et al., 1980; Young et al., 1980; Tai and Warner, 1980). However, none of these markers have been shown to be restricted to NK cells. Further, in contrast to LGL, which account for virtually all of the natural cytotoxic reactivity against a wide range of target cells (Landazuri et al., 1981), most of the alloantigenic markers on mouse NK cells have not been found on the related natural cytotoxic (NC) effector cells that react with some solid tumor target cells (Stutman et al., 1980b; Burton, 1980).

In regard to their functional characteristics, NK cells share a number of features with macrophages and PMNs. As with these other effector cells, NK cells have spontaneous activity in normal individuals and their activity can be rapidly augmented, particularly by interferon (Herberman et al., 1980; Saksela et al., 1980) but also by other stimuli (Goldfarb and Herberman (1982; Herberman et al., 1982). However, like T cells, and in contrast to macrophages and PMNs, NK cells can proliferate in response to TCGF. As with all of the other types of effector cells, the activity of NK cells appears to be well regulated, subject to a variety of inhibitory cells and factors (Herberman et al., 1982). The nature of the target cell recognition by NK cells seems to be intermediate between the exquisite specificity of T cells and the ill-defined or absent specificity of macrophages or PMNs (Ortaldo and Herberman, 1982). NK cells can react against a wide variety of syngeneic, allogeneic and xenogeneic cells. Susceptibility to cytotoxic activity is not restricted to malignant cells, with fetal cells, virus-infected cells, and some subpopulations of thymus cells, bone marrow cells and macrophages also being sensitive to lysis. It appears that NK cells can recognize at least several, widely distributed antigenic specificities, and that such recognition is clonally distributed (Ortaldo and Herberman, 1982). Despite this analogy with antigen recognition by T cells, recognition by NK cells does not seem to require expression of products of the major histocompatibility complex on target cells and there is no evidence for a memory response by NK cells. However, some similarity to a memory response has been seen with NK cells, since in vivo or in vitro exposure to NK-susceptible cell lines can rapidly activate NK cells via induction of interferon (Djeu et al., 1981). The nature of this recognition for interferon production and for cytotoxic interactions of NK cells with target cells is not clear. Some investigators have suggested that NK cells have T cell-like receptors (Kaplan and Callewaert, 1980), whereas others have postulated lectin-like receptors (Stutman et al., 1980a).

Similar to each of the other effector cell types, NK cells have been found to have not only direct cytotoxic effects against target cells, but also to produce and release soluble factors. Best documented is the ability of NK cells to produce interferon (Trinichieri and Santoli, 1978; Saksela et al., 1980; Djeu et al., 1981). In recent studies with highly enriched populations of human LGL, various tumor cell lines, viruses, mitogens and bacterial and other adjuvants were shown to induce considerable production of interferon after culture overnight (Djeu et al., 1981). Of particular note was that during these short-term incubations, only the LGL and not T cells or monocytes produced interferon in response to most of the stimuli. Human LGL, upon incubation with concanavalin A plus phorbol ester, also were found to produce low levels of TCGF (Domzig et al., 1981). These observations are of considerable interest from at least three standpoints. First, they indicate that NK cells may be able to serve as important immunoregulatory cells, providing accessory function for a variety of immune responses that are affected by interferon or TCGF. Secondly, it appears that NK cells may be able to react with foreign materials in a multifaceted way, by producing soluble factors that can induce antiviral resistance and cytostasis of tumor cells, as well as by direct cytotoxic effects. Further, the ability of NK cells to rapidly produce interferon and possibly TCGF provides a mechanism for positive self regulation.

Until recently, most attention has been focused on a central role of T cells in immune surveillance, particularly against cancer. However, it has become increasingly clear that T cell-mediated immunity alone cannot account for resistance against develpment of tumors or against infection by various microbial agents. For example, athymic nude or neonatally thymectomized mice don't have particularly high incidences of various types of spontaneous or carcinogen-induced tumors (Stutman, 1979), and are quite resistant, at least during the initial phases of infection, to growth of some microbial agents (Cutler, 1976; Cauley and Murphy, 1979; Newborg and North, 1980). These exceptions to a central role for T cells have led to much general skepticism and pessimism as to whether there is any type of immunological protection against cancer (Prehn, 1971). However, rather than rejecting the basic hypothesis of immune surveillance (Thomas, 1959; Burnet, 1970), it seems more realistic to consider the possible involvement of other effector cells, including NK cells. In view of the nature of the processes required for development of T cell-mediated immunity, it's not surprising that they alone would not be sufficient for protection against disease. There is a requisite lag period between exposure to foreign materials, be they cancer cells or microbes, and development of specific immunity. Also, some invaders have poorly expressed or even absent antigenic structures that can trigger T cell immunity. It seems reasonable therefore to postulate a primary, broader range defense system that can respond almost immediately to foreign materials and at least partially control them, until the more potent and specific immune system begins to adequately respond. The natural cellular immune system, consisting of NK cells, macrophages and PMNs, seems to be well-suited to play important roles in the postulated primary line of defense. It is not possible, and perhaps is not even reasonable, to try to decide which of the various effector cells is most important. Each may have an appreciable role and their relative contributions may vary with different types of tumors or microbial agents and with the particular situation. Also, the various effector cells can interact with each other in a complex variety of ways and thereby influence each other's activities.

Most of the evidence for a role of NK cells *in vivo* relates to resistance against the growth of NK-susceptible tumor cell lines. The major approach has been to look for correlations between *in vivo* resistance to the growth of the tumor cell lines and the levels of NK activity in the recipients. In a variety of different situations, tumors have grown less well in recipients with high NK activity than in those with low activity (Kiessling et al., 1975b; Hanna, 1980; Riesenfeld et al., 1980, Talmadge et al., 1980; Karre et al., 1980; Habu et al., 1981). Furthermore, it has been possible to transfer increased resistance against tumor growth, and increased clearance of intravenously or subcutaneously inoculated radiolabeled tumor cells, by transfer of NK cell-enriched populations or of bone marrow precursors of NK cells (Haller et al., 1977; Kasai et al., 1979; Cheever et al., 1980; Tam et al., 1980; Riccardi et al., 1981).

Although such results are encouraging, they don't indicate whether NK cells also can have a similar role in defense against growth and metastasis of spontaneous or carcinogen-induced primary tumors. Much less evidence for this important issue is available. However, some data have been accumulated in this direction. The majority of spontaneous mammary tumors of C3H mice (Serrate and Herberman, 1981) and of spontaneous lymphomas in AKR mice (Nunn et al., 1977) have been found to have detectable, albeit low, susceptibility to lysis by NK cells. Similarly, some human leukemias, a myeloma, and some carcinomas, sarcomas, and melanomas (Rosenberg et al., 1972; Axberg et al., 1980; Zarling et al., 1979; Vanky et al., 1981; Mantovani et al., 1982) have been significantly lysed by NK cells. Such lysis has been appreciably augmented, and thereby evident with a higher proportion of tumors, when the effector cells were pretreated with interferon (Axberg et al., 1980; Zarling et al., 1979; Vanky et al., 1980; Mantovani et al., 1982). As further support for the ability of NK cells to recognize primary tumor cells, Ortaldo et al. (1977) showed that a variety of human tumor cells could cold target inhibit the lysis of radiolabeled K562 cells.

Most of these positive results were obtained with NK cells from normal allogeneic donors. In fact Vanky et al. (1980) detected NK reactivity only against allogeneic human tumor cells and concluded that the NK cells of the tumor-bearing individual lacked the ability to recognize the autologous tumor cells. They postulated that recognition of foreign histocompatibility antigens was involved in lysis by NK cells, particularly those stimulated by interferon. If correct, their hypothesis would virtually preclude a role for NK cells in resistance against primary tumor growth. However, such restriction of NK reactivity to allogeneic tumors does not fit the many examples of tumor cell lines being susceptible to syngeneic NK cells (see, for example Herberman et al., 1975; Kiessling et al., 1975a). Similarly, normal C3H mice have been found to be reactive against some syngeneic mammary tumors (Serrate and Herberman, 1981), and some cancer patients also have had detectable, interferon-augmentable, NK activity against their autologous tumor cells (Mantovani et al., 1982).

The reasons for the discrepancies among the human studies are not clear. The positive results were obtained with ovarian carcinoma cells, mainly in 20 hr cytotoxicity assays (Mantovani et al., 1982)), whereas the allo-restricted results involved other types of tumors, tested only in 4 hr assays. The greater sensitivity of the prolonged assay would seem sufficient to account for the differences. In addition, it is possible that the subpopulation of NK cells that are required to interact with certain types of tumors may be selectively inhibited in the autologous tumor-bearing host.

Another line of evidence indicating that NK cells may interact in vivo with autologous primary tumor cells is the demonstration that NK cells can enter and accumulate at the site of tumor growth. NK cells have been detected in small spontaneous mouse mammary carcinomas (Gerson et al., 1980) and in small primary mouse tumors induced by murine sarcoma virus (Gerson et al., 1980; Becker, 1980). In contrast, NK activity has usually been undetectable in large tumors in mice (Gerson et al., 1980) or in clinical tumor specimens. This may be due, at least in part, to the presence of suppressor cells, which have been demonstrated in some cell suspensions from some tumors (Gerson et al., 1980; Vose, 1980; Eremin, 1980; Allavena et al., 1981).

Several pieces of evidence suggest that NK cells may be involved in surveillance against primary tumors. One of the major predictions of the immune surveillance theory is that tumor development would be associated with, and in fact be preceded by, depressed immunity. Several observations fit this prediction: a) Patients with the Chediak-Higashi syndrone, who have a selective and marked deficit in NK activity (Roder et al., 1980), have a high incidence of lymphoproliferative diseases (Dent et al, 1966). b) Similarly in a colony of beige mice, which have an analogous selective deficit in NK activity (Roder and Duwe, 1979), a high incidence of lymphomas was noted (Loutit et al., 1980). c) Kidney allograft recipients, who received immunosuppressive drugs and have a high risk of developing lymphoproliferative and other tumors, have been found to have severely depressed NK activity (Lipinski et al., 1980).

A related prediction of the immune surveillance theory is that carcinogenic agents would cause depressed immune function, thereby impairing the ability of the host to reject the transformed cells. This postulate has been examined by many investigators in regard to the possible role of mature T cells and humoral immunity, and conflicting results have been obtained (Stutman, 1975). In contrast, the initial and still fragmentary data on this point in relation to NK cells are promising: a) Urethane, which produces lung tumors in only some strains of mice, caused transient and marked depression of NK activity in a susceptible strain but not in resistant strains (Gorelik and Herberman, 1981a and 1981b). Administration of normal bone marrow, which can reconstitute NK activity, to urethane-treated susceptible mice reduced the subsequent development of lung tumors (Kraskovsky et al., 1973; Gorelik and Herberman, unpublished observations). b) Multiple, low doses of irradiation of C57BL mice, that has been highly effective in inducing leukemia in this strain, produced a substantial deficit in NK activity (Parkinson et al, 1981). The depressed NK activity could be restored by transfer of normal bone marrow cells from C57BL mice but not from beige mice (Gorelik and Herberman, unpublished observations), and such transfer of normal C57BL bone marrow has been reported to interfere with radiation-induced leukemogenesis (Kaplan et al., 1953). c) Carcinogenic doses of dimethylbenzanthracene in vivo (Ehilich et al., 1980), and in vitro treatment with two different classes of tumor promoters, phorbol esters and teleocidin (Goldfarb and Herberman, 1982), have produced inhibition of NK activity. Each of these observations support the possibility that one of the requisites for tumor induction by carcinogenic agents may be interference with host defenses, including those mediated by NK cells.

## EVIDENCE FOR EFFECTS OF CENTRAL NERVOUS SYSTEM (CNS) ON NK CELL ACTIVITY

Particularly because of the above evidence for an important role of NK cells in host defenses against cancer, it is of interest to consider the possibility that some effects of the CNS on tumor growth are mediated via influences on the activity of NK cells. Although this issue has not been studied extensively, there are several pieces of evidence in support of such an association:

1) Some intriguing evidence has come from the studies of Locke and his associates, summarized in detail elsewhere in this volume. In a study of healthy male student volunteers, they observed a significant correlation between low NK cell activity and psychiatric symptomatology associated with chronic stress. In a more detailed evaluation of the volunteers, those with low NK activity were found to have a high need for power, with frequent life events challenging their power status (McClelland and Jemmott, 1980).

2) In studies of mouse NK cells, low activity has been consistently associated with transportation stress (Herberman and Holden, 1978). Between one and five days after shipment of mice, or even movement from one building to another, a significant reduction in NK activity has been observed. By seven days, NK activity returned to the normal range.

3) Although the mechanism for transportation stress-induced depression of NK activity has not been determined, it seems likely that it is due to elevated levels of adrenocortical hormones. In vivo treatment of mice, rats or human donors with such hormones caused substantial but transient reduction in NK and antibody-dependent cell-mediated cytotoxic activities (Oehler and Herberman, 1978; Djeu et al., 1979; Parrillo and Fauci, 1978). It seems likely that this depression in reactivity is due to an effect of the hormones on the function of the effector cells rather than a direct cytotoxic effect, since normal levels of activity could be restored by stimulation with interferon-inducers (Oehler and Herberman, 1978; Djeu et al., 1979). Similarly, in vitro depression of mouse NK activity by corticosteroids was shown to be rapidly reversible after removal of the hormone (Santoni et al., 1979). Stress might also affect NK activity by induction of elevated levels of adrenergic hormones. Such hormones can cause increased levels of cyclic AMP within cells and such elevations have been shown to be associated with inhibition of NK activity (Goldfarb and Herberman, 1982).

4) Direct evidence for effects of the CNS on NK activity has come from neurosurgical ablation studies. Bardos et al (1982) have reported that removal of the left cerebral cortex of mice caused a severe depression in NK activity as well as T cell functions, but had no detectable effect on the function of macrophages or other immune cells. In contrast, removal of the right cerebral cortex had no significant effect on NK activity. Similarly, Sobue et al. (1982) have found that ablation of a portion of the hypothalamus also caused a marked depression of NK activity and of T cell functions (See Chapter 3, this volume, for an extensive review of this area). Saxena et al. (1982) have also shown

that hypophysectomy of newborn mice resulted in a profound depression of the subsequent levels of NK activity. It seems likely that the effects of hypophysectomy were mediated by loss of growth hormone production, since that hormone has been shown to be able to restore NK activity.

PROSPECTS FOR FUTURE STUDIES

Although the above evidence points to some role of the central nervous system in regulating the activity of NK cells, much more information is needed on the mechanism(s) and extent of such effects. In view of recent advances in knowledge about the subpopulation of lymphocytes mediating NK activity and factors such as interferon which regulate their activity (Herberman et al., 1982), it should be possible to design studies to obtain detailed information on the effects of neuroendocrine manipulations. After various treatments or under conditions of various types of stress, one could separately look for changes in the number of large granular lymphocytes, the levels of spontaneous NK activity, and the degree of augmentation of NK activity by interferon or interferon-inducers. Because of the likelihood of considerable spontaneous fluctuations in levels of NK activity from day to day, due at least in part to technical variations among experiments, it will be important to rigorously control such studies to ensure that any observed changes are in fact due to the treatments.

Although NK activity is probably not the sole mediator of host defenses against development and progressive growth of tumors, the likelihood of some important anti-neoplastic role for these cells would indicate the importance of obtaining a clear understanding of the modulation of this effector function by the central nervous system.

REFERENCES

Allavena P, Introna M, Mangioni C, Mantovani A (1981) Inhibition of natural killer activity by tumor-associated lymphoid cells from ascitic ovarian carcinomas. J Natl Cancer Inst, in press.
Ault KA, Springer TA (1981) Cross-reaction of a rat-anti-mouse phagocyte-specific monoclonal antibody (anti-Mac-1) with human monocytes and natural killer cells. J Immunol 126:359-364.
Axberg I, Gidlund M, Orn A, Pattengale P, Riesenfeld I., Stern P. Wigzell H (1980) In Aiuti F (ed.), Thymus, Thymic Hormones and T Lymphocytes. New York: Academic Press.
Bardos P, Biziere K, Degenne D, Renoux G (1982) Regulation of NK activity by the cerebral neocortex. In Serrou B, Herberman RB (eds.), NK Cells: Fundamental Aspects and Role in Cancer. Human Cancer Immunology, Vol. 6. Amsterdam: Elsevier North-Holland, in press.
Becker S (1980) Intratumor NK reactivity. In Herberman RB (ed.), Natural Cell-Mediated Immunity Against Tumors. New York: Academic Press.
Breard J, Reinherz EL, O'Brien C, Schlossman SF (1981) Delineation of an effector population responsible for natural killing and antibody-dependent cellu-

lar cytotoxicity in man. Clin Immunol Immunopathol 124:2682-2687.
Burnet FM (1970) The concept of immunological surveillance. Progr Exp Tumor Res 13:1-27.
Burton RC (1980) Alloantisera selectively reactive with NK cells: characterization and use in defining NK cell classes. In Herberman RB (ed.), Natural Cell-Mediated Immunity Against Tumors. New York: Academic Press.
Cantor H, Kasai M, Shen HW, LeClerc JC, Glimcher, L (1979) Immunogenetic analysis of natural killer activity in the mouse. Immunol Rev 44:1-32.
Cauley LK, Murphy JW (1979) Response of congenitally athymic (nude) and phenotypically normal mice to Cryptococcus neoformans infection. Infect Immun 23:644-651, 1979.
Cheever MA, Greenberg PD, Fefer A (1980) Therapy of leukemia by nonimmune syngeneic spleen cells. J Immunol 124:2137-2142.
Cutler JE (1976) Acute systemic Candidiasis in normal and congenitally thymic-deficient (nude) mice. J Reticuloendothel Soc 19:121-124, 1976.
Dennert G (1980) Cloned lines of natural killer cells. Nature 287:47-49.
Dent PB, Fish LA, White JF, Good RA (1966) Chediak-Higashi syndrome. Observations on the nature of the associated malignancy. Lab Invest 15:1634-1641.
Djeu JY, Heinbaugh J, Vieira WD, Holden HT, Herberman RB (1979) The effect of immunopharmacological agents on mouse natural cell-mediated cytotoxicity and on its augmentation by poly I:C. Immunopharmacology 1:231-244.
Djeu JY, Timonen T, Herberman RB (1981) Augmentation of natural killer cell activity and induction of interferon by tumor cells and other biological response modifiers. In Chirigos M (ed.), Role of Natural Killer Cells, Macrophages and Antibody Dependent Cellular Cytotoxicity in Tumor Rejection and as Mediators of Biological Response Modifiers Activity. New York: Raven Press.
Domzig W, Timonen TT, Stadler BM (1981) Human natural killer (NK) cells produce interleukin-2 (IL-2). Proc Amer Assoc Cancer Res 22:309.
Ehrlich R, Efrati M, Witz IP (1980) Cytotoxicity and cytostasis mediated by splenocytes of mice subjected to chemical carcinogens and of mice bearing primary tumors. In Herberman RB (ed.), Natural Cell-Mediated Immunity Against Tumors. New York: Academic Press.
Eremin O (1980) NK cell activity in the blood, tumour-draining lymph nodes and primary tumors of women with mammary carcinoma. In Herberman RB (ed.), Natural Cell-Mediated Immunity Against Tumors. New York: Academic Press.
Ferrarini M, Cadoni A, Franzi T, Ghigliotti C, Leprini A, Zicca A, Grossi CE (1980) Ultrastructural and cytochemical markers of human lymphocytes. In Aiuti FA (ed.), Thymus, Thymic Hormones and T Lymphocytes. New York: Academic Press.
Gerson JM (1980) Systemic and in situ natural killer activity in tumor-bearing mice and patients with cancer. In Herberman, RB (ed.), Natural Cell-Mediated Immunity Against Tumors. New York: Academic Press.
Glimcher L, Shen FW, Cantor H (1977) Identification of a cell-surface antigen selectively expressed on the natural killer cell. J Exp Med 145:1-9.
Goldfarb RH, Herberman RB (1982) Characteristics of natural killer cells and possible mechanisms for their cytotoxic activity. In Weissman G (ed.), Advances in Inflammation Research. New York: Raven Press, in press.
Gorelik E, Herberman RB (1981a) Inhibition of the activity of mouse NK cells by urethane. J Natl Cancer Inst 66:543-548.
Gorelik E, Herberman RB (1981b) Carcinogen-induced inhibition of NK activity in mice. Fed Proc 40:1093.
Habu S, Fukui H, Shimamura K, Kasai M, Nagai Y, Okumura K, Tamaoki N. (1981) In vivo effects of anti-asialo GM1. I. Reduction of NK activity and enhancement of transplanted tumor growth in nude mice. J Immunol 127:34-42.
Haller O, Kiessling R, Orn A, Wigzell H (1977) Generation of natural killer cells: an autonomous function of the bone marrow. J Exp Med 145:1411-1416.

Hanna N (1980) Expression of metastatic potential of tumor cells in young nude mice is correlated with low levels of natural killer cell-mediated cytotoxicity. Int J Cancer 16:674-680.

Herberman RB (ed.) (1980) Natural Cell-Mediated Immunology Against Tumors. New York: Academic Press.

Herberman RB, Brunda MJ, Djeu JY, Domzig W, Goldfarb RH, Holden HT, Ortaldo JR, Reynolds CW, Riccardi C, Santoni A, Stadler BM, Timonen T (1982) Immunoregulation and natural killer cells. In Serrou B, Herberman RB (ed.), NK Cells: Fundamental Aspects and Role in Cancer. Human Cancer Immunology, Vol. 6. Amsterdam: Elsevier North-Holland, in press.

Herberman RB, Holden HT (1978) Natural cell-mediated immunity. Adv Cancer Res 27:305-377.

Herberman RB, Nunn ME, Lavrin DH (1975) Natural cytotoxic reactivity of mouse lymphoid cells against syngeneic and allogeneic tumors. I. Distribution of reactivity and specificity. Int J Cancer 16:216-229.

Herberman RB, Ortaldo JR, Djeu JY, Holden HT, Jett J, Lang NP, Pestka S (1980) Role of Interferon in regulation of cytotoxicity by natural killer cells and macrophages. Ann NY Acad Sci 350:63-71.

Kaplan HS, Brown MB, Paull J (1953) Influence of bone marrow injections on involution and neoplasia of mouse thymus after systemic irradiation. J Natl Cancer Inst 14:303-316.

Kaplan J, Callewaert DM (1980) Are natural killer cells germ line V-gene encoded prothymocytes specific for self and nonself histocompatibility antigens? In Herberman RB (ed.), Natural Cell-Mediated Immunity Against Tumors. New York: Academic Press.

Karre K, Klein GO, Kiessling R, Klein G, Roder JC (1980) Low natural in vivo resistance to syngeneic leukemias in natural killer-deficient mice. Nature 284:624-626.

Kasai M, Iwamori M, Nagai Y, Okumura K, Tada T (1980) A glycolipid on the surface of mouse natural killer cells. Eur J Immunol 10:175-180.

Kasai M, Leclerc JC, McVay-Boudreau L, Shen FW, Cantor H (1979) Direct evidence that natural killer cells in nonimmune spleen cell populations prevent tumor growth in vivo. J Exp Med 149:1260-1264.

Kay HD, Horwitz DA (1980) Evidence by reactivity with hybridoma antibodies for a possible myeloid origin of peripheral blood cells active in natural cytotoxicity and antibody-dependent cell-mediated cytotoxicity. J Clin Invest 66:847-851.

Kiessling R, Klein E, Wigzell H (1975a) "Natural" killer cells in the mouse. I. Cytotoxic cells with specificity for mouse Moloney leukemia cells. Specificity and distribution according to genotype. Eur J Immunol 5:112-117.

Kiessling R, Petranyi G, Klein G, Wigzell H (1975b) Genetic variation of in vitro cytolytic activity and in vivo rejection potential of nonimmunized semisyngeneic mice against a mouse lymphoma line. Int J Cancer 15:933-940.

Koo GC, Hatzfeld A (1980) Antigenic phenotype of mouse natural killer cells. In Herberman RB (ed.), Natural Cell-Mediated Immunity Against Tumors. New York: Academic Press.

Kraskovsky G, Gorelik L, Kagan L (1973) Abrogration of the immunosuppressive and carcinogenic action of urethan by transplantation of syngeneic bone marrow cells from normal mice. Proc Acad Sci BSSR 11:1052-1053.

Landazuri MO, Lopez-Botet M, Timonen T, Ortaldo JR, Herberman RB (1981) Human large granular lymphocytes: Spontaneous and interferon-boosted NK activity against adherent and nonadherent tumor cell lines. J Immunol 127:1380-1383.

Landazuri MO, Silva A, Alvarez J, Herberman RB (1979) Evidence that natural cytotoxicity and antibody dependent cellular cytotoxicity are mediated in humans by the same effector cell populations. J Immunol 123:252-258.

Lipinski M, Tursz T, Kreis H, Finale Y, Amiel JL (1980) Dissociation of natural killer cell activity and antibody-dependent cell-mediated cytotoxicity in

246

kidney allograft recipients receiving high-dose immunosuppressive therapy. Transplantation 29:214-218.

Lohmann-Matthes M-L, Domzig W (1980) Natural cytotoxicity of macrophage precursor cells and of mature macrophages. In Herberman RB (ed.), Natural Cell-Mediated Immunity Against Tumors. New York: Academic Press.

Loutit JF, Towsend KMS, Knowles JF (1980) Tumour surveillance in beige mice. Nature 272:634-636.

Mantovani A, Allavena P, Biondi A, Sessa C, Introna M (1982) Natural killer activity in human ovarian carcinoma. In Serrou B, Herberman RB (ed.), NK Cells: Fundamental Aspects and Role in Cancer. Human Cancer Immunology, Vol. 6. Amsterdam: Elsevier North-Holland, in press.

Mattes MJ, Sharrow SO, Herberman RB, Holden HT (1979) Identification and separation of Thy-1 positive mouse spleen cells active in natural cytotoxicity antibody-dependent cell-mediated cytotoxicity. J Immunol 123:2851-2860.

McCelland DC, Jemmott JB (1980) Power motivation, stress and physical illness. J Human Stress 6:6-15.

Newborg MF, North RJ (1980) On the mechanism of T cell-independent anti-Listeria resistance in nude mice. J Immunol 124:571-176.

Nunn ME, Herberman RB, Holden HT (1977) Natural cell-mediated cytotoxicity in mice against non-lymphoid tumor cells and some normal cells. Int J Cancer 20:381-387.

Oehler JR, Herberman RB (1978) Natural cell-mediated cytotoxicity in rats. III. Effects of immunopharmacologic treatments on natural reactivity and on reactivity augmented by polyinosinic-polycytidylic acid. Int J Cancer 21: 221-229.

Ojo E, Wigzell H (1978) Natural killer cells may be the only cells in normal mouse lymphoid populations endowed with cytolytic ability for antibody-coated tumor target cells. Scand J Immunol 7:297-306.

Ortaldo JR, Herberman RB (1982) Specificity of natural killer cells. In Serrou B, Herberman RB (ed.), Fundamental Aspects and Role in Cancer. Human Cancer Immunology, Vol. 6. Amsterdam: Elsevier North-Holland, in press.

Ortaldo JR, Oldham RK, Cannon GB, Herberman RB (1977) Specificity of natural cytotoxic reactivity of normal human lymphocytes against a myeloid leukemia cell line. J Natl Cancer Inst 59:77-82.

Ortaldo JR, Sharrow SO, Timonen T, Herberman RB (1982) Analysis of surface antigens on highly purified human NK cells by flow cytometry with monoclonal antibodies. J Immunol, in press.

Ortaldo JR, Timonen TT (1982) Modification of antigen expression and surface receptors on human NK cells grown in vitro. In Proceedings of the 14th International Leukocyte Culture Conference.

Parkinson DR, Brightman RP, Waksal SD (1981) Altered natural killer cell biology in C57BL/6 mice after leukemogenic split-dose irradiation. J Immunol 126: 1460-1464.

Parrillo JE, Fauci AS (1978) Comparison of the effector cells in human spontaneous cellular cytotoxicity and antibody-dependent cellular cytotoxicity: differential sensitivity of effector cells to in vivo and in vitro corticosteroids. Scand J Immunol 8:99-107.

Prehn, RT (1971) Immunosurveillance, regeneration and oncogenesis. Progr Exp Tumor Res 14:1-24.

Reinherz EL, Kung PC, Goldstein G, Levey RH, Schlossman SF (1980a) Discrete stages of human intrathymic differentiation: analysis of normal thymocytes and leukemic lymphoblasts of T-cell lineage. Proc Natl Acad Sci USA 77:1588-1592.

Reinherz EL, Moretta L, Roper M, Breard JM, Mingari MC, Cooper MD, Schlossman SF (1980b) Human T lymphocyte subpopulations defined by Fc receptors and monoclonal antibodies. A comparison. J Exp Med 151:969-974.

Riesenfeld I, Orn A Gidlund M, Axberg I, Alm GV, Wigzell H (1980) Positive correlation between in vitro NK activity and in vivo resistance towards AKR lymphoma cells. Int J Cancer 25:399-403.

Reynolds CW, Sharrow SO, Ortaldo JR, Herberman RB (1981a) Natural killer activity in the rat. II. Analysis of surface antigens on LGL by flow cytometry. J Immunol, in press.

Reynolds CW, Timonen T, Herberman RB (1981b) Natural killer (NK) cell activity in the rat. I. Isolation and characterization of the effector cell. J Immunol 127:282-287.

Riccardi C, Barlozzari T, Santoni A, Herberman RB, Cesarini C (1981) Transfer to cyclophosphamide-treated mice of natural killer (NK) cells and in vivo natural reactivity against tumors. J Immunol 126:1284-1289.

Roder J, Duwe A (1979) The beige mutation in the mouse selectively impairs natural killer cell function. Nature 278:451-453.

Roder, JC, Haliotis T, Klein M, Korec S, Jett JR, Ortaldo J, Herberman RB, Katz P, Fauci AS (1980) A new immunodeficiency disorder in humans involving NK cells. Nature 284:553-555.

Rosenberg, EB, Herberman RB, Levine PH, Halterman RH, McCoy JL, Wunderlich JR (1972) Lymphocyte cytotoxicity reactions to leukemia-associated antigens in identical twins. Int J Cancer 9:648-658.

Saksela E, Timonen T, Virtanen I, Cantell K (1980) Regulation of human natural killer activity by interferon. In Herberman RB (ed.), Natural Cell-Mediated Immunity Against Tumors. New York: Academic Press.

Santoni A, Herberman RB, Holden HT (1979) Correlation between natural and antibody-dependent cell-mediated cytotoxicity against tumor targets in the mouse. II. Characterization of the effector cells. J Natl Cancer Inst 63:995-1003.

Saxena QB, Saxena RK, Adler WH (1982) Regulation of natural killer activity in vivo. III. Effect of hypophysectomy and growth hormone treatment on the natural killer activity of the mouse spleen cell population. Int Arch Allergy Appl Immunol, in press.

Serrate S, Herberman RB (1981) Natural cell-mediated cytotoxicity against primary mammary tumors. Fed Proc 40:1007.

Sobue H, Ueki K, Tanaka R, Aoki T (1982) Immune response-influencing regions in the brain. In Aoki T (ed.), Manipulation of Host Defense Mechanisms, in press.

Stutman O (1975) Immunodepression and malignancy. In Klein G, Weinhouse S, Haddow A (eds.), Advances in Cancer Research, Vol. 22. New York: Academic Press.

Stutman O (1979) Chemical carcinogenesis in nude mice: Comparison between nude mice from homozygous matings and heterozygous matings and effect of age and carcinogen dose. J Natl Cancer Inst 62:353-358.

Stutman O, Dien P, Wisun R, Pecoraro G, Lattime EC (1980a) Natural cytotoxic (NC) cells against solid tumors in mice: some target cell characteristics and blocking of cytotoxicity by D-mannose. In Herberman RB (ed.), Natural Cell-Mediated Immunity Against Tumors. New York: Academic Press.

Stutman O, Figarella, EF, Paige CJ, Lattime EC (1980b) Natural cytotoxic (NC) cells against solid tumors in mice: general characteristics and comparison to natural killer (NK) cells. In Herberman RB (ed.), Natural Cell-Mediated Immunity Against Tumors. New York: Academic Press.

Tai A, Warner NL (1980) Biophysical and serological characterization of murine NK cells. In Herberman RB (ed.), Natural Cell-Mediated Immunity Against Tumors. New York: Academic Press.

Talmadge JE, Meyers KM, Prieur DJ, Starkey JR (1980) Role of NK cells in tumour growth and metastasis in beige mice. Nature 284:622-624.

Tam MR, Emmons SL, Pollack SB (1980) FACS analysis and enrichment of NK effector cells. In Herberman RB (ed.), Natural Cell-Mediated Immunity Against Tumors. New York: Academic Press.

Thomas L (1959) Discussion. In Lawrence HS (ed.), Cellular and Humoral Aspects of the Hypersensitive State. New York: Harper.

Timonen T, Ortaldo JR, Bonnard GD, Herberman RB (1981a) Cultures of human natural killer cells in the presence of T cell growth factor (TCGF) containing medium (CM). In Proceedings of the 14th International Leukocyte Culture Conference, in press.

Timonen T, Ortaldo JR, Herberman RB (1981b) Characteristics of human large granular lymphocytes and relationship to natural killer and K cells. J Exp Med 153:569-582.

Timonen T, Saksela E (1980) Isolation of human natural killer cells by discontinuous gradient centrifugation. J Immunol Methods 36:285-291.

Trinchieri G, Santoli D (1978) Anti-viral activity induced by culturing lymphocytes with tumor-derived or virus-transformed cells. Enhancement of human natural killer cell activity by interferon and antagonistic inhibition of susceptibility of target cells to lysis. J Exp Med 147:1314-1333.

Vanky FT, Argov SA, Einhorn SA, Klein E (1980) Role of alloantigens in natural killing. Allogeneic but not autologous tumor biopsy cells are sensitive for interferon-induced cytotoxicity of human blood lymphocytes. J Exp Med 151: 1151-1165.

Vose BM (1980) Natural killers in human cancer: activity of tumor-infiltrating and draining nude lymphocytes. In Herberman RB (ed.), Natural Cell-Mediated Immunity Against Tumors. New York: Academic Press.

West, WH, Cannon GB, Kay HD, Bonnard GD, Herberman RB (1977) Natural cytotoxic reactivity of human lymphocytes against a myeloid cell line: characterization of effector cells. J Immunol 118:355-361.

Young WW Jr, Hakomori S-I, Durdik JM, Henney CS (1980) Identification of ganglio-N-tetrasylceramide as a new cell surface marker for murine natural killer (NK) cells. J Immunol 124:199-201.

Zarling JM, Eskra L, Borden EC, Horoszewicz J, Carter WA (1979) Activation of human natural killer cells cytotoxic for human leukemia cells by purified interferon. J Immunol 123:63-70.

Zarling JM, Kung PC (1980) Monoclonal antibodies which distinguish between human NK cells and cytotoxic T lymphocytes. Nature 288:394-396.

# DISCUSSION

DR. VERNON RILEY:  There are answers to two of Dr. Wunderlich's questions. One, concerned with the communication between the tumor and CNS, we have demonstrated quite conclusively and repeatedly that as a tumor grows, the food consumption decreases. The tumor induces an anorexia and it seems reasonable that the anorexia could be traced to hunger centers in the central nervous system. In the experiments that we've done, we don't see any possible means of explaining it by taste aversion. It looks like the tumor excretes something that communicates with the taste centers or with the hunger centers. So, perhaps that is communication.

Does the tumor communicate with the immune system?  Another effect as the tumor grows is that the thymus involutes. Again, this phenomenon apparently is a consequence of the milieu interior. Something that is produced by the tumor causes the thymus involution. In this case we don't think that it's corticosterone. So those are two examples of possible communication links between the tumor and those two systems.

DR. LOCKE:  This is a quick question. I wondered with respect to the question mark between the CNS and the tumor, we discussed possible ways in which the tumor might affect the CNS, and short of operating through the immune system can anybody think of any examples of ways in which the CNS can affect the tumor?

DR. WUNDERLICH:  He's basically asking the question of whether or not tumors are known to have receptors for, for example, hormones that could change their form of metastastes or division?

DR. LOCKE:  Well, am I correct in saying that tumors don't develop nerves? Nerve supplies, it that right?

DR. MILLER:  Obviously if the tumor is of a tissue that is affected by corticosterone, the nervous system can do that. And that was the explanation of some of the negative results. So--

DR. LOCKE:  Yes. That would be an example.

DR. MILLER:  I think there are some other possibilities, but not with a tumor. It's just conceivable that the nervous system could affect the liver in such a way that is wouldn't detoxify certain carcinogens as much or could affect intestinal motility in such a way that you'd be more or less likely to get a tumor, just like I guess that fiber in the diet is supposed to do something, isn't it? So I think there are other pathways other than those we've been discussing that haven't been looked at. Whether they'd be any good or not, I don't know.

DR. FOX:  There is one other possibility. It is true, I believe, that tumors have almost no catecholamines in the substance, itself. Now, with that low level, if you get a proliferation from the nervous system, it's possible that the tumor is reactive to circulating catecholamines, and that might be something to look at because that's strongly under the control of the nervous system.

DR. ANISMAN: To what extent might, say, stress influence peripheral epinephrine or corticosterone, which in turn influences the tumor, not by immune fuction per se, but by providing it with an energy supply?

DR. FOX: It's possible. But because there are practically no catecholamines at all in the tumor itself.

DR. ANISMAN: I was thinking of something in a different way, thinking of this from the naive point of view. I assume that one limiting factor for tumor growth is that is needs a greater source of energy. Corticosterone and epinephrine will, I believe, cause the release of free fatty acids. Would this be a source of food, energy, for the tumor? And stress could have this effect.

DR. FOX: It's possible. There was an article in Science by a Russian who describes that mechanism that you just talked about.

DR. HERBERMAN: There are many things that one could possibly do in looking at how the CNS might interact with the immune system. But if the objective is to understand finally how the CNS would be affecting tumor growth, then I would think the main question would be to pick out something in the immune system, or some other mechanistic intermediary, that would seem to be most relevant to host defenses or resistance against tumor growth. And I think as one candidate for that, certainly, the natural killer cells are quite relevant. As I've said to some of you earlier, I certainly wouldn't state my position that I think that the natural killer cells are The Mechanism on which to focus. I think it is a complex situation in which various parts of the immune system may be involved. But there seems to be enough suggested evidence for an important role of natural killer cells, and this could be one direct area for studies to develop information about how there is an interaction between the CNS and natural killer cells.

DR. ADER: I'd like to address a question to you about this. I'm really not trying to be facetious. I have a problem with this, as I think all behaviorists would under the circumstances. I work with an immunologist, and I'm more fortunate than most in that regard. I'm frequently asked, "Well, how does one go about doing this?" And my answer is, find an immunologist that finds this interesting and truly collaborate. My experience has been that--and I've predicted--that what they will tell you to measure--

DR. HERBERMAN: Is what they do.

DR. ADER: --is what they do. That's right. You know, since, at the moment, most of the initiatives in this area are coming from the behavioral sciences rather than from immunology, I think there is very little to go on to make a rational judgement about, "You should look here rather than there because--" There just aren't any "becauses." Other than NK cells, would you kind of free associate to what other possibilities might be interesting? I think it's a critical question in terms of initiating research.

DR. HERBERMAN: Well, I think the two other main compartments that I would single out would be the other major natural defense mechanisms, namely, monocytes and macrophages, and T-cell mediated immunity. But the last is actually the most complicated, because there is heterogeneity within the T-cell compartment, and it becomes very difficult to really say what would be the most appropriate assay. Even if you are going to say "All right, I want to measure T-cell mediated immunity," well what aspect of it and what subpopulation of cells? In an animal system, my own preference would be to study T-cell mediated immunity against tumor, the development of these cells, and the levels of their activity. Among all of the various parts of the immune system, that might be the most likely aspect of that system to be linked with host defenses. But that's just a guess.

DR. BORYSENKO: In humans it's much harder though.

DR. HERBERMAN: In humans it is almost impossible.

DR. BORYSENKO: The T-cell measures are really difficult and very varied.

DR. HERBERMAN: Well to have a good specific anti-tumor measure in humans like cytotoxic T-cells, you get into immense logistical problems. There's only a couple of labs in the world that have been doing these studies, you know.

DR. ANISMAN: Right.

DR. FOX: Dr. Anisman, related to your group-caged versus isolated animals, you may want to consider the possibility that animals that live in a group have a different hormonal distribution from those that live in isolation. And it has been suggested in humans that during a certain "window" in the life of girls, particularly during menarche, they are at extremely high risk of much, much later cancer if they are exposed to a carcinogen at that time. Before the window and after the window, there is relatively little, if any, increase in relative risk many later years for breast cancer. But during that window they are at high risk, and the question is, whether you might find some distribution of hormones, sex hormones, that differs among the isolates and the group-living?

DR. ANISMAN: Yes. You've published data dealing with different developmental phases and the effects of stress at different developmental phases. What precisely is happening isn't clear. On the one hand, not only are there differences in hormonal levels, but the maturation of the nervous system has to be considered. So, for example, in the mouse or the rat models, the cholinergic system isn't fully mature, until approximately 21 days of age. A manipulation that's done prior to 20 or 21 days of age might have a very much different effect than one which is done after 20 days of age. The same thing would hold true with seratonin, which is mature at about 15 days of age, or seems to be mature at that point. There are all sorts of factors which have to be considered here with respect to these developmental windows. How we go about analyzing the relationship between a pathology such as cancer and these developemental windows, given that there are so many of them, becomes a very tedious problem.

DR. VERNON RILEY: There are a number of interesting things that occur as a function of population density and some of these are metabolic. For example, the food consumption will be quite different in cages where there are one or two animals, as compared with 5, 10, or 15. And this presumably is tied to the homeostatic caloric temperature control system. So, with a different caloric intake, we know that that influences the malignant process and may influence other important parameters, also. We found that these factors have to be very closely controlled and taken into consideration in the interpretation of results.

DR. BORYSENKO: One of the kinds of things that has come out that I'd like to ask you to comment on, Dr. Ader, is the effect of early handling. Many critical studies have suggested that there seems to be something early in the background of the child that impaired his or her ability to cope or perhaps set up a conditioned kind of response so that when they came across a stress later in life, their ability to cope was impaired. Regardless of what the intervening mechanism might be, could you comment on that?

DR. ADER: From lots of points of view, because I think that's an exceedingly important area on the grounds that studies indicate that there is a parallel in the development of neuroendocrine function and immune function. And there is a whole literature on manipulation of early life experiences and chronic alterations in neuroendocrine function. I should think it awfully surprising if there were not also parallel changes in immune function.

Now, in one sense, part of that literature started because there was at the time only one viable candidate as a mediator, and this gets us back to the issue of "reductionism." Where reductionism gets in the way of this kind of research is in the premature quest for mechanisms or phenomena which have not been adequately evaluated in the first place, under the supposition that if you can't explain it, it is not real. I think that's the reductionism that Dr. Cunningham is fighting. We don't have a lot of data here yet, and yet we are getting a lot of attention. Then somebody asks you the question, "How do you account for that?" I'm frankly always amused by the question because it usually comes from a reductionist philosophy that says if you can't explain it, it isn't real. And yet they wouldn't ask you the question at all if they hadn't accepted your original premise in the first place. So that part washes.

But the only existing hypothesis at the time essentially was that the early experience effects were mediated by alterations in corticosteroid levels, again following from an orientation to stress the typical circular response that what is stress is whatever elicits an adrenal response. When the adrenocortical mediation hypothesis fell through, people were left high and dry. "Well, where do I go now?" because there wasn't any rationale.

Now, there's clearly evidence that manipulating early life experience will chronically alter neuroendocrine function, will chronically alter the animal in such a way that it will respond differently to stimuli, not stressors, stimuli that have the capacity to induce manifest disease. Of those manifest diseases, some of them presumably may involve immunologic competence. Some of them certainly do, because there have been at least two involving the direct measurement of antibody. Most of the studies are old. I know of only one direct early experience study with immunologic parameters as dependent variables, and that was, I guess, in the '50's. The second one was published this year in Physiology and Behavior. Those are essentially the only two.

I think that development, the study of ontogeny, should become a primary focus of concern in this area for just the reasons you've hinted at, and because I think it provides a rationale for where to look in terms of the parellel changes in neuroendocrine function. I'm just guessing, but I think it's a good guess.

DR. LEVY: Dr. Anisman, I had wanted to ask you earlier, in your Psych Bulletin review, you differentiated the adaptation that seems to occur with respect to physical stress, acute versus chronic, and there seems to be some kind of an adaptation in the chronic application of physical stress that doesn't seem to happen if the stress is social. Chronic social stress still seems to have an effect on various biological systems.

DR. ANISMAN: In our own studies, at least, when we applied a physical stress uncontrollably we got adaptations. When we looked at isolation as a social stress, we didn't see any adaptation at all. In the original studies, we isolated animals for either one day, seven days, 28 days—I can't even remember them all—and in each instance there was an increase in the turnover of catecholamines with as little as 24 hours of isolation. And we assumed that because it continued in the same fashion through more than 28 days—it could have been 56 days, I just can't recall now—that adaptation didn't occur.

Since writing that paper we found that isolation of one hour was sufficient to give a very great increase in turnover. With from one hour to 24 hours, you actually get a decline toward control values, toward the non-isolated animals, and then it flattens out.

So there does, in fact, seem to be some adaptation, but it occurs very very rapidly.

Okay, given this adaptation, why you get enhanced tumor growth, for example, in isolated animals, I haven't got a clue. Our original statement saying there was no adaptation with isolation was clearly incorrect; there is some sort of adaptation.

DR. LOCKE: I was trying to imagine the effect of a large hand reaching into this room and grabbing me and putting me in a room by myself. And I would imagine that as time went on I probably would relax; but I think initially I'd be quite frightened.

DR. ANISMAN: It's not a pure handling effect. Our grouped animals are handled as well. But I should say that more than that, these studies started not because we were interested in the short-term isolation effect, but because we were trying to get mice to fight. And one way to get mice to engage in fighting is to isolate them for 24 hours. We had thought that this isolation for 24 hours would increase the fighting and we wanted to see if that modified the stress effects on norepinephrine induced by electric shock. We found at that point that if you isolate the animals for this one hour period that that was sufficient to induce the fighting. In fact, you got less fighting if you isolated them for three days. Between one day and three days there was no further adaptation. There was far less fighting at three days than there was at one day.

DR. VERNON RILEY: A general comment. I sort of hate to be a spoilsport this late in the afternoon, but one point I think I did not make clearly, and that is within the limits of our animal studies we have concluded that stress does not cause cancer; that it cannot cause cancer. It can only exploit an incipient situation that is present. And now the work of Jim Henry and others may demonstrate that stress can cause cardiovascular or other diseases directly, but we've seen no evidence whatsoever of an induction of cancer by controlled stress.

DR. CUNNINGHAM: But isn't there a semantic point there, depending on whether you believe that the neoplastic transformation is common, in which case stress might either deter or enhance the development of these cancers. This would be similar to viewing all of us as having incipient hypertension. In a sense we all do have arterial tension.

DR. VERNON RILEY: Exactly. But in our mammary tumor situation where we examined them for two years or more, there we know that there is a transforming factor, and the transformed cells undoubtedly exist. We're able to prevent them from maturing into overt tumors as long as they were young and had an immunological system that we were able to protect and to augment. Once the animals were old and had a natural immunological deficiency, we could not protect them from the disease, even though we protected them from stress.

DR. MILLER: Well, I don't know if that should be so alarming. I mean it certainly is a possible limitation. But if I understand your studies correctly, what you've done is primarily taken the natural mouse room, which is quite stressful, and developed an environment that is much less stressful.

DR. VERNON RILEY: Right.

DR. MILLER: And your stress have been like rotating mice, which may be very stressful for them, I don't know, but have you tried subjecting them to very severe stresses, and if not why? Have you found that you are at asymptote, and that it doesn't take any more, or that it causes other bad factors that confound your experiments?

DR. VERNON RILEY: We've intentionally tried to avoid heavy stress, partially on the grounds that we didn't want to complicate our relatively simplified experimental picture by activating metabolic processes, or by even maybe activating the adrenal medulla. We wanted to keep the changes insofar as feasible confined to the adrenal cortex. And we're able to activate that with relatively mild stress; the rotation, the handling, the noises in the room, and so forth.

DR. MILLER: Now, then probably your conclusion about not being able to initiate cancer, which as I say isn't a disturbing conclusion to me at all, might be--

DR. VERNON RILEY: It's reassuring in a way.

DR. MILLER: --Yes, might be limited a little bit to the range of manipulations you've made. But on your side I would say that the evidence that I know of anyhow in the cardiovascular area seems to indicate that with the exception I guess of Henry's procedure, which is a pretty drastic and long-lasting procedure, that you can't very well induce hypertension unless, "A", you combine it with something like a high salt diet that tends to push the animal that way; or "B", get a strain of mice that is susceptible to it. So, you wouldn't get much of an effect by itself, but rather that stress might be a potentiating factor. This is not astonishing nor disturbing. These findings could still have quite a bit of practical importance.

# Subject Index

Acetylcholine, 125
Activity Inhibition, 45
Ader, R., vii, ix, 93
Adrenal cortex, 175
Adrenalectomy, 67, 76
Adrenal medulla, 178
Adrenocorticotropic hormone
    (ACTH), 58, 128
Age, 127, 210
Agression, expression of, 116
Allogenic model, xii
Amines, 126
Anaphylaxis, 150, 164, 165
    passive, 154
Androgens, 58, 68, 74
Animal studies, 31, 42
    experimental design, 179
Anisman, H., xi
Autochthonous tumors, 197
Autonomic nervous system, 17,
    39, 167
Aversive stimulation, 124

Bacterial lipopolysaccharides,
    xi
Ball, G.G., 115
Bartrop, R.W., 85
B-cells, 132, 137
Beatson, G., 55
Beecher, H.K., 115
Behavior
    and cancer, 29, 46, 79, 228
    and ectopic hormones, 79
    and immune system, 33
Benign stressing device, 187
Bereavement, x, 10, 67, 85
Beta-adrenergic stimulation,
    167
Beta-endorphin, 17
Bittner oncogenic virus, x, 31
Body, effects on, by mind, 83,
    93

Bowers, K.S., 84
Brain
    and cell-mediated immunity,
        158
    and humoral immunity, 150
    -immune system link, 10
    lesions, 150
Breast cancer, xiii, 65
    hormones and, 59
Burnet, F.M., 87

Cancer. See also Cancer
        patients; Neoplasia;
        Tumor growth
    behavior and, 29, 113, 228
    hormones produced ectopically
        by, 59, 78
    and mental state, 86, 93
    and psychoneuroimmunology,
        43
    regulation of, 87
    stress of diagnosis and
        treatment of, 118
Cancer patients, 30, 90, 229
Cassel, J., 85
Catecholamines, 36, 126, 129,
    135
Cell-mediated immunity, brain
    and, 158
Central nervous system, 124,
    226
    and immune system, vii, 42
    and NK cells, 241
Central neurochemical changes,
    135
Chemotherapy, 103
Chirigos, M., xi
Circadian rhythms, 167
Circulating serum factors, xiii
Cochran, N., xiii
Conditioning, x, 183
Coping, 11, 32, 36, 89, 124,

260